AUTHOR'S GUIDE TO JOURNALS
IN NURSING & RELATED FIELDS

Author's Guide to Journals Series

Author's Guide to Journals in the Health Field
  Edited by Donald B. Ardell, Ph.D., and John Y. James, M.P.H.

Author's Guide to Journals in Law, Criminal Justice, & Criminology
  *Edited by Roy M. Mersky, J.D., M.L.S., Robert C. Berring, J.D.,
  M.L.S., and James K. McCue, J.D., M.L.S.*

Author's Guide to Journals in Library & Information Science
  Edited by Norman D. Stevens, Ph.D., and Nora B. Stevens, M.L.S.

Author's Guide to Journals in Nursing & Related Fields
  Edited by Steven D. Warner and Kathryn D. Schweer, R.N., Ph.D.

Author's Guide to Journals in Psychology, Psychiatry, & Social Work
  Edited by Allan Markle, Ph.D., and Roger C. Rinn, Ph.D.

Author's Guide to Journals in Sociology & Related Fields
  Edited by Marvin B. Sussman, Ph.D.

AUTHOR'S GUIDE TO JOURNALS

in nursing
& related fields

Edited by
Steven D. Warner
Kathryn D. Schweer, R.N., Ph.D.

THE HAWORTH PRESS, NEW YORK

The Haworth Press, 28 East 22 Street, New York, New York 10010

Library of Congress Cataloging in Publication Data
Main entry under title:

Author's guide to journals in nursing & related
  fields.

  (Author's guide to journals series)
  Includes index.
  1. Nursing literature—Marketing. 2. Medical
literature—Marketing. 3. Nursing—Periodicals—
Directories. 4. Medicine—Periodicals—Directories.
I. Warner, Steven D. II. Schweer, Kathryn D.
III. Series.
RT24.A97   070.5'2   82-1058
ISBN 0-917724-11-9   AACR2

Printed in the United States of America

To nurses, for whom this book was prepared

To secretaries, without whom research would not find its way to print

CONTENTS

ACKNOWLEDGMENTS

We would like to thank the editors and publishers of the journals we have included, whose cooperation was necessary to make this book possible.

Our very special thanks to Ruth Lewis, Librarian, Health Sciences Library, the University of Iowa, whose suggestions and expertise made everything so much easier.

We would also like to acknowledge Kathy Thiemann and Kay Weiler for their help in researching much of the information included herein.

Finally, we wish to express our thanks to Bill Cohen and Faye Zucker of The Haworth Press for their encouragement, patience, and guidance.

EDITORS' NOTE: The text of this book was initially processed and printed using a CPT 8000 Word Processor.

INTRODUCTION

Since the beginning of modern nursing, nurse authors have contributed to the development of the profession. However, for nearly a century relatively few nurses followed Florence Nightingale's example of publishing ideas, procedures, and reports of studies. Although it was common for physicians, sociologists, lawyers, and others to write articles intended for nurses, it was rare for a nurse to publish anything outside the field of nursing.

In the last two to three decades, there have been quantitative and qualitative changes in the authorship of articles for journals in nursing and related fields. Many nurses are entering the "publish or perish" world of academia. More nurses have the educational background that fosters the knowledge and ability to communicate, in writing, their findings in education, research, or practice. Nursing has become more specialized and nurses have become members of interdisciplinary health teams. This dichotomy has resulted in the need for information sharing on many levels, not only with nurses in general, but with consumers, among specialty groups, and with professionals in other disciplines.

The Author's Guide to Journals in Nursing and Related Fields is intended to provide useful information on publishing opportunities for nurse authors and others who write for a nursing audience. The number of people writing for nursing and the number of periodicals in nursing and related fields are both growing at an exponential rate. This has greatly increased the difficulty of finding the right journal for a particular article. Authors fear rejection slips, while journal editors dread reviewing stacks of manuscripts which are not relevant for their journals.

INFORMATION INCLUDED

The Author's Guide provides over 350 profiles of scholarly journals in nursing and related fields. Each profile includes detailed information about the types of articles usually selected, the percentage of manuscripts accepted, major content areas, preferred topics, inappropriate topics, review procedures, by which indexing or abstracting services the information published will be listed, and important practical information such as: publication lag time; addresses of journals; style requirements; and subscription, circulation, and other publication information (See Table 1). In most cases, this information comes directly from questionnaires sent to the journal editors. Additional information, and information not provided by the journal editors, was obtained from recent copies of the journals and/or major periodical indexes.

Major Content Areas

One hundred and twenty content areas relating to nursing were provided to journal editors. Editors selected those content areas which were most likely to be the focus of articles published by their journals. This information was compiled and is presented as part of the index. A list of these major content areas can be found in Appendix A.

Indexing Abstracting Information

Knowing who will have access to information that is published is of great importance to an author. Therefore, special care was taken in collecting this information by 1) the report of editors as to where their journals are indexed or abstracted, 2) checking *Cumulative Index to Nursing and Allied Health Literature* and *International Nursing Index*, and 3) checking the 1980 edition of *Ulrich's International Guide to Periodicals* (R. R. Bowker Company).

Recent Changes

Information on journals is constantly changing. Titles, addresses, scope and foci change frequently in an effort to meet the needs of demanding readerships; some journals incorporate with others or may cease publication. In an effort to provide accurate profiles of the journals included in this book, the editors checked information on titles, subscription and manuscript submission addresses early in 1982. Title changes and cessations are listed in Appendix B. In the text, a dagmar (†) identifies those journals which have had title changes. When reviewing journal profiles, the reader is encouraged to refer to Appendix B and make note of these changes which could not be included in the text at the time of publication. Also included in Appendix B is a list of new journals which were not being published when data were originally collected.

SELECTION STRATEGY

The basic and applied sciences have always formed a foundation for nursing. Therefore, nursing scholars 1) may not be nurses, 2) often hold higher degrees in fields other than nursing, and 3) may want to report their research findings to other disciplines. Since compiling information on all journals relevant to the disciplines associated with nursing would be far beyond the scope of this book, a selection strategy was devised to select those journals most pertinent to the nursing profession. The strategy for inclusion and exclusion of journals is outlined in Table 2. Some journals may have appeared on the market after the data for this book were gathered in 1980 and could not be included. A brief list of new journals which have come to the attention of the editors is included in Appendix B.

The Author's Guide to Journals in Nursing and Related Fields is intended to help novices and experienced writers find the appropriate journals for their articles. Similar author's guides have provided this service in sociology, psychology, and other fields. The future of professional development in nursing depends upon the publication of ideas, research findings, critiques, activities, discoveries, philosophies, and analyses of all of these writings. As nursing becomes more fully a part of academia, publishing becomes more imperative for more and more people. It is our hope that *The Author's Guide* will serve in a useful, practical way to meet the needs of authors and the needs of the nursing profession. In addition, we hope that it proves to be a useful reference for students, librarians, secretaries, research assistants, and other adjunct support personnel.

— Kathryn D. Schweer, RN, PhD
— Steven D. Warner, BFA

TABLE 1

INFORMATION INCLUDED FOR EACH JOURNAL

JOURNAL TITLE: The correct current title of the journal.

MANUSCRIPT ADDRESS: The correct address for submitting manuscripts.

TYPES OF ARTICLES: The types of articles (e.g., research, review, theoretical, case studies) which according to the present editor are most likely to be accepted for publication. Preferences for particular types of articles are cited in ranked order.

MAJOR CONTENT AREAS: The major subjects which are of primary interest to the journal. (See Appendix A for a list of content areas provided to the journal editors.) This information was used to prepare the subject index found at the end of this book.

TOPICS PREFERRED: A list of topics cited by the journal's editor as being of particular interest to the journal.

INAPPROPRIATE TOPICS: Topics or types of articles which the journal editor identified as frequently received "but wish I hadn't."
Inappropriate submissions usually deal with content, but other reasons may also be explained in this entry.

REVIEW PROCEDURE: The type of procedure used in reviewing manuscripts (e.g., editorial board, external review).

REVIEW PERIOD: The average amount of time, as estimated by the journal editor, it takes from receipt of a manuscript until the author is notified whether it has been accepted or rejected. It should be noted that these are averages; a manuscript may require more or less time for review.

MANUSCRIPT WORD LENGTH: The editor's estimate of the average length of manuscripts acceptable for publication given in words per manuscript. (Estimates were based on 250 words per double-spaced page.)

MANUSCRIPT COPIES: The number of copies of a manuscript required for review purposes.

PUBLICATION LAG TIME: The editor's estimate of the amount of time it takes from the time an article is accepted until it is published.

EARLY PUBLICATION OPTION: Whether a journal will publish an article sooner than its normal publication lag time. If this option is desired, additional information should be obtained from the journal editor.

ACCEPTANCE RATE: The editor's estimate of the approximate percentage of manuscripts accepted for publication.

AUTHORSHIP RESTRICTIONS: Whether the journal has any policies which would restrict certain persons from publishing in that particular journal (e.g., society members only, nurses only).

PAGE CHARGES: Whether the author incurs any charges for the publication of an article.

STYLE REQUIREMENTS: The style requirements followed by the journal. A list of abbreviations used for this entry are listed in Table 4. If the journal has unique style requirements, the designation "Own" is used.

STYLE SHEET: Whether the editor will send a copy of the journal's style requirements to prospective authors. The notation "SASE" means that a self-addressed stamped envelope must accompany the request.

REVISED THESES: Whether M.A./Ph.D. graduates are encouraged to submit theses/dissertations for publication.

STUDENT PAPERS: Whether as a matter of policy the journal "seeks one or two 'student papers'" every year for publication.

REPRINT POLICY: The journal's policy regarding article reprints and the provision of reprints to authors. "None free" indicates that reprints are not provided free of charge. "Author purchase" indicates that the author is required to purchase reprints. If a quantity of free reprints are provided to the author, the number is indicated.

SUBSCRIPTION ADDRESS: The correct address for ordering subscriptions.

ANNUAL SUBSCRIPTION RATE: The cost of an annual subscription in U.S. dollars.

FREQUENCY: How often the journal is published (e.g., monthly, quarterly, bimonthly).

CIRCULATION: The approximate circulation of the journal.

AFFILIATION: Whether the journal is affiliated with any society.

INDEXED/ABSTRACTED IN: A listing of where the journal is indexed or abstracted. A list of abbreviations used can be found in Table 3.

TABLE 2
JOURNAL SELECTION STRATEGY

JOURNALS INCLUDED IN THE AUTHOR'S GUIDE

1. Journals covered by *Cumulative Index to Nursing and Allied Health Literature*
2. Journals covered by *International Nursing Index*
3. Journals listed under the section "Medicine—Nursing" in the 1980 edition of *Ulrich's International Guide to Periodicals* (R. R. Bowker Company)
4. Journals not covered by 1, 2, or 3 but known to accept articles by or for nurses

JOURNALS EXCLUDED FROM THE AUTHOR'S GUIDE

1. Non-English language journals
2. Most newsletters
3. Journals which, according to questionnaires returned, only rarely accept articles written by nurses
4. Minor state and local periodicals

TABLE 3

ABBREVIATIONS USED

Indexing and Abstracting Services

AA	Abstracts in Anthropology
ACP	Abstracts of Criminology & Penology
ACSR	Aged Care & Services Review
AHCMS	Abstracts of Health Care Management Studies
AHM	Abstracts of Hospital Management Studies
AMR	Applied Mechanics Review
API	Alternative Press Index
ASCA	Automatic Subject Citation Alert
ASTI	Applied Science & Technology Index
BA	Biological Abstracts
BAI	Biological & Agricultural Index
BD	Biology Digest
BEA	Bioengineering Abstracts
BPI	Business Periodicals Index
BRD	Book Review Digest
BRI	Book Review Index
BS	Bulletin Signaletique
CA	Chemical Abstracts
CAAL	Classified Abstract Archive of the Alcohol Literature
CBPI	Canadian Business Periodical Index
CC	Current Contents
CC(ABES)	Current Contents: Agriculture, Biology & Environment
CC(CP)	Current Contents: Clinical Practice
CC(LS)	Current Contents: Life Sciences
CC(SBS)	Current Contents: Social & Behavioral Sciences
CDA	Child Development Abstracts
CDL	Crime & Delinquency Abstracts
CEI	Canadian Education Index
CIJE	Current Index to Journals in Education
CINAHL	Cumulative Index to Nursing & Allied Health Literature
CMHR	Community Mental Health Review
CPI	Canadian Periodical Literature Index
CSPA	College Student Personnel Abstracts
CWHM	Current Work in the History of Medicine
DA	Dental Abstracts
DI	Index to Dental Literature

DSHA	DSH Abstracts
EA	Environmental Abstracts
EAA	Educational Administration Abstracts
ECER	Exceptional Child Education Resources
EI	Education Index
EM	Excerpta Medica
Engl	Engineering Index
EPB	Environmental Periodicals Bibliography
GA	Genetics Abstracts
GSSRPL	Guide to Social Science & Religion in Periodical Literature
HA	Historical Abstracts
HAS	Hospital Abstracts Services
HLI	Hospital Literature Index
HosA	Hospital Abstracts
HRA	Human Resources Abstracts
IHD	Industrial Hygiene Digest
IM	Index Medicus
IndPA	Indian Psychological Abstracts
INI	International Nursing Index
IPA	International Pharmaceutical Abstracts
IPSA	International Political Science Abstracts
ISI	Institute for Scientific Information
IUSGP	Index to U.S. Government Periodicals
JEL	Journal of Economic Literature
KES	Key to Economic Science
LLBA	Language & Language Behavior Abstracts
MA	Microbiology Abstracts
MCR	Medical Care Review
MeA	Metal Abstracts
MGA	Meteorological & Geoastrophysical Abstracts
MHBRI	Mental Health Book Review Index
MR	Mathematical Reviews
MRA	Mental Retardation Abstracts
MRD	Media Review Digest
MSRS	Medical Socioeconomic Research Sources
NAR	Nutrition Abstracts & Reviews
NR	Nursing Research
NSA	Nuclear Science Abstracts
OA	Oceanic Abstracts
OSHA	Occupational Safety & Health Abstracts
PA	Psychological Abstracts
PAIS	Public Affairs Information Service Bulletin
PCC	Pastoral Care & Counseling Abstracts
PHR	Public Health Reviews

PI	Philosophers Index
PMA	Personnel Management Abstracts
PolA	Pollution Abstracts
PPA	Psychopharmacology Abstracts
PRG	Psychological Readers Guide
PSIBR	Population Sciences: Index of Biomedical Research
RGPL	Reader's Guide to Periodical Literautre
RL	Rehabilitation Literature
RPR	Review of Population Reviews
RTA	Religious & Theological Abstracts
SA	Science Abstracts
SCI	Science Citation Index
SocA	Sociological Abstracts
SPAA	Sage Public Administration Abstracts
SSA	Safety Science Abstracts Journal
SSCI	Social Science Citation Index
SSI	Social Sciences Index
SUSA	Sage Urban Studies Abstracts
SWRA	Social Work Research & Abstracts
WSA	Women's Study Abstracts

TABLE 4
ABBREVIATIONS USED
Style Manuals

AA	American Anthropological Association
AIBS	American Institute for Biological Sciences
AMA	American Medical Association Style Book
AP	The Associated Press Style Book
APA	Publication Manual of the American Psychological Association
ASA	American Sociological Association
ASM	American Society for Microbiology
C	A Manual of Style, Chicago University Press
CBE	Council of Biological Editors Style Manual, 4th Edition
GPO	Government Printing Office Style Manual
H	Harvard System
IM	Index Medicus
NT	New York Times Manual of Style & Usage
SW	The Elements of Style, 3rd Edition, Strunk & White
T	Manual for Writers of Term Papers, Theses, & Dissertations, 4th Edition, K. Turabian
WT	Words into Type, 3rd Edition

ALPHABETICAL LISTING OF JOURNALS

JOURNAL TITLE: AANA Journal

MANUSCRIPT ADDRESS: Betty A. Colitti
216 Higgins Road
Park Ridge IL 60068
TYPES OF ARTICLES: Research, theoretical, case studies, unsolicited
book reviews
MAJOR CONTENT AREAS: anesthesiology

TOPICS PREFERRED: Anesthesiology

INAPPROPRIATE TOPICS: None cited

REVIEW PROCEDURE:	Editorial board		
REVIEW PERIOD:	2 months		
MANUSCRIPT WORD LENGTH:	2500	**PAGE CHARGES:**	No
MANUSCRIPT COPIES:	3	**STYLE REQUIREMENTS:**	C, Own
PUBLICATION LAG TIME:	1-8 months	**STYLE SHEET:**	Yes
EARLY PUBLICATION OPTION:	No	**REVISED THESES:**	Yes
ACCEPTANCE RATE:	75%	**STUDENT PAPERS:**	Yes
AUTHORSHIP RESTRICTIONS:	Yes	**REPRINT POLICY:**	25 free

SUBSCRIPTION ADDRESS: AANA Journal
216 Higgins Road
Park Ridge IL 60068
ANNUAL SUBSCRIPTION RATE: $20
FREQUENCY: Bimonthly   **CIRCULATION:** 23,000
AFFILIATION: American Association of Nurse Anesthetists
INDEXED/ABSTRACTED IN: INI, CINAHL, EM, HLI

◆

JOURNAL TITLE: Acupuncture and Electrotherapeutics Research
The International Journal
MANUSCRIPT ADDRESS: Yoshiaki Omura, M.D., Sc.D., FACA
800 Riverside Drive (8-I)
New York NY 10032
TYPES OF ARTICLES: Research, theoretical, review, case studies,
letters to the editor
MAJOR CONTENT AREAS: acupuncture and electrotherapeutics, electro-
analgesia, Shiatsu, kinesiology, moxibustion, her-
bal medicine; biofeedback, biorhythms; nursing:
diagnosis, history, research; perception; medical
problems throughout the life span
TOPICS PREFERRED: Promotion of basic and clinical research in acupuncture, electrotherapeutics, and related fields
INAPPROPRIATE TOPICS: None cited

REVIEW PROCEDURE:	Editorial board		
REVIEW PERIOD:	1-3 months		
MANUSCRIPT WORD LENGTH:	1000-10,000	**PAGE CHARGES:**	No
MANUSCRIPT COPIES:	4	**STYLE REQUIREMENTS:**	Own
PUBLICATION LAG TIME:	3-10 months	**STYLE SHEET:**	No
EARLY PUBLICATION OPTION:	Yes	**REVISED THESES:**	Yes
ACCEPTANCE RATE:	50%	**STUDENT PAPERS:**	No
AUTHORSHIP RESTRICTIONS:	No	**REPRINT POLICY:**	Author purchase

SUBSCRIPTION ADDRESS: Pergamon Press, Inc.
Fairview Park
Elmsford NY 10523
ANNUAL SUBSCRIPTION RATE: Individuals: $30   Institutions: $60
FREQUENCY: Quarterly   **CIRCULATION:** 2000
AFFILIATION: None
INDEXED/ABSTRACTED IN: Not cited (new journal)

JOURNAL TITLE: Administration in Mental Health

MANUSCRIPT ADDRESS: Saul Feldman, Editor
P.O. Box 2088
Rockville MD 20852

TYPES OF ARTICLES: Theoretical, case studies, review, research, commentaries

MAJOR CONTENT AREAS: emergency services, epidemiology, ethics, leadership, mental health/illness, psychology, psychopathology, psychiatric/mental health nursing, public health

TOPICS PREFERRED: Mental health administration

INAPPROPRIATE TOPICS: None cited

REVIEW PROCEDURE: External review
REVIEW PERIOD: 4 months
MANUSCRIPT WORD LENGTH: 4000
MANUSCRIPT COPIES: 3
PUBLICATION LAG TIME: 4 months
EARLY PUBLICATION OPTION: No
ACCEPTANCE RATE: 25%
AUTHORSHIP RESTRICTIONS: No

PAGE CHARGES: No
STYLE REQUIREMENTS: APA
STYLE SHEET: Yes
REVISED THESES: Yes
STUDENT PAPERS: No
REPRINT POLICY: Not cited

SUBSCRIPTION ADDRESS: Human Sciences Press
72 Fifth Avenue
New York NY 10011
ANNUAL SUBSCRIPTION RATE: Individuals: $23   Institutions: $48
FREQUENCY: Quarterly   CIRCULATION: 2000
AFFILIATION: None
INDEXED/ABSTRACTED IN: IM, SWRA, CC(SBS), SSCI, AHCMS, SPAA, EAA, EM, PA, CIJE

◆

JOURNAL TITLE: Administrative Science Quarterly

MANUSCRIPT ADDRESS: Editor, ASQ, Graduate School of Business & Public Administration
Cornell University, Ithaca NY 14853

TYPES OF ARTICLES: Theoretical, research, case studies, commentaries, review, unsolicited book reviews

MAJOR CONTENT AREAS: change theory, leadership, nursing service administration, systems theory, organizational behavior, work conditions, i.e. stress, decision making, phsyical settings, growth/development of organizations

TOPICS PREFERRED: Organizational behavior, theories of management and leader styles

INAPPROPRIATE TOPICS: Practitioner-oriented topics

REVIEW PROCEDURE: Editorial board and external review
REVIEW PERIOD: 3 months
MANUSCRIPT WORD LENGTH: 7500
MANUSCRIPT COPIES: 4
PUBLICATION LAG TIME: 3-5 months
EARLY PUBLICATION OPTION: Not cited
ACCEPTANCE RATE: 10%
AUTHORSHIP RESTRICTIONS: No

PAGE CHARGES: No
STYLE REQUIREMENTS: C, Own
STYLE SHEET: Yes
REVISED THESES: No
STUDENT PAPERS: No
REPRINT POLICY: 50 free

SUBSCRIPTION ADDRESS: Business Manager, ASQ, Graduate School of Business & Public Administration, Cornell University
Ithaca NY 14853
ANNUAL SUBSCRIPTION RATE: Individuals: $16   Institutions: $32
FREQUENCY: Quarterly   CIRCULATION: 4900
AFFILIATION: None
INDEXED/ABSTRACTED IN: ISI, BPI, EAA, IPSA, PAIS, PA, PMA, SocA, KES, SSCI

JOURNAL TITLE: Adolescence

MANUSCRIPT ADDRESS: Libra Publishers, Inc.
P.O. Box 165, 391 Willets Road
Roslyn Heights, L.I., NY 11577

TYPES OF ARTICLES: Research, case studies, theoretical

MAJOR CONTENT AREAS: adolescence

TOPICS PREFERRED: Any related to adolescence

INAPPROPRIATE TOPICS: None cited

REVIEW PROCEDURE: Editorial board		
REVIEW PERIOD: 3 weeks		
MANUSCRIPT WORD LENGTH: 4000	PAGE CHARGES:	Yes
MANUSCRIPT COPIES: 2	STYLE REQUIREMENTS:	Own
PUBLICATION LAG TIME: 1-3 years	STYLE SHEET:	Yes
EARLY PUBLICATION OPTION: Yes	REVISED THESES:	Yes
ACCEPTANCE RATE: 25%	STUDENT PAPERS:	No
AUTHORSHIP RESTRICTIONS: No	REPRINT POLICY:	None free

SUBSCRIPTION ADDRESS: Libra Publishers, Inc.
P.O. Box 165, 391 Willets Road
Roslyn Heights, L.I., NY 11577

ANNUAL SUBSCRIPTION RATE: Individuals: $16   Institutions: $20
FREQUENCY: Quarterly   CIRCULATION: 3000
AFFILIATION: None
INDEXED/ABSTRACTED IN: BA, EI, PA, SSCI, SSI, IM

◆

JOURNAL TITLE: Advances in Nursing Science

MANUSCRIPT ADDRESS: Aspen Systems Corporation
1600 Research Boulevard
Rockville MD 20850

TYPES OF ARTICLES: Research, review, theoretical, applied research

MAJOR CONTENT AREAS: nursing diagnosis, nursing philosophy, nursing
research, nursing science, nursing theory

TOPICS PREFERRED: Applied research--articles, not papers only

INAPPROPRIATE TOPICS: Most commissioned

REVIEW PROCEDURE: Editorial board, external review, and referee		
REVIEW PERIOD: 60 days		
MANUSCRIPT WORD LENGTH: 4500-6000	PAGE CHARGES:	No
MANUSCRIPT COPIES: 3	STYLE REQUIREMENTS:	C
PUBLICATION LAG TIME: 60-120 days	STYLE SHEET:	Yes
EARLY PUBLICATION OPTION: No	REVISED THESES:	Yes
ACCEPTANCE RATE: 2%	STUDENT PAPERS:	Yes
AUTHORSHIP RESTRICTIONS: No	REPRINT POLICY:	None free

SUBSCRIPTION ADDRESS: Aspen Systems Corporation
16792 Oakmont Avenue
Gaithersburg MD 20877

ANNUAL SUBSCRIPTION RATE: $32.75 Interns, Students, Residents: $18.00
FREQUENCY: Quarterly   CIRCULATION: 5000-6000
AFFILIATION: None
INDEXED/ABSTRACTED IN: CINAHL

JOURNAL TITLE: Age - Journal of the American Aging Association

MANUSCRIPT ADDRESS: 42nd and Dewey Avenue
Omaha NB 68105

TYPES OF ARTICLES: Research, review, theoretical

MAJOR CONTENT AREAS: aging & aged, biochemistry, biology, biomedical research, biomedical aging research

TOPICS PREFERRED: All aspects of biomedical aging research

INAPPROPRIATE TOPICS: None cited

REVIEW PROCEDURE: Editorial Board		
REVIEW PERIOD: 4 weeks		
MANUSCRIPT WORD LENGTH: 600-1200	**PAGE CHARGES:** Yes, optional
MANUSCRIPT COPIES: 3	**STYLE REQUIREMENTS:** CBE
PUBLICATION LAG TIME: 3 months	**STYLE SHEET:** Yes
EARLY PUBLICATION OPTION: Yes	**REVISED THESES:** Yes
ACCEPTANCE RATE: 75%	**STUDENT PAPERS:** No
AUTHORSHIP RESTRICTIONS: No	**REPRINT POLICY:** None free

SUBSCRIPTION ADDRESS: University of Nebraska Medical Center
42nd and Dewey Avenue
Omaha NB 68105

ANNUAL SUBSCRIPTION RATE: $20
FREQUENCY: Quarterly   **CIRCULATION:** 400
AFFILIATION: American Aging Association
INDEXED/ABSTRACTED IN: CC, CA

◆

JOURNAL TITLE: AJOT: American Journal of Occupational Therapy

MANUSCRIPT ADDRESS: Elaine Viseltear, Editor
616 Tanner Marsh Road
Guilford CT 06437
TYPES OF ARTICLES: Research, review, theoretical, case studies

MAJOR CONTENT AREAS: Many areas listed in Appendix A including: adaptation, chronicity, crisis, family planning, growth/development, health promotion, loss/grief, mental health, public health, pain, quality of life, rehabilitation, stress

TOPICS PREFERRED: Practice of occupational therapy as a profession emphasizing research; problems in practice
INAPPROPRIATE TOPICS: None cited

REVIEW PROCEDURE: Editorial Board		
REVIEW PERIOD: 4-6 weeks		
MANUSCRIPT WORD LENGTH: 1600-1900	**PAGE CHARGES:** No
MANUSCRIPT COPIES: 3	**STYLE REQUIREMENTS:** Own
PUBLICATION LAG TIME: 2-12 months	**STYLE SHEET:** Yes
EARLY PUBLICATION OPTION: No	**REVISED THESES:** Yes
ACCEPTANCE RATE: 60%	**STUDENT PAPERS:** Yes
AUTHORSHIP RESTRICTIONS: No	**REPRINT POLICY:** None free

SUBSCRIPTION ADDRESS: Subscription Secretary
6000 Executive Boulevard
Rockville MD 20852
ANNUAL SUBSCRIPTION RATE: Individuals: $20 Institutions: $25
FREQUENCY: Monthly   **CIRCULATION:** 32,500
AFFILIATION: American Occupational Therapy Association, Inc.
INDEXED/ABSTRACTED IN: CC(SBS), CIJE, CINAHL, IM, BA, ECER, PA, SSCI, HLI

JOURNAL TITLE: Alcoholism: Clinical and Experimental Research

MANUSCRIPT ADDRESS: Jeanette Mason, Managing Editor
733 Third Avenue
New York NY 10017
TYPES OF ARTICLES: Research

MAJOR CONTENT AREAS: alcoholism & drug abuse, anatomy & physiology,
biochemistry, psychology, research methodology

TOPICS PREFERRED: Alcoholism, other categories as they pertain to
alcoholism, e.g., biochemistry of alcoholism
INAPPROPRIATE TOPICS: None cited

REVIEW PROCEDURE: Editorial board and external review
REVIEW PERIOD: 4-6 weeks
MANUSCRIPT WORD LENGTH: 3000-4000   PAGE CHARGES: No
MANUSCRIPT COPIES: 3   STYLE REQUIREMENTS: C, IM
PUBLICATION LAG TIME: Varies   STYLE SHEET: Yes
EARLY PUBLICATION OPTION: No   REVISED THESES: Not cited
ACCEPTANCE RATE: Not cited   STUDENT PAPERS: Not cited
AUTHORSHIP RESTRICTIONS: No   REPRINT POLICY: 50 free

SUBSCRIPTION ADDRESS: Grune & Stratton
111 Fifth Avenue
New York NY 10003
ANNUAL SUBSCRIPTION RATE: $38
FREQUENCY: Quarterly   CIRCULATION: 1500
AFFILIATION: National Council on Alcoholism
INDEXED/ABSTRACTED IN: IM

◆

JOURNAL TITLE: Allied Health and Behavioral Sciences †

MANUSCRIPT ADDRESS: School of Allied Health Professions
University of Wisconsin - Milwaukee, P.O. Box 413
Milwaukee WI 53201
TYPES OF ARTICLES: Research, theoretical, commentaries

MAJOR CONTENT AREAS: Many areas listed in Appendix A including: adaptation, biofeedback, communication, counseling,
health promotion, & rehabilitation of all age
groups; health sciences for all medical & allied
health personnel, continuing & patient education
TOPICS PREFERRED: Topical and related to allied health

INAPPROPRIATE TOPICS: None cited

REVIEW PROCEDURE: Editorial board and external review
REVIEW PERIOD: 3-4 months
MANUSCRIPT WORD LENGTH: 3000-4000   PAGE CHARGES: No
MANUSCRIPT COPIES: 5   STYLE REQUIREMENTS: APA
PUBLICATION LAG TIME: 8-10 months   STYLE SHEET: Yes
EARLY PUBLICATION OPTION: No   REVISED THESES: Yes
ACCEPTANCE RATE: 50%   STUDENT PAPERS: No
AUTHORSHIP RESTRICTIONS: No   REPRINT POLICY: 1 free

SUBSCRIPTION ADDRESS: School of Allied Health Professions
University of Wisconsin - Milwaukee, P.O. Box 413
Milwaukee WI 53201
ANNUAL SUBSCRIPTION RATE: Individuals: $20   Institutions: $34
FREQUENCY: Quarterly   CIRCULATION: 1000
AFFILIATION: None
INDEXED/ABSTRACTED IN: CINAHL

JOURNAL TITLE: Ambulatory Nursing Administration

MANUSCRIPT ADDRESS: Evelyn La Rocque, Editor
20 S. Quaker Lane
Alexandria VA 22314

TYPES OF ARTICLES: Theoretical, commentaries

MAJOR CONTENT AREAS: emergency services, hospitals, nursing: care, community/public health, diagnosis, process, service administration, theory, occpuational, patient teaching, professionalism, trauma; management issues in the ambulatory care center

TOPICS PREFERRED: Topics pertinent to ambulatory nursing and/or nurse management

INAPPROPRIATE TOPICS: None cited

REVIEW PROCEDURE: Editorial board
REVIEW PERIOD: Not cited
MANUSCRIPT WORD LENGTH: 1500-2000
MANUSCRIPT COPIES: 1
PUBLICATION LAG TIME: Not cited
EARLY PUBLICATION OPTION: No
ACCEPTANCE RATE: Not cited
AUTHORSHIP RESTRICTIONS: Not cited

PAGE CHARGES: No
STYLE REQUIREMENTS: Own
STYLE SHEET: Yes
REVISED THESES: No
STUDENT PAPERS: No
REPRINT POLICY: Not cited

SUBSCRIPTION ADDRESS: American Academy of Ambulatory Nursing Administration, 20 So. Quaker Lane
Alexandria VA 22314

ANNUAL SUBSCRIPTION RATE: Not cited
FREQUENCY: Bimonthly
CIRCULATION: Not cited
AFFILIATION: Ame. Academy of Ambulatory Nursing Administration
INDEXED/ABSTRACTED IN: Not cited

◆

JOURNAL TITLE: American Family Physician

MANUSCRIPT ADDRESS: American Academy of Family Physicians
1740 W. 92nd Street
Kansas City MO 64114

TYPES OF ARTICLES: Review, case studies, research, theoretical, commentaries, unsolicited book reviews

MAJOR CONTENT AREAS: accidents, adolescence, cancer, circulatory diseases, family planning, human behavior, immunization, medicine, mental retardation, nutrition, physical therapy, respiratory diseases

TOPICS PREFERRED: AFP is interested in any clinical topic which is of interest and value to family physicians

INAPPROPRIATE TOPICS: Most articles are assigned

REVIEW PROCEDURE: Editorial Board and external review
REVIEW PERIOD: 2-3 weeks
MANUSCRIPT WORD LENGTH: 2500-3000
MANUSCRIPT COPIES: 1
PUBLICATION LAG TIME: 3-6 months
EARLY PUBLICATION OPTION: No
ACCEPTANCE RATE: 30-35%
AUTHORSHIP RESTRICTIONS: No

PAGE CHARGES: No
STYLE REQUIREMENTS: Own
STYLE SHEET: Yes
REVISED THESES: No
STUDENT PAPERS: No
REPRINT POLICY: 100 free

SUBSCRIPTION ADDRESS: American Family Physician
1740 W. 92nd Street
Kansas City MO 64114

ANNUAL SUBSCRIPTION RATE: $20
FREQUENCY: Monthly
CIRCULATION: 130,000
AFFILIATION: American Academy of Family Physicians
INDEXED/ABSTRACTED IN: CA, IM

JOURNAL TITLE: American Health Care Association Journal

MANUSCRIPT ADDRESS: 1200 15th Street NW
Washington DC 20005

TYPES OF ARTICLES: Commentaries, case studies, research, theoretical, review, unsolicited book reviews

MAJOR CONTENT AREAS: aging, allied health, chronicity, continuing education, continuity of care, death, health promotion, mental retardation, nursing: assessment, audit, care, clinical, diagnosis, geriatric, occupational, psychiatric; nursing homes

TOPICS PREFERRED: Nursing homes

INAPPROPRIATE TOPICS: None cited

REVIEW PROCEDURE: Editorial board
REVIEW PERIOD: 4 weeks
MANUSCRIPT WORD LENGTH: 3000
MANUSCRIPT COPIES: 2
PUBLICATION LAG TIME: 4 months
EARLY PUBLICATION OPTION: No
ACCEPTANCE RATE: 70%
AUTHORSHIP RESTRICTIONS: No

PAGE CHARGES: No
STYLE REQUIREMENTS: Own
STYLE SHEET: Yes
REVISED THESES: Yes
STUDENT PAPERS: No
REPRINT POLICY: As requested

SUBSCRIPTION ADDRESS: American Health Care Association Journal
1200 15th Steet NW
Washington DC 20005
ANNUAL SUBSCRIPTION RATE: $12
FREQUENCY: Bimonthly
AFFILIATION: None
INDEXED/ABSTRACTED IN: INI, CINAHL

CIRCULATION: 8000

◆

JOURNAL TITLE: American Heart Journal

MANUSCRIPT ADDRESS: Dean T. Mason, M.D.
132 E Street, Suite 3E
Davis CA 95616
TYPES OF ARTICLES: Research, review, case studies, theoretical, unsolicited book reviews
MAJOR CONTENT AREAS: circulatory diseases, medicine, vascular diseases

TOPICS PREFERRED: All aspects of heart disease and circulatory disorders
INAPPROPRIATE TOPICS: None cited

REVIEW PROCEDURE: Editorial Board
REVIEW PERIOD: Not cited
MANUSCRIPT WORD LENGTH: 3600
MANUSCRIPT COPIES: 2
PUBLICATION LAG TIME: 6-8 months
EARLY PUBLICATION OPTION: No
ACCEPTANCE RATE: 42%
AUTHORSHIP RESTRICTIONS: No

PAGE CHARGES: No
STYLE REQUIREMENTS: AMA, IM
STYLE SHEET: Yes
REVISED THESES: No
STUDENT PAPERS: No
REPRINT POLICY: None free

SUBSCRIPTION ADDRESS: The C.V. Mosby Company, Circulation Department
11830 Westline Industrial Drive
St. Louis MO 63141
ANNUAL SUBSCRIPTION RATE: Individuals: $25.50 Institutions: $40.50
FREQUENCY: Monthly
AFFILIATION: None
INDEXED/ABSTRACTED IN: IM, CC, BA, CA, IPA, NAR, CINAHL

CIRCULATION: 11,000

JOURNAL TITLE: American Industrial Hygiene Association Journal

MANUSCRIPT ADDRESS: 475 Wolf Ledges Parkway
Akron OH 44311
Attention: R.S. Lee

TYPES OF ARTICLES: Research, case studies, review, theoretical,
practical applications

MAJOR CONTENT AREAS: biochemistry, compliance, continuing education,
epidemiology, instructional technology, micro-
biology, occupational nursing, professionalism,
systems theory

TOPICS PREFERRED: Topics applicable to industrial hygiene/
occupational health

INAPPROPRIATE TOPICS: Pure medical information

REVIEW PROCEDURE: Editorial board and external review
REVIEW PERIOD: 60 days
MANUSCRIPT WORD LENGTH: 2500-4500   PAGE CHARGES: Yes
MANUSCRIPT COPIES: 3   STYLE REQUIREMENTS: Own
PUBLICATION LAG TIME: 6-8 months   STYLE SHEET: Yes
EARLY PUBLICATION OPTION: No   REVISED THESES: No
ACCEPTANCE RATE: 80%   STUDENT PAPERS: No
AUTHORSHIP RESTRICTIONS: No   REPRINT POLICY: 100 free

SUBSCRIPTION ADDRESS: American Industrial Hygiene Association Journal
475 Wolf Ledges Parkway
Akron OH 44311
ANNUAL SUBSCRIPTION RATE: $30
FREQUENCY: Monthly   CIRCULATION: 7100
AFFILIATION: American Industrial Hygiene Association
INDEXED/ABSTRACTED IN: BA, CA, OA, PoIA, IHD, IM

◆

JOURNAL TITLE: American Journal of Clinical Biofeedback

MANUSCRIPT ADDRESS: c/o Department of Psychology
George Peabody College for Teachers
Nashville TN 37203

TYPES OF ARTICLES: Research, case studies, review, theoretical,
commentaries, unsolicited book reviews

MAJOR CONTENT AREAS: biofeedback, health sciences, pain, professionalism, rehabilitation, relaxation, stress, psychosomatic disorders, self-control

TOPICS PREFERRED: Treatment of stress related disorders, behavior
therapy, stress management and behavioral medicine

INAPPROPRIATE TOPICS: None cited

REVIEW PROCEDURE: Editorial Board
REVIEW PERIOD: 2-3 months
MANUSCRIPT WORD LENGTH: Varies   PAGE CHARGES: No
MANUSCRIPT COPIES: 3   STYLE REQUIREMENTS: APA
PUBLICATION LAG TIME: 4-6 months   STYLE SHEET: Yes
EARLY PUBLICATION OPTION: No   REVISED THESES: Yes
ACCEPTANCE RATE: 25%   STUDENT PAPERS: May submit
AUTHORSHIP RESTRICTIONS: No   REPRINT POLICY: None free

SUBSCRIPTION ADDRESS: F.N. Anchor, Psychology - 319
Peabody College
Nashville TN 37203
ANNUAL SUBSCRIPTION RATE: Individuals: $8 Institutions: $12
FREQUENCY: Semianually   CIRCULATION: 1400
AFFILIATION: American Association of Biofeedback Clinicians
INDEXED/ABSTRACTED IN: PA

JOURNAL TITLE: American Journal of Clinical Hypnosis

MANUSCRIPT ADDRESS: Sheldon B. Cohen, M.D., Editor
401 Peachtree Street, N.E. - Suite 804
Atlanta GA 30308

TYPES OF ARTICLES: Clinical, research, theoretical, review, case studies, commentaries, unsolicited book reviews

MAJOR CONTENT AREAS: adaptation, adolescence, adulthood, aging, counseling, crisis, death, dependency, eating disorders, human behavior & sexuality, loss/grief, marriage & divorce, psychopathology, quality of life, rehabilitation, relaxation, sleep, stress

TOPICS PREFERRED: Hypnosis

INAPPROPRIATE TOPICS: None cited

REVIEW PROCEDURE: Editorial board
REVIEW PERIOD: 1-4 months

MANUSCRIPT WORD LENGTH: 2000-4000	PAGE CHARGES: No	
MANUSCRIPT COPIES: 3	STYLE REQUIREMENTS: APA	
PUBLICATION LAG TIME: 6-12 months	STYLE SHEET: In journal	
EARLY PUBLICATION OPTION: No	REVISED THESES: No	
ACCEPTANCE RATE: 30%	STUDENT PAPERS: No	
AUTHORSHIP RESTRICTIONS: No	REPRINT POLICY: None free	

SUBSCRIPTION ADDRESS: Business Manager
2400 E. Devon Avenue, Suite 218
Des Plaines IL 60018

ANNUAL SUBSCRIPTION RATE: Individuals: $18 Institutions: $28
FREQUENCY: Quarterly   CIRCULATION: 3500
AFFILIATION: The American Society of Clinical Hypnosis
INDEXED/ABSTRACTED IN: IM, BA, PA

◆

JOURNAL TITLE: American Journal of Clinical Nutrition

MANUSCRIPT ADDRESS: Editor
9650 Rockville Pike
Bethesda MD 20014

TYPES OF ARTICLES: Research

MAJOR CONTENT AREAS: biochemistry, biomedical research, nutrition

TOPICS PREFERRED: None cited

INAPPROPRIATE TOPICS: None cited

REVIEW PROCEDURE: Editorial board and external review
REVIEW PERIOD: 2 months

MANUSCRIPT WORD LENGTH: Varies	PAGE CHARGES: No	
MANUSCRIPT COPIES: 3	STYLE REQUIREMENTS: CBE	
PUBLICATION LAG TIME: 2-4 months	STYLE SHEET: Yes	
EARLY PUBLICATION OPTION: No	REVISED THESES: No	
ACCEPTANCE RATE: 65%	STUDENT PAPERS: No	
AUTHORSHIP RESTRICTIONS: No	REPRINT POLICY: None free	

SUBSCRIPTION ADDRESS: Subscription Department
9650 Rockville Pike
Bethesda MD 20014

ANNUAL SUBSCRIPTION RATE: Individuals: $35 Institutions: $50
FREQUENCY: Monthly   CIRCULATION: 5900
AFFILIATION: American Society for Clinical Nutrition, Inc.
INDEXED/ABSTRACTED IN: CA, IM, BA, NAR, PA, ASTI, INI

JOURNAL TITLE: American Journal of Diseases of Children

MANUSCRIPT ADDRESS: Gilbert B. Forbes, M.D., Chief Editor
Department of Pediatrics, Box 777, University of
Rochester Medical Center, Rochester NY 14642
TYPES OF ARTICLES: Clinical studies, research, case studies

MAJOR CONTENT AREAS: Any area of interest to pediatricians and others
involved in child health

TOPICS PREFERRED: Topics of interest to pediatricians and others
involved in child health
INAPPROPRIATE TOPICS: None cited

REVIEW PROCEDURE: Editorial board and external review
REVIEW PERIOD: 2-4 months
MANUSCRIPT WORD LENGTH: 1000-5000　　　　　PAGE CHARGES: No
MANUSCRIPT COPIES: 3　　　　STYLE REQUIREMENTS: AMA, Own
PUBLICATION LAG TIME: 4-10 months　　　　STYLE SHEET: Yes
EARLY PUBLICATION OPTION: Yes　　　　REVISED THESES: No
ACCEPTANCE RATE: 35%　　　　STUDENT PAPERS: No
AUTHORSHIP RESTRICTIONS: No　　　　REPRINT POLICY: None free

SUBSCRIPTION ADDRESS: American Journal of Diseases of Children
535 N. Dearborn St.
Chicago IL 60610
ANNUAL SUBSCRIPTION RATE: $25
FREQUENCY: Monthly　　　　CIRCULATION: 26,000
AFFILIATION: American Medical Association
INDEXED/ABSTRACTED IN: BA, CC, CA, EM, IPA, IM, NAR, PA, CINAHL

◆

JOURNAL TITLE: American Journal of Drug & Alcohol Abuse

MANUSCRIPT ADDRESS: Dr. Edward Kaufman, Editor-in-Chief
University of California, Irvine Medical Center
101 City Drive South, Orange CA 92668
TYPES OF ARTICLES: Research, case studies, commentaries

MAJOR CONTENT AREAS: alcoholism & drug abuse

TOPICS PREFERRED: Preclinical, clinical & social modalities involved
in the study & treatment of drug abuse & alcoholism
INAPPROPRIATE TOPICS: None cited

REVIEW PROCEDURE: Editorial board
REVIEW PERIOD: Not cited
MANUSCRIPT WORD LENGTH: 2500-7500　　　　PAGE CHARGES: No
MANUSCRIPT COPIES: 3　　　　STYLE REQUIREMENTS: Own, IM
PUBLICATION LAG TIME: Not cited　　　　STYLE SHEET: Not cited
EARLY PUBLICATION OPTION: Not cited　　　　REVISED THESES: Not cited
ACCEPTANCE RATE: Not cited　　　　STUDENT PAPERS: Not cited
AUTHORSHIP RESTRICTIONS: Not cited　　　　REPRINT POLICY: Not cited

SUBSCRIPTION ADDRESS: Marcel Dekker Journals
270 Madison Avenue
New York NY 10016
ANNUAL SUBSCRIPTION RATE: Individuals: $34　　Institutions: $68
FREQUENCY: Quarterly　　　　CIRCULATION: Not cited
AFFILIATION: None
INDEXED/ABSTRACTED IN: IPA, IM, SWRA, CAAAL, CA, CC(SBS), EM, PA

JOURNAL TITLE: American Journal of Epidemiology

MANUSCRIPT ADDRESS: 550 N. Broadway, Suite 201
Baltimore MD 21205

TYPES OF ARTICLES: Research, theoretical, review, commentaries, case
studies

MAJOR CONTENT AREAS: epidemiology of infectious & non-infectious acute
& chronic diseases, accidents, aging & aged,
genetics, handicapping conditions, immunization,
loss/grief, microbiology, nutrition, pharmacology,
stress, suicide

TOPICS PREFERRED: Epidemiology of any and all diseases; need more
articles on infectious diseases

INAPPROPRIATE TOPICS: Case studies and clinical articles are not of
interest, emphasis must be epidemiologic

REVIEW PROCEDURE: Editorial board and external review
REVIEW PERIOD: 3 months

MANUSCRIPT WORD LENGTH: 4000	PAGE CHARGES:	Yes
MANUSCRIPT COPIES: 3	STYLE REQUIREMENTS:	CBE, IM
PUBLICATION LAG TIME: 6 months	STYLE SHEET:	Yes
EARLY PUBLICATION OPTION: Yes	REVISED THESES:	No
ACCEPTANCE RATE: 55%	STUDENT PAPERS:	No
AUTHORSHIP RESTRICTIONS: No	REPRINT POLICY:	None free

SUBSCRIPTION ADDRESS: American Journal of Epidemiology
550 N. Broadway, Suite 201
Baltimore MD 21205

ANNUAL SUBSCRIPTION RATE: Individuals: $25 Institutions: $47.50
FREQUENCY: Monthly   CIRCULATION: 3500
AFFILIATION: Society for Epidemiologic Research
INDEXED/ABSTRACTED IN: IM, BA, CC, CA, SSCI

JOURNAL TITLE: American Journal of Infection Control

MANUSCRIPT ADDRESS: Mary Castle, R.N., M.P.H.
P.O. Box 6090
Boulder CO 80206

TYPES OF ARTICLES: Research, review, case studies

MAJOR CONTENT AREAS: biomedical research, epidemiology, health
sciences, health policies, hospitals, inservice
education, medicine, microbiology, nursing: care,
maternal/child, medical/surgical, pediatric,
research; nursing homes, respiratory diseases

TOPICS PREFERRED: Infection control: nursing & medical care of infec-
tions, housekeeping, antiseptics, quality of care

INAPPROPRIATE TOPICS: None cited

REVIEW PROCEDURE: External review
REVIEW PERIOD: 3-4 Weeks

MANUSCRIPT WORD LENGTH: 2000-2500	PAGE CHARGES:	No
MANUSCRIPT COPIES: 3	STYLE REQUIREMENTS:	CBE, IM
PUBLICATION LAG TIME: 1-2 months	STYLE SHEET:	Yes
EARLY PUBLICATION OPTION: No	REVISED THESES:	No
ACCEPTANCE RATE: 50%	STUDENT PAPERS:	No
AUTHORSHIP RESTRICTIONS: No	REPRINT POLICY:	None free

SUBSCRIPTION ADDRESS: Journal Circulation Department, The C.V. Mosby Co.
11830 Westline Industrial Drive
St. Louis MO 63141

ANNUAL SUBSCRIPTION RATE: Not cited (new journal)
FREQUENCY: Quarterly   CIRCULATION: 5000
AFFILIATION: Association for Practitioners in Infection Control
INDEXED/ABSTRACTED IN: CINAHL

JOURNAL TITLE: American Journal of Intravenous Therapy &
Clinical Nutrition
MANUSCRIPT ADDRESS: Salvatore J. Turco
3307 N. Broad St.
Philadelphia PA 19104
TYPES OF ARTICLES: Review, case studies, commentaries

MAJOR CONTENT AREAS: Practical articles dealing with IV therapy and
pharmacy

TOPICS PREFERRED: None cited

INAPPROPRIATE TOPICS: None cited

REVIEW PROCEDURE: Editorial Board	
REVIEW PERIOD: 30-60 days	
MANUSCRIPT WORD LENGTH: 3000-4000	**PAGE CHARGES:** No
MANUSCRIPT COPIES: 3	**STYLE REQUIREMENTS:** AMA
PUBLICATION LAG TIME: 6-12 months	**STYLE SHEET:** Yes
EARLY PUBLICATION OPTION: No	**REVISED THESES:** Yes
ACCEPTANCE RATE: 75%	**STUDENT PAPERS:** No
AUTHORSHIP RESTRICTIONS: No	**REPRINT POLICY:** None free

SUBSCRIPTION ADDRESS: 121 S. Gertrude Avenue
Paramus NJ 07652

ANNUAL SUBSCRIPTION RATE: $14
FREQUENCY: Bimonthly   **CIRCULATION:** 10,000
AFFILIATION: American, NY, Canadian Associations of IV Therapy
INDEXED/ABSTRACTED IN: IM, CINAHL, IPA

◆

JOURNAL TITLE: American Journal of Medical Genetics

MANUSCRIPT ADDRESS: John M. Opitz, Editor-in-Chief
Shodair Children's Hospital, P.O. Box 5539,
840 Helena Avenue, Helena MT 59601
TYPES OF ARTICLES: Research, theoretical, review, case studies,
commentaries, solicited book reviews, clinical
MAJOR CONTENT AREAS: biomedical research, counseling, epidemiology,
ethics, family planning, genetics, growth/develop-
ment, handicapping conditions, life span, medicine,
mental health/illness, mental retardation, quality
of life, rehabilitation, research methodology
TOPICS PREFERRED: Clinical genetics

INAPPROPRIATE TOPICS: None cited

REVIEW PROCEDURE: Editorial board and external review	
REVIEW PERIOD: 2 1/2 months	
MANUSCRIPT WORD LENGTH: 2500	**PAGE CHARGES:** No
MANUSCRIPT COPIES: 3	**STYLE REQUIREMENTS:** IM
PUBLICATION LAG TIME: 8 months	**STYLE SHEET:** Yes
EARLY PUBLICATION OPTION: No	**REVISED THESES:** Yes
ACCEPTANCE RATE: 80%	**STUDENT PAPERS:** Yes
AUTHORSHIP RESTRICTIONS: No	**REPRINT POLICY:** 50 free

SUBSCRIPTION ADDRESS: Alan R. Liss, Inc.
150 Fifth Avenue
New York NY 10011
ANNUAL SUBSCRIPTION RATE: $45
FREQUENCY: Monthly   **CIRCULATION:** Not cited
AFFILIATION: None
INDEXED/ABSTRACTED IN: GA, CC

JOURNAL TITLE: American Journal of Nursing

MANUSCRIPT ADDRESS: 555 West 57th Street
New York NY 10019

TYPES OF ARTICLES: Authoritative descriptions of care, research,
case studies
MAJOR CONTENT AREAS: Nearly all areas listed in Appendix A ranging
from new devices for improving patient care to
well-tested plans for administering nursing
service

TOPICS PREFERRED: Nursing practice

INAPPROPRIATE TOPICS: School papers

REVIEW PROCEDURE: Staff review and external review by consultants
REVIEW PERIOD: 2-4 months
MANUSCRIPT WORD LENGTH: 1500-2500   PAGE CHARGES: No
MANUSCRIPT COPIES: 2   STYLE REQUIREMENTS: C
PUBLICATION LAG TIME: 3 months-2 years   STYLE SHEET: Yes
EARLY PUBLICATION OPTION: No   REVISED THESES: No
ACCEPTANCE RATE: 5%   STUDENT PAPERS: No
AUTHORSHIP RESTRICTIONS: No   REPRINT POLICY: $20/page or
100 free

SUBSCRIPTION ADDRESS: American Journal of Nursing
555 West 57th Street
New York NY 10019
ANNUAL SUBSCRIPTION RATE: $18
FREQUENCY: Monthly   CIRCULATION: 350,000
AFFILIATION: American Nurses' Association
INDEXED/ABSTRACTED IN: INI, CINAHL, IM, CA, HLI, IPA, PAIS, SSI, PA

◆

JOURNAL TITLE: American Journal of Ophthalmology

MANUSCRIPT ADDRESS: Tribune Tower, Suite 1415
435 North Michigan Avenue
Chicago IL 60611
TYPES OF ARTICLES: Research, case studies, unsolicited book reviews,
theoretical
MAJOR CONTENT AREAS: adaptation, basic medical sciences, diseases
related to opthalmology, epidemiology, genetics,
growth/development, handicapping conditions, immun-
ization, mental retardation, pain, perception,
sensory deprivation, stigma, testing/measurement
TOPICS PREFERRED: Topics relating to clinical and research aspects
of ophthalmology
INAPPROPRIATE TOPICS: Review articles, animal studies, multi-part
articles
REVIEW PROCEDURE: Editorial board, internal editor
REVIEW PERIOD: 3-4 weeks
MANUSCRIPT WORD LENGTH: 5000   PAGE CHARGES: No
MANUSCRIPT COPIES: 3   STYLE REQUIREMENTS: AMA, C, CBE, IM, SW
PUBLICATION LAG TIME: 6-12 months   STYLE SHEET: Yes
EARLY PUBLICATION OPTION: No   REVISED THESES: No
ACCEPTANCE RATE: 25%   STUDENT PAPERS: No
AUTHORSHIP RESTRICTIONS: No   REPRINT POLICY: 50 free

SUBSCRIPTION ADDRESS: Ophthalmic Publishing Company
Tribune Tower, Suite 1415, 435 North Michigan Ave.
Chicago IL 60611
ANNUAL SUBSCRIPTION RATE: $18 domestic, $22 foreign
FREQUENCY: Monthly   CIRCULATION: 18,000
AFFILIATION: None
INDEXED/ABSTRACTED IN: ISI, IM, BA, CA, NAR, PA

JOURNAL TITLE: American Journal of Orthopsychiatry

MANUSCRIPT ADDRESS: 1775 Broadway
New York NY 10019

TYPES OF ARTICLES: Research, theoretical, review, case studies

MAJOR CONTENT AREAS: abuse (child/spouse), adaptation, adolescence, adulthood, aging and aged, children, epidemiology, growth/development, health promotion, human behavior, marriage & divorce, mental health/illness, mental retardation, parenting

TOPICS PREFERRED: Topics in the areas listed that best inform public policy and professional practice

INAPPROPRIATE TOPICS: None cited

REVIEW PROCEDURE: Editorial board	
REVIEW PERIOD: 3-4 months	
MANUSCRIPT WORD LENGTH: 5000	**PAGE CHARGES:** No
MANUSCRIPT COPIES: 3	**STYLE REQUIREMENTS:** Own
PUBLICATION LAG TIME: 3-4 months	**STYLE SHEET:** Yes
EARLY PUBLICATION OPTION: No	**REVISED THESES:** No
ACCEPTANCE RATE: 12%	**STUDENT PAPERS:** No
AUTHORSHIP RESTRICTIONS: No	**REPRINT POLICY:** 1 free journal

SUBSCRIPTION ADDRESS: 49 Sheridan Avenue
Albany NY 12210

ANNUAL SUBSCRIPTION RATE: $20
FREQUENCY: Quarterly   **CIRCULATION:** 11,500
AFFILIATION: American Orthopsychiatric Association
INDEXED/ABSTRACTED IN: BA, CA, CDL, EI, HLI, IM, INI, LLBA, MRA, NAR, PA, SCI, SSI, SSCI, CINAHL

◆

JOURNAL TITLE: American Journal of Physical Medicine

MANUSCRIPT ADDRESS: H.D. Bouman, M.D., Editor
P.O. Box 617, Downtown Station
Phoenix AZ 85001

TYPES OF ARTICLES: Research, clinical research, theoretical, review, case studies

MAJOR CONTENT AREAS: anatomy and physiology, biofeedback, biomedical research, handicapping conditions, medicine, physical therapy, rehabilitation, testing/measurement

TOPICS PREFERRED: Physical medicine, rehabilitation, physiology

INAPPROPRIATE TOPICS: None cited

REVIEW PROCEDURE: Editorial board	
REVIEW PERIOD: 3 months	
MANUSCRIPT WORD LENGTH: Depends on content	**PAGE CHARGES:** No
MANUSCRIPT COPIES: 3	**STYLE REQUIREMENTS:** Minimal
PUBLICATION LAG TIME: 8-15 months	**STYLE SHEET:** Yes
EARLY PUBLICATION OPTION: No	**REVISED THESES:** Depends on quality
ACCEPTANCE RATE: 60%	**STUDENT PAPERS:** No
AUTHORSHIP RESTRICTIONS: No	**REPRINT POLICY:** None free

SUBSCRIPTION ADDRESS: Williams and Wilkins Company
428 East Preston St.
Baltimore MD 21202
ANNUAL SUBSCRIPTION RATE: Individuals: $17   Institutions: $23
FREQUENCY: Bimonthly   **CIRCULATION:** 2600
AFFILIATION: None
INDEXED/ABSTRACTED IN: BA, CA, IM, PA, CINAHL

JOURNAL TITLE: American Journal of Public Health

MANUSCRIPT ADDRESS: 1015 15th Steet NW
Washington DC 20005

TYPES OF ARTICLES: Research, review, commentaries, methodology,
evaluative studies

MAJOR CONTENT AREAS: Many areas listed in Appendix A including: all
age groups and health problems, continuity of
care, discharge planning, epidemiology, health
promotion, nursing, public health, quality of
life, research methodology

TOPICS PREFERRED: Significant articles covering the current aspects
of public health

INAPPROPRIATE TOPICS: None cited

REVIEW PROCEDURE:	Editorial board, external & peer review		
REVIEW PERIOD:	2 months		
MANUSCRIPT WORD LENGTH:	1000-5000	**PAGE CHARGES:**	No
MANUSCRIPT COPIES:	3	**STYLE REQUIREMENTS:**	CBE, IM
PUBLICATION LAG TIME:	6 months	**STYLE SHEET:**	Yes
EARLY PUBLICATION OPTION:	Yes	**REVISED THESES:**	No
ACCEPTANCE RATE:	15%	**STUDENT PAPERS:**	No
AUTHORSHIP RESTRICTIONS:	No	**REPRINT POLICY:**	None free

SUBSCRIPTION ADDRESS: Publication Sales Division
American Public Health Association
1015 15th Street NW, Washington DC 20005

ANNUAL SUBSCRIPTION RATE: $40

FREQUENCY:	Monthly	**CIRCULATION:**	35,000

AFFILIATION: American Public Health Association

INDEXED/ABSTRACTED IN: IM, BA, CA, PAIS, HLI, EPB, PHR, CINAHL, MSRS,
EM, SSA, NSA, SWRA, ASTI, BRD, Engl, IPA, INI,
NAR, OA, PAIS, PolA, SSCI, SSI

◆

JOURNAL TITLE: American Journal of Roentgenology

MANUSCRIPT ADDRESS: Editorial Office
4545 15th Avenue NE   Room 403
Seattle WA 98105

TYPES OF ARTICLES: Research, review, theoretical, case studies,
technical notes, commentaries

MAJOR CONTENT AREAS: biomedical research, cancer, research methodology,
all phases of diagnostic radiology, nuclear
medicine, computed tomography, ultrasound

TOPICS PREFERRED: All phases of diagnostic radiology

INAPPROPRIATE TOPICS: None cited

REVIEW PROCEDURE:	External review		
REVIEW PERIOD:	3-4 months		
MANUSCRIPT WORD LENGTH:	Varies	**PAGE CHARGES:**	No
MANUSCRIPT COPIES:	2	**STYLE REQUIREMENTS:**	C, CBE, IM, Own
PUBLICATION LAG TIME:	3-4 months	**STYLE SHEET:**	Not cited
EARLY PUBLICATION OPTION:	No	**REVISED THESES:**	No
ACCEPTANCE RATE:	40%	**STUDENT PAPERS:**	No
AUTHORSHIP RESTRICTIONS:	No	**REPRINT POLICY:**	50 free

SUBSCRIPTION ADDRESS: Williams and Wilkins, Publisher
428 East Preston Street
Baltimore MD 21202

ANNUAL SUBSCRIPTION RATE: Individuals: $40   Institutions: $50

FREQUENCY:	Monthly	**CIRCULATION:**	15,000

AFFILIATION: American Roentgen Ray and American Radium Societies

INDEXED/ABSTRACTED IN: IM, BA, CA, INI, NAR

JOURNAL TITLE: American Laboratory

MANUSCRIPT ADDRESS: International Scientific Communications, Inc.
808 Kings Highway
Fairfield CT 06430

TYPES OF ARTICLES: Research

MAJOR CONTENT AREAS: biochemistry, biomedical research, microbiology,
nutrition, pharmacology, research methodology

TOPICS PREFERRED: Laboratory instrumentation, separations techniques, research technique in analytical chemistry

INAPPROPRIATE TOPICS: None cited

REVIEW PROCEDURE: Editorial board		
REVIEW PERIOD: 8 weeks		
MANUSCRIPT WORD LENGTH: 1500-2000	PAGE CHARGES: No	
MANUSCRIPT COPIES: 3	STYLE REQUIREMENTS: Own	
PUBLICATION LAG TIME: 3-5 months	STYLE SHEET: Yes	
EARLY PUBLICATION OPTION: No	REVISED THESES: No	
ACCEPTANCE RATE: 60%	STUDENT PAPERS: No	
AUTHORSHIP RESTRICTIONS: No	REPRINT POLICY: 2 free	

SUBSCRIPTION ADDRESS: International Scientific Communications, Inc.
808 Kings Highway
Fairfield CT 06430

ANNUAL SUBSCRIPTION RATE: $36

FREQUENCY: Monthly   CIRCULATION: 103,000

AFFILIATION: None

INDEXED/ABSTRACTED IN: CA, CINAHL, BA

◆

JOURNAL TITLE: American Lung Association Bulletin

MANUSCRIPT ADDRESS: Editor
1740 Broadway
New York NY 10019

TYPES OF ARTICLES: Articles for broad readership publication

MAJOR CONTENT AREAS: allied health personnel, community/public health
nursing, continuity of care, occupational nursing,
rehabilitation, respiratory diseases

TOPICS PREFERRED: Pediatric lung disease, respiratory disease,
smoking, occupational lung disease

INAPPROPRIATE TOPICS: Research articles in journal style, most articles
commissioned

REVIEW PROCEDURE: Staff review		
REVIEW PERIOD: 4 weeks		
MANUSCRIPT WORD LENGTH: 1200	PAGE CHARGES: No	
MANUSCRIPT COPIES: 1	STYLE REQUIREMENTS: C, WT	
PUBLICATION LAG TIME: 5-6 months	STYLE SHEET: Yes	
EARLY PUBLICATION OPTION: No	REVISED THESES: No	
ACCEPTANCE RATE: Not cited	STUDENT PAPERS: No	
AUTHORSHIP RESTRICTIONS: No	REPRINT POLICY: 25-100 free	

SUBSCRIPTION ADDRESS: American Lung Association Bulletin
1740 Broadway
New York NY 10019

ANNUAL SUBSCRIPTION RATE: Not cited

FREQUENCY: 10 times yearly   CIRCULATION: 45,000

AFFILIATION: American Lung Association

INDEXED/ABSTRACTED IN: CINAHL, INI

JOURNAL TITLE: Anaesthesia & Intensive Care

MANUSCRIPT ADDRESS: Dr. B.J. Barry
P.O. Box 345
Paddington NSW 2021 Australia
TYPES OF ARTICLES: Research, case studies, personal experiences

MAJOR CONTENT AREAS: anesthesiology, intensive care, clinical practice

TOPICS PREFERRED: Educational journal; topics associated with anaesthesia, intensive care & related subjects
INAPPROPRIATE TOPICS: None cited

REVIEW PROCEDURE: Editorial board		
REVIEW PERIOD: Not cited		
MANUSCRIPT WORD LENGTH: Not cited	**PAGE CHARGES:** Not cited	
MANUSCRIPT COPIES: Not cited	**STYLE REQUIREMENTS:** Own	
PUBLICATION LAG TIME: Not cited	**STYLE SHEET:** Not cited	
EARLY PUBLICATION OPTION: Not cited	**REVISED THESES:** Not cited	
ACCEPTANCE RATE: Not cited	**STUDENT PAPERS:** Not cited	
AUTHORSHIP RESTRICTIONS: Not cited	**REPRINT POLICY:** Author purchase	

SUBSCRIPTION ADDRESS: P.O. Box 345
Paddington NSW 2021 Australia

ANNUAL SUBSCRIPTION RATE: $28 Australian
FREQUENCY: Quarterly   **CIRCULATION:** 1600
AFFILIATION: Australian Society of Anaesthetists
INDEXED/ABSTRACTED IN: IM, CC(CP), CINAHL

◆

JOURNAL TITLE: Anesthesia and Analgesia

MANUSCRIPT ADDRESS: Nicholas M. Green, M.D.,Editor-in-Chief
Yale University School of Medicine
333 Cedar St., New Haven, CT 06510
TYPES OF ARTICLES: Research, case studies, review, unsolicited book reviews
MAJOR CONTENT AREAS: anesthesiology, biomedical research, pain, pharmacology, respiratory diseases

TOPICS PREFERRED: Anesthesiology, intensive care of critically ill, pain, pharmacology, physiology
INAPPROPRIATE TOPICS: None cited

REVIEW PROCEDURE: Editorial board and external review		
REVIEW PERIOD: 5 weeks		
MANUSCRIPT WORD LENGTH: 800-2000	**PAGE CHARGES:** No	
MANUSCRIPT COPIES: 3	**STYLE REQUIREMENTS:** CBE, IM	
PUBLICATION LAG TIME: 4-5 months	**STYLE SHEET:** Yes	
EARLY PUBLICATION OPTION: No	**REVISED THESES:** No	
ACCEPTANCE RATE: 30%	**STUDENT PAPERS:** No	
AUTHORSHIP RESTRICTIONS: No	**REPRINT POLICY:** 2 free journals	

SUBSCRIPTION ADDRESS: International Anesthesia Research Society
3645 Warrensville Center Road
Cleveland OH 44122
ANNUAL SUBSCRIPTION RATE: $30
FREQUENCY: Bimonthly   **CIRCULATION:** 12,000
AFFILIATION: International Anesthesia Research Society
INDEXED/ABSTRACTED IN: IM, CC, BA, CA, EM, INI

JOURNAL TITLE: Annals of Allergy

MANUSCRIPT ADDRESS: M. Coleman Harris, M.D.
31561 Table Rock Drive
South Laguna Beach CA 92677
TYPES OF ARTICLES: Clinical articles, research articles, case reports, editorials, news, book reviews
MAJOR CONTENT AREAS: allergies

TOPICS PREFERRED: Allergic disorders in adults & children; otolaryngology and other specialties
INAPPROPRIATE TOPICS: None cited

REVIEW PROCEDURE: Not cited
REVIEW PERIOD: Not cited
MANUSCRIPT WORD LENGTH: 3000   PAGE CHARGES: Not cited
MANUSCRIPT COPIES: Not cited   STYLE REQUIREMENTS: Own
PUBLICATION LAG TIME: Not cited   STYLE SHEET: Not cited
EARLY PUBLICATION OPTION: Not cited   REVISED THESES: Not cited
ACCEPTANCE RATE: Not cited   STUDENT PAPERS: Not cited
AUTHORSHIP RESTRICTIONS: Not cited   REPRINT POLICY: None free

SUBSCRIPTION ADDRESS: Annals of Allergy
P.O. Box 20671
Bloomington MN 55420
ANNUAL SUBSCRIPTION RATE: $20
FREQUENCY: Monthly   CIRCULATION: 4550
AFFILIATION: American College of Allergists
INDEXED/ABSTRACTED IN: BA, CA, IM

◆

JOURNAL TITLE: Annals of Clinical and Laboratory Science

MANUSCRIPT ADDRESS: Institute for Clinical Science
230 North Broad Street
Philadelphia PA 19102
TYPES OF ARTICLES: Review, case studies, research studies

MAJOR CONTENT AREAS: No particular content areas cited

TOPICS PREFERRED: Clinical science

INAPPROPRIATE TOPICS: None cited

REVIEW PROCEDURE: Editorial board
REVIEW PERIOD: 1 month
MANUSCRIPT WORD LENGTH: None specified   PAGE CHARGES: No
MANUSCRIPT COPIES: 3   STYLE REQUIREMENTS: IM
PUBLICATION LAG TIME: 8 months   STYLE SHEET: No
EARLY PUBLICATION OPTION: No   REVISED THESES: No
ACCEPTANCE RATE: 66%   STUDENT PAPERS: No
AUTHORSHIP RESTRICTIONS: No   REPRINT POLICY: None free

SUBSCRIPTION ADDRESS: Institute for Clinical Science
230 North Broad Street
Philadelphia PA 19102
ANNUAL SUBSCRIPTION RATE: $33
FREQUENCY: Bimonthly   CIRCULATION: 2000
AFFILIATION: Association of Clinical Scientists
INDEXED/ABSTRACTED IN: CC(CP), CC(LS), SCI, CA, BA, IM

JOURNAL TITLE: Annals of Emergency Medicine

MANUSCRIPT ADDRESS: P.O. Box 61911
Dallas TX 75261

TYPES OF ARTICLES: Research, case studies, review, theoretical,
commentaries, unsolicited book reviews
MAJOR CONTENT AREAS: accidents, emergency services, pain, primary care

TOPICS PREFERRED: Topics dealing with emergency medicine

INAPPROPRIATE TOPICS: None cited

REVIEW PROCEDURE: Editorial board
REVIEW PERIOD: 3 months
MANUSCRIPT WORD LENGTH: Not cited   PAGE CHARGES: Not cited
MANUSCRIPT COPIES: 3   STYLE REQUIREMENTS: AMA, IM
PUBLICATION LAG TIME: 8 months   STYLE SHEET: Yes
EARLY PUBLICATION OPTION: Yes   REVISED THESES: No
ACCEPTANCE RATE: 50%   STUDENT PAPERS: Not cited
AUTHORSHIP RESTRICTIONS: No   REPRINT POLICY: 1 free

SUBSCRIPTION ADDRESS: Annals of Emergency Medicine
P.O. Box 61911
Dallas TX 75261
ANNUAL SUBSCRIPTION RATE: $34
FREQUENCY: Monthly   CIRCULATION: 13,000
AFFILIATION: American College of Emergency Physicians
INDEXED/ABSTRACTED IN: IM, CINAHL

◆

JOURNAL TITLE: Annals of Human Biology

MANUSCRIPT ADDRESS: Department of Growth and Development
Institute of Child Health
30 Guilford Street, London WC1N 1EH England
TYPES OF ARTICLES: Research

MAJOR CONTENT AREAS: anatomy and physiology, anesthesiology,
anthropology, biology, biomedical research,
epidemiology, genetics, growth/development,
research methodology

TOPICS PREFERRED: Population genetics, growth, all aspects of human
biology
INAPPROPRIATE TOPICS: Clinical

REVIEW PROCEDURE: Editorial board, external review
REVIEW PERIOD: 2 months
MANUSCRIPT WORD LENGTH: 3000-4000   PAGE CHARGES: No
MANUSCRIPT COPIES: 2   STYLE REQUIREMENTS: CBE
PUBLICATION LAG TIME: 4-6 months   STYLE SHEET: Yes
EARLY PUBLICATION OPTION: Yes   REVISED THESES: Yes
ACCEPTANCE RATE: 40%   STUDENT PAPERS: No
AUTHORSHIP RESTRICTIONS: No   REPRINT POLICY: 50 free

SUBSCRIPTION ADDRESS: Taylor & Francis, Ltd.
10 Macklen Street
London WC2B 5NF England
ANNUAL SUBSCRIPTION RATE: $46
FREQUENCY: Bimonthly   CIRCULATION: 1000
AFFILIATION: Society for the Study of Human Biology
INDEXED/ABSTRACTED IN: CC, IM, EM

JOURNAL TITLE: AORN Journal

MANUSCRIPT ADDRESS: Elinor S. Schrader, Editor
10170 E. Mississippi Avenue
Denver CO 80231

TYPES OF ARTICLES: Not applicable

MAJOR CONTENT AREAS: nursing: assessment, audit, care, diagnosis, education, history, medical/surgical, operating room, philosophy, process, research, science, service administration, theory; women's issues

TOPICS PREFERRED: Topics of relevance and interest to nurses practicing in the operating room and recovery room
INAPPROPRIATE TOPICS: None cited

REVIEW PROCEDURE: Editorial Board		
REVIEW PERIOD: 1-6 months		
MANUSCRIPT WORD LENGTH: 2000-5000	PAGE CHARGES: No	
MANUSCRIPT COPIES: 2	STYLE REQUIREMENTS: AMA, C, T	
PUBLICATION LAG TIME: 2-12 months	STYLE SHEET: Yes	
EARLY PUBLICATION OPTION: No	REVISED THESES: Yes	
ACCEPTANCE RATE: 75%	STUDENT PAPERS: No	
AUTHORSHIP RESTRICTIONS: No	REPRINT POLICY: None free	

SUBSCRIPTION ADDRESS: Members: Rosalie Retzer Nonmembers: Sonia Visness
10170 E. Mississippi Avenue
Denver CO 80231
ANNUAL SUBSCRIPTION RATE: Members: free Nonmembers: $32
FREQUENCY: 13 times yearly   CIRCULATION: 31,100
AFFILIATION: Association of Operating Room Nurses, Inc.
INDEXED/ABSTRACTED IN: IM, CINAHL, HLI, INI

◆

JOURNAL TITLE: Applied Radiology

MANUSCRIPT ADDRESS: 825 S. Barrington Avenue
Los Angeles CA 90049

TYPES OF ARTICLES: Research, theoretical, review, case studies, equipment surveys, commentaries
MAJOR CONTENT AREAS: anesthesiology, radiologists and technologists, diagnostic radiology, nuclear medicine, radiation therapy, computed tomography, thermography, ultrasound

TOPICS PREFERRED: Case history, equipment use and administrative management
INAPPROPRIATE TOPICS: None cited

REVIEW PROCEDURE: Editorial board, external review, in-house review		
REVIEW PERIOD: 2-3 weeks		
MANUSCRIPT WORD LENGTH: 3500	PAGE CHARGES: No	
MANUSCRIPT COPIES: 2	STYLE REQUIREMENTS: C	
PUBLICATION LAG TIME: Varies	STYLE SHEET: Yes	
EARLY PUBLICATION OPTION: Yes	REVISED THESES: Yes	
ACCEPTANCE RATE: 75%	STUDENT PAPERS: Yes	
AUTHORSHIP RESTRICTIONS: No	REPRINT POLICY: 1 free	

SUBSCRIPTION ADDRESS: Applied Radiology
825 S. Barrington Avenue
Los Angeles CA 90049
ANNUAL SUBSCRIPTION RATE: $30
FREQUENCY: Bimonthly   CIRCULATION: 30-40,000
AFFILIATION: None
INDEXED/ABSTRACTED IN: CINAHL

JOURNAL TITLE: Archives of Andrology

MANUSCRIPT ADDRESS: C.S. Mott Center for Human Growth & Development
Wayne State University School of Medicine
275 E. Hancock, Detroit MI 48201
TYPES OF ARTICLES: Research, review, unsolicited book reviews

MAJOR CONTENT AREAS: Many areas listed in Appendix A including: health
problems of all age groups; basic medical sciences;
nursing: clinical specialties, maternal/child,
geriatric; biofeedback, continuity of care, counseling, family planning, human behavior & sexuality
TOPICS PREFERRED: Andrology

INAPPROPRIATE TOPICS: None cited

REVIEW PROCEDURE: Editorial board and external review
REVIEW PERIOD: 4 months
MANUSCRIPT WORD LENGTH: 2500
MANUSCRIPT COPIES: 3
PUBLICATION LAG TIME: 4 months
EARLY PUBLICATION OPTION: Yes
ACCEPTANCE RATE: 50%
AUTHORSHIP RESTRICTIONS: No

PAGE CHARGES: Yes
STYLE REQUIREMENTS: Own
STYLE SHEET: Yes
REVISED THESES: Yes
STUDENT PAPERS: No
REPRINT POLICY: 25 free

SUBSCRIPTION ADDRESS: C.S. Mott Center for Human Growth & Development
Wayne State University School of Medicine
275 E. Hancock, Detroit MI 48201
ANNUAL SUBSCRIPTION RATE: Individuals: $60   Institutions: $120
FREQUENCY: 8 times yearly   CIRCULATION: 1000
AFFILIATION: None
INDEXED/ABSTRACTED IN: Not cited (new journal)

◆

JOURNAL TITLE: Archives of General Psychiatry

MANUSCRIPT ADDRESS: Daniel Freedman, M.D.
University of Chicago Hospitals and Clinics
950 East 59th Street, Box 2011, Chicago IL 60637
TYPES OF ARTICLES: Research, review

MAJOR CONTENT AREAS: abuse (child/spouse, alcoholism/drug), epidemiology, genetics, human behavior, marriage and
divorce, mental health/illness, mental retardation, psychopathology, psychiatric/mental health
nursing, research methodology, stress, suicide
TOPICS PREFERRED: Psychiatry and neuropharmacology

INAPPROPRIATE TOPICS: None cited

REVIEW PROCEDURE: Editorial board and external review
REVIEW PERIOD: 3-4 months
MANUSCRIPT WORD LENGTH: 5000
MANUSCRIPT COPIES: 3
PUBLICATION LAG TIME: 8-12 months
EARLY PUBLICATION OPTION: Yes
ACCEPTANCE RATE: 15%
AUTHORSHIP RESTRICTIONS: No

PAGE CHARGES: No
STYLE REQUIREMENTS: AMA
STYLE SHEET: Yes
REVISED THESES: Yes
STUDENT PAPERS: No
REPRINT POLICY: None free

SUBSCRIPTION ADDRESS: AMA - Division of Specialty Journals
535 North Dearborn Street
Chicago IL 60637
ANNUAL SUBSCRIPTION RATE: $24
FREQUENCY: Monthly   CIRCULATION: 24,000
AFFILIATION: American Medical Association
INDEXED/ABSTRACTED IN: IM, ACP, BA, CA, EM, IPA, NAR, PA, SSCI, CINAHL

JOURNAL TITLE: Archives of Physical Medicine and Rehabilitation

MANUSCRIPT ADDRESS: Suite 922
30 North Michigan
Chicago IL 60602

TYPES OF ARTICLES: Research, case studies, review, commentaries

MAJOR CONTENT AREAS: allied health sciences, cancer, circulatory & respiratory diseases, nursing: clinical specialties, education, geriatric, orthopedic, pediatric, research; physical therapy, rehabilitation, adaptation to handicapping conditions

TOPICS PREFERRED: Any topic related to restoration of function in the physically handicapped

INAPPROPRIATE TOPICS: None cited

REVIEW PROCEDURE: External review		
REVIEW PERIOD: 90 days		
MANUSCRIPT WORD LENGTH: 6500 maximum	**PAGE CHARGES:** No	
MANUSCRIPT COPIES: 3	**STYLE REQUIREMENTS:** AMA, Own	
PUBLICATION LAG TIME: 8-12 months	**STYLE SHEET:** Yes	
EARLY PUBLICATION OPTION: No	**REVISED THESES:** No	
ACCEPTANCE RATE: 40%	**STUDENT PAPERS:** Yes	
AUTHORSHIP RESTRICTIONS: No	**REPRINT POLICY:** None free	

SUBSCRIPTION ADDRESS: Suite 922
30 North Michigan Avenue
Chicago IL 60602

ANNUAL SUBSCRIPTION RATE: $20

FREQUENCY: Monthly   **CIRCULATION:** 6500

AFFILIATION: American Congress of Rehabilitation Medicine

INDEXED/ABSTRACTED IN: IM, CC, CINAHL, BA, CA, HLI, INI

JOURNAL TITLE: ARN Journal †

MANUSCRIPT ADDRESS: Editor
2506 Gross Point Road
Evanston IL 60201

TYPES OF ARTICLES: Research, case studies, review, theoretical, commentaries, unsolicited book reviews

MAJOR CONTENT AREAS: Many areas listed in Appendix A including: adaptation to chronicity & handicapping conditions; discharge planning; nursing: community/public health, geriatric, homes, assessment, audit, research; patient teaching/counseling; rehabilitation

TOPICS PREFERRED: Topics relating to rehabilitation

INAPPROPRIATE TOPICS: None cited

REVIEW PROCEDURE: Editorial board		
REVIEW PERIOD: 2-3 months		
MANUSCRIPT WORD LENGTH: 2000-3000	**PAGE CHARGES:** No	
MANUSCRIPT COPIES: 2	**STYLE REQUIREMENTS:** C	
PUBLICATION LAG TIME: 2-6 months	**STYLE SHEET:** Yes	
EARLY PUBLICATION OPTION: No	**REVISED THESES:** Yes	
ACCEPTANCE RATE: 75%	**STUDENT PAPERS:** Yes	
AUTHORSHIP RESTRICTIONS: No	**REPRINT POLICY:** 4 free	

SUBSCRIPTION ADDRESS: ARN Journal †
2506 Gross Point Road
Evanston IL 60201

ANNUAL SUBSCRIPTION RATE: $18

FREQUENCY: Bimonthly   **CIRCULATION:** 2000

AFFILIATION: Association of Rehabilitation Nurses

INDEXED/ABSTRACTED IN: CINAHL, INI

JOURNAL TITLE: Arthritis and Rheumatism

MANUSCRIPT ADDRESS: Nathan J. Zvaifler, M.D., Editor
H-229, Univ. of California Med. Cntr.
225 West Dickinson St., San Diego CA 92103
TYPES OF ARTICLES: Research, case studies, review, theoretical

MAJOR CONTENT AREAS: biochemistry, biomedical research, epidemiology, genetics, microbiology

TOPICS PREFERRED: Research and clinical articles related to patients with arthritis
INAPPROPRIATE TOPICS: None cited

REVIEW PROCEDURE: Editorial board
REVIEW PERIOD: 4-6 weeks
MANUSCRIPT WORD LENGTH: 3000   **PAGE CHARGES:** No
MANUSCRIPT COPIES: 2   **STYLE REQUIREMENTS:** AMA
PUBLICATION LAG TIME: 4-5 months   **STYLE SHEET:** Yes
EARLY PUBLICATION OPTION: No   **REVISED THESES:** No
ACCEPTANCE RATE: 45%   **STUDENT PAPERS:** No
AUTHORSHIP RESTRICTIONS: No   **REPRINT POLICY:** None free

SUBSCRIPTION ADDRESS: Arthritis and Rheumatism
3400 Peachtree Road NE
Atlanta GA 30326
ANNUAL SUBSCRIPTION RATE: $35
FREQUENCY: Monthly   **CIRCULATION:** 7000
AFFILIATION: American Rheumatism Association
INDEXED/ABSTRACTED IN: CC, IM

◆

JOURNAL TITLE: Asian Journal of Infectious Diseases

MANUSCRIPT ADDRESS: Crawford P.O. Box 666
Singapore 9119
Republic of Singapore
TYPES OF ARTICLES: Research, review, case studies

MAJOR CONTENT AREAS: biology, biomedical research, epidemiology, health sciences, immunization, medicine, microbiology, pathology, public health, research methodology, respiratory diseases

TOPICS PREFERRED: Medical microbiology, clinical immunology, and infectious diseases
INAPPROPRIATE TOPICS: None

REVIEW PROCEDURE: Editorial board and external review
REVIEW PERIOD: 3 months
MANUSCRIPT WORD LENGTH: 4000   **PAGE CHARGES:** No
MANUSCRIPT COPIES: 2   **STYLE REQUIREMENTS:** IM
PUBLICATION LAG TIME: 6 months   **STYLE SHEET:** Yes
EARLY PUBLICATION OPTION: No   **REVISED THESES:** Yes
ACCEPTANCE RATE: 50%   **STUDENT PAPERS:** Yes
AUTHORSHIP RESTRICTIONS: No   **REPRINT POLICY:** 25 free

SUBSCRIPTION ADDRESS: Crawford P.O. Box 666
Singapore 9119
Republic of Singapore
ANNUAL SUBSCRIPTION RATE: $18
FREQUENCY: Quarterly   **CIRCULATION:** 3000
AFFILIATION: None
INDEXED/ABSTRACTED IN: BA, CA, MA

JOURNAL TITLE: Association for the Care of Children's Health
Journal †
MANUSCRIPT ADDRESS: Mary C. Cerretto, Ph.D.
Child Development Div., Univ. of Texas
Medical Branch, Galveston TX 77550
TYPES OF ARTICLES: Research, theoretical, review, case studies,
commentaries, unsolicited book reviews
MAJOR CONTENT AREAS: Most areas in Appendix A including: nursing:
assessment, care, community/public health, criti-
cal care, diagnosis, education, maternal/child,
medical/surgical, philosophy, research, theory,
operating room, pediatric, school, trauma
TOPICS PREFERRED: Articles on children and their families in health
care settings
INAPPROPRIATE TOPICS: None

REVIEW PROCEDURE: Editorial board
REVIEW PERIOD: 8-10 weeks
MANUSCRIPT WORD LENGTH: 2500-4000   PAGE CHARGES: No
MANUSCRIPT COPIES: 3   STYLE REQUIREMENTS: APA
PUBLICATION LAG TIME: 2-6 months   STYLE SHEET: Yes
EARLY PUBLICATION OPTION: Yes   REVISED THESES: Yes
ACCEPTANCE RATE: 50%   STUDENT PAPERS: Yes
AUTHORSHIP RESTRICTIONS: No   REPRINT POLICY: 2-5 free journals

SUBSCRIPTION ADDRESS: Charles B. Slack
6900 Grove Road
Thorofare NJ 08086
ANNUAL SUBSCRIPTION RATE: $19
FREQUENCY: Quarterly   CIRCULATION: 2500
AFFILIATION: Association for the Care of Children in Hospitals
INDEXED/ABSTRACTED IN: PA, CINAHL

◆

JOURNAL TITLE: The Australasian Nurses Journal

MANUSCRIPT ADDRESS: Managing Editor
P.O. Box 197
Pt. Adelaide 5015, Australia
TYPES OF ARTICLES: Research, case studies

MAJOR CONTENT AREAS: Nearly all areas listed in Appendix A

TOPICS PREFERRED: Nursing, medical, community and general

INAPPROPRIATE TOPICS: None cited

REVIEW PROCEDURE: Not cited
REVIEW PERIOD: 1 month
MANUSCRIPT WORD LENGTH: 2000-3000   PAGE CHARGES: No
MANUSCRIPT COPIES: 1   STYLE REQUIREMENTS: Own
PUBLICATION LAG TIME: 1-2 months   STYLE SHEET: Yes
EARLY PUBLICATION OPTION: Not cited   REVISED THESES: Not cited
ACCEPTANCE RATE: Not cited   STUDENT PAPERS: Yes
AUTHORSHIP RESTRICTIONS: No   REPRINT POLICY: 6 free journals

SUBSCRIPTION ADDRESS: Australasian Nurses Journal
P.O. Box 197
Pt. Adelaide 5015 Australia
ANNUAL SUBSCRIPTION RATE: $8.00 Australian
FREQUENCY: 11 times yearly   CIRCULATION: 18,000
AFFILIATION: None
INDEXED/ABSTRACTED IN: INI, CINAHL

JOURNAL TITLE: Australian Nurses' Journal

MANUSCRIPT ADDRESS: 132-136 Albert Rd.
South Melbourne
Victoria Australia 3205
TYPES OF ARTICLES: Research, theoretical, case studies, commentaries

MAJOR CONTENT AREAS: Most areas listed in Appendix A including:
nursing education, professional standards, tech-
nical systems, industrial matters, women's issues

TOPICS PREFERRED: None cited

INAPPROPRIATE TOPICS: None cited

REVIEW PROCEDURE: Not cited		
REVIEW PERIOD: Not cited		
MANUSCRIPT WORD LENGTH: Not cited	**PAGE CHARGES:** Not cited	
MANUSCRIPT COPIES: Not cited	**STYLE REQUIREMENTS:** Own	
PUBLICATION LAG TIME: Not cited	**STYLE SHEET:** Yes	
EARLY PUBLICATION OPTION: Not cited	**REVISED THESES:** Not cited	
ACCEPTANCE RATE: Not cited	**STUDENT PAPERS:** Not cited	
AUTHORSHIP RESTRICTIONS: Not cited	**REPRINT POLICY:** Not cited	

SUBSCRIPTION ADDRESS: 132-136 Albert Rd.
South Melbourne
Victoria Australia 3205
ANNUAL SUBSCRIPTION RATE: $23 Australian
FREQUENCY: Monthly   **CIRCULATION:** 50,000
AFFILIATION: Royal Australian Nursing Federation
INDEXED/ABSTRACTED IN: CINAHL, INI

◆

JOURNAL TITLE: Australian Paediatric Journal

MANUSCRIPT ADDRESS: Royal Children's Hospital
Flemington Rd.
Parkville Victoria 3052 Australia
TYPES OF ARTICLES: Research, case studies, review

MAJOR CONTENT AREAS: abuse (child/spouse), accidents, adolescence,
children, genetics, growth/development, han-
dicapping conditions, health promotion, human
behavior, nutrition, parenting

TOPICS PREFERRED: Scientific papers of paediatric medical and
surgical topics
INAPPROPRIATE TOPICS: Case reports that are already well covered by
the literature
REVIEW PROCEDURE: External review
REVIEW PERIOD: 2-3 months

MANUSCRIPT WORD LENGTH: 6000	**PAGE CHARGES:** No	
MANUSCRIPT COPIES: 2	**STYLE REQUIREMENTS:** Not cited	
PUBLICATION LAG TIME: 1-6 months	**STYLE SHEET:** Yes	
EARLY PUBLICATION OPTION: No	**REVISED THESES:** No	
ACCEPTANCE RATE: 60%	**STUDENT PAPERS:** No	
AUTHORSHIP RESTRICTIONS: No	**REPRINT POLICY:** None free	

SUBSCRIPTION ADDRESS: Royal Children's Hospital
Flemington Road
Parkville, Victoria 3052, Australia
ANNUAL SUBSCRIPTION RATE: $37.50
FREQUENCY: Quarterly   **CIRCULATION:** 925
AFFILIATION: Australian College of Paediatrics
INDEXED/ABSTRACTED IN: IM, CC(CP), CA

JOURNAL TITLE: Aviation, Space, and Environmental Medicine

MANUSCRIPT ADDRESS: Sidney D. Leverett, Jr., Ph.D.
103 Encino Blanco
San Antonio TX 78232

TYPES OF ARTICLES: Research, review, case studies, theoretical, commentaries, unsolicited book reviews

MAJOR CONTENT AREAS: accidents, adaptation, alcoholism & drug abuse, basic medical sciences, biorhythms, circulatory & respiratory diseases, human behavior, nursing: care, medical/surgical, science, theory, trauma; research methodology, sensory deprivation, sleep

TOPICS PREFERRED: Clinical aerospace and aviation medicine and nursing

INAPPROPRIATE TOPICS: Equipment descriptions

REVIEW PROCEDURE: Editorial board and external review

REVIEW PERIOD: 2 months

MANUSCRIPT WORD LENGTH: 3000

MANUSCRIPT COPIES: 3

PUBLICATION LAG TIME: 6 months

EARLY PUBLICATION OPTION: No

ACCEPTANCE RATE: 65%

AUTHORSHIP RESTRICTIONS: No

PAGE CHARGES: No

STYLE REQUIREMENTS: APA, CBE, IM

STYLE SHEET: Yes

REVISED THESES: No

STUDENT PAPERS: No

REPRINT POLICY: None free

SUBSCRIPTION ADDRESS: Aerospace Medical Association
Washington National Airport
Washington DC 20001

ANNUAL SUBSCRIPTION RATE: $35

FREQUENCY: Monthly

CIRCULATION: 7000

AFFILIATION: Aerospace Medical Association

INDEXED/ABSTRACTED IN: IM, CC, BA, CA, NAR, PA, CINAHL

JOURNAL TITLE: Behavior Research Methods & Instrumentation

MANUSCRIPT ADDRESS: Joseph B. Sidowski, Editor
Psychology Department, University of South Florida
Tampa FL 33620

TYPES OF ARTICLES: Research, review

MAJOR CONTENT AREAS: biofeedback, biomedical research, communication,
fatigue, groups, human behavior, instructional
technology, mental health/illness, pain, research
methodology, sensory deprivation, sleep, stress,
systems theory, testing/measurement

TOPICS PREFERRED: Experimental methods & designs, instrumentation &
techniques, computer technology

INAPPROPRIATE TOPICS: Statistics

REVIEW PROCEDURE: Editorial board, external review
REVIEW PERIOD: 15-45 days

MANUSCRIPT WORD LENGTH: No limit	PAGE CHARGES: No	
MANUSCRIPT COPIES: 4	STYLE REQUIREMENTS: APA	
PUBLICATION LAG TIME: 60 days	STYLE SHEET: Yes	
EARLY PUBLICATION OPTION: No	REVISED THESES: Will review	
ACCEPTANCE RATE: 50%	STUDENT PAPERS: Will review	
AUTHORSHIP RESTRICTIONS: No	REPRINT POLICY: None free	

SUBSCRIPTION ADDRESS: Psychonomic Society Journals
1108 W. 34th St.
Austin TX 78705

ANNUAL SUBSCRIPTION RATE: Individuals: $15   Institutions: $30
FREQUENCY: Bimonthly   CIRCULATION: 1100
AFFILIATION: Psychonomic Society
INDEXED/ABSTRACTED IN: BA, PA, SSCI

◆

JOURNAL TITLE: Behavior Research & Therapy

MANUSCRIPT ADDRESS: Professor S. Rachman, Institute of Psychiatry
De Crespigny Park Rd.
Denmark Hill London SE5 8AF England

TYPES OF ARTICLES: Research, theoretical, case studies

MAJOR CONTENT AREAS: behavior therapy

TOPICS PREFERRED: Experimental clinical research in behavior
therapy

INAPPROPRIATE TOPICS: None

REVIEW PROCEDURE: Editorial board
REVIEW PERIOD: 3 months

MANUSCRIPT WORD LENGTH: Not cited	PAGE CHARGES: Not cited	
MANUSCRIPT COPIES: Not cited	STYLE REQUIREMENTS: APA	
PUBLICATION LAG TIME: 9 months	STYLE SHEET: Yes	
EARLY PUBLICATION OPTION: No	REVISED THESES: Not cited	
ACCEPTANCE RATE: 15%	STUDENT PAPERS: Not cited	
AUTHORSHIP RESTRICTIONS: Not cited	REPRINT POLICY: 25 free	

SUBSCRIPTION ADDRESS: Pergamon Press
Headington Hall
Oxford   England

ANNUAL SUBSCRIPTION RATE: Individuals: $25   Institutions: $50
FREQUENCY: Bimonthly   CIRCULATION: Not cited
AFFILIATION: None
INDEXED/ABSTRACTED IN: Not cited

JOURNAL TITLE: Behavioral and Neural Biology

MANUSCRIPT ADDRESS: Department of Psychobiology
University of California
Irvine CA 92717

TYPES OF ARTICLES: Research, review, rapid communication, commentaries

MAJOR CONTENT AREAS: anatomy & physiology, biochemistry, biology, genetics, psychology, sleep; neural and endocrine bases of behavior

TOPICS PREFERRED: Neurobiological bases of behavior

INAPPROPRIATE TOPICS: Purely descriptive behavioral studies

REVIEW PROCEDURE: External review		
REVIEW PERIOD: 1 month		
MANUSCRIPT WORD LENGTH: 800-7000	PAGE CHARGES: No	
MANUSCRIPT COPIES: 4	STYLE REQUIREMENTS: Own	
PUBLICATION LAG TIME: 4 months	STYLE SHEET: Yes	
EARLY PUBLICATION OPTION: No	REVISED THESES: Possibly	
ACCEPTANCE RATE: 40%	STUDENT PAPERS: No	
AUTHORSHIP RESTRICTIONS: No	REPRINT POLICY: 50 Free	

SUBSCRIPTION ADDRESS: Academic Press, Inc.
111 Fifth Avenue
New York NY 10003

ANNUAL SUBSCRIPTION RATE: $52.50
FREQUENCY: Monthly   CIRCULATION: 1000
AFFILIATION: None
INDEXED/ABSTRACTED IN: BA, PA, CC

◆

JOURNAL TITLE: Behavioral Science

MANUSCRIPT ADDRESS: Building 446
University of California at Santa Barbara
Santa Barbara CA 93106

TYPES OF ARTICLES: Theoretical, research, review, unsolicited book reviews

MAJOR CONTENT AREAS: adaptation, anthropology, biology, communication, cultural diversity, health sciences, perception, psychology, research methodology, sociology; general systems science articles

TOPICS PREFERRED: Most articles are inter- or multidisciplinary; systems science

INAPPROPRIATE TOPICS: Articles involving only one discipline

REVIEW PROCEDURE: Editorial board and external review		
REVIEW PERIOD: 4 months		
MANUSCRIPT WORD LENGTH: 7000	PAGE CHARGES: No	
MANUSCRIPT COPIES: 5	STYLE REQUIREMENTS: APA	
PUBLICATION LAG TIME: 6-8 months	STYLE SHEET: Yes	
EARLY PUBLICATION OPTION: No	REVISED THESES: No	
ACCEPTANCE RATE: 25%	STUDENT PAPERS: No	
AUTHORSHIP RESTRICTIONS: No	REPRINT POLICY: None free	

SUBSCRIPTION ADDRESS: P.O. Box 64025
Baltimore MD 21264

ANNUAL SUBSCRIPTION RATE: Individuals: $25   Institutions: $40
FREQUENCY: Bimonthly   CIRCULATION: 2500
AFFILIATION: Society for General Systems Research
INDEXED/ABSTRACTED IN: BA, IM, MR, PA, SocA, SSCI

JOURNAL TITLE: Bioethics Quarterly

MANUSCRIPT ADDRESS: Jane A. (Raible) Boyajian, D. Min.
3000 5th St., N.W.
New Brighton MN 55112

TYPES OF ARTICLES: Research, theoretical, case studies, commentaries, book reviews

MAJOR CONTENT AREAS: Most areas listed in Appendix A including: bioethics in general, all areas pertaining to nursing, all age groups, teaching/learning, women's issues

TOPICS PREFERRED: Bioethical topics

INAPPROPRIATE TOPICS: None cited

REVIEW PROCEDURE: Editorial board and external review
REVIEW PERIOD: Not cited
MANUSCRIPT WORD LENGTH: Not cited
MANUSCRIPT COPIES: 3
PUBLICATION LAG TIME: Not cited
EARLY PUBLICATION OPTION: No
ACCEPTANCE RATE: Not cited
AUTHORSHIP RESTRICTIONS: Not cited

PAGE CHARGES: No
STYLE REQUIREMENTS: C, T
STYLE SHEET: Yes
REVISED THESES: No
STUDENT PAPERS: Not cited
REPRINT POLICY: None free

SUBSCRIPTION ADDRESS: Human Sciences Press
72 Fifth Avenue
New York NY 10014
ANNUAL SUBSCRIPTION RATE: Individuals: $20   Institutions: $40
FREQUENCY: Quarterly   **CIRCULATION:** 400
AFFILIATION: The Northwest Institute of Ethics & Life Sciences
INDEXED/ABSTRACTED IN: None cited

JOURNAL TITLE: Biomedical Communications

MANUSCRIPT ADDRESS: 475 Park Avenue South
New York NY 10016

TYPES OF ARTICLES: "How-to", case studies, research, theoretical, review, commentaries, unsolicited book reviews

MAJOR CONTENT AREAS: communication, compliance, continuing & inservice education, counseling, emergency services, hospitals, instructional technology, nursing: clinical specialties, community/public health, assessment, education, service administration

TOPICS PREFERRED: Continuing education, inservice training, communications

INAPPROPRIATE TOPICS: Clinical subject matter

REVIEW PROCEDURE: Editorial board
REVIEW PERIOD: 1-6 months
MANUSCRIPT WORD LENGTH: 1500
MANUSCRIPT COPIES: 2
PUBLICATION LAG TIME: 15 months
EARLY PUBLICATION OPTION: No
ACCEPTANCE RATE: 60%
AUTHORSHIP RESTRICTIONS: No

PAGE CHARGES: No
STYLE REQUIREMENTS: Own
STYLE SHEET: Yes
REVISED THESES: No
STUDENT PAPERS: No
REPRINT POLICY: 2 free

SUBSCRIPTION ADDRESS: Biomedical Communications
475 Park Avenue South
New York NY 10016
ANNUAL SUBSCRIPTION RATE: $7.50
FREQUENCY: Bimonthly   **CIRCULATION:** 23,000
AFFILIATION: None
INDEXED/ABSTRACTED IN: BA

JOURNAL TITLE: Birth and the Family Journal

MANUSCRIPT ADDRESS: 110 El Camino Real
Berkeley CA 94705

TYPES OF ARTICLES: Review, research, unsolicited book reviews,
letters to the editor
MAJOR CONTENT AREAS: Many areas listed in Appendix A including: all
topics and nursing specialties related to child-
birth and child rearing, health policies,
genetics, patient teaching, research methodology,
and women's issues
TOPICS PREFERRED: None cited

INAPPROPRIATE TOPICS: None cited

REVIEW PROCEDURE: Editorial board and external review
REVIEW PERIOD: 1-3 months
MANUSCRIPT WORD LENGTH: 2500   PAGE CHARGES: No
MANUSCRIPT COPIES: 3   STYLE REQUIREMENTS: AMA
PUBLICATION LAG TIME: 3-6 months   STYLE SHEET: Yes
EARLY PUBLICATION OPTION: Yes   REVISED THESES: Yes
ACCEPTANCE RATE: 20%   STUDENT PAPERS: Yes
AUTHORSHIP RESTRICTIONS: No   REPRINT POLICY: Author purchase

SUBSCRIPTION ADDRESS: Birth and the Family Journal
110 El Camino Real
Berkeley CA 94705
ANNUAL SUBSCRIPTION RATE: Individuals: $10   Institutions: $12
FREQUENCY: Quarterly   CIRCULATION: 5500
AFFILIATION: International Childbirth Education Association
INDEXED/ABSTRACTED IN: CC(SBS), CC(CP), EM, PA, CINAHL, INI, SSCI, IM

◆

JOURNAL TITLE: British Journal of Anaesthesia

MANUSCRIPT ADDRESS: Editor, University of Glasgow
Dept. of Anaesthesia, Western Infirmary
Glasgow   G11 GNT Scotland
TYPES OF ARTICLES: Research, review, case studies

MAJOR CONTENT AREAS: accidents, anesthesiology, biochemistry,
medicine, pain, pharmacology, physics, respiratory
diseases

TOPICS PREFERRED: None cited

INAPPROPRIATE TOPICS: None cited

REVIEW PROCEDURE: Editorial board and external review
REVIEW PERIOD: Not cited
MANUSCRIPT WORD LENGTH: 5000   PAGE CHARGES: No
MANUSCRIPT COPIES: 2   STYLE REQUIREMENTS: Own
PUBLICATION LAG TIME: Not cited   STYLE SHEET: Not cited
EARLY PUBLICATION OPTION: No   REVISED THESES: No
ACCEPTANCE RATE: Not cited   STUDENT PAPERS: No
AUTHORSHIP RESTRICTIONS: No   REPRINT POLICY: 25 free

SUBSCRIPTION ADDRESS: MacMillan Journals Ltd.
Houndsmills Estate
Baskinstoke, Hants   England
ANNUAL SUBSCRIPTION RATE: $49
FREQUENCY: Monthly   CIRCULATION: 7500
AFFILIATION: None
INDEXED/ABSTRACTED IN: CC, BA, CA, IM, INI

JOURNAL TITLE: British Journal of Radiology

MANUSCRIPT ADDRESS: The Honorary Editors
32 Welbeck Street
London W1M 7PG England

TYPES OF ARTICLES: Research, review, case studies

MAJOR CONTENT AREAS: cancer, physics, X-ray diagnosis, radiation
oncology, nuclear medicine, ultrasound, radiological physics, radiobiology, radiation protection
and related disciplines

TOPICS PREFERRED: As cited under content areas

INAPPROPRIATE TOPICS: Not cited

REVIEW PROCEDURE: Editorial board, external review
REVIEW PERIOD: 2-3 months
MANUSCRIPT WORD LENGTH: Varies   PAGE CHARGES: No
MANUSCRIPT COPIES: 2   STYLE REQUIREMENTS: H
PUBLICATION LAG TIME: 4-6 months   STYLE SHEET: Yes
EARLY PUBLICATION OPTION: No   REVISED THESES: No
ACCEPTANCE RATE: 35-40%   STUDENT PAPERS: No
AUTHORSHIP RESTRICTIONS: No   REPRINT POLICY: 25 free

SUBSCRIPTION ADDRESS: Subscription Department
32 Welbeck Street
London W1M 7PG England

ANNUAL SUBSCRIPTION RATE: $40
FREQUENCY: Monthly   CIRCULATION: 5500
AFFILIATION: British Institute of Radiology
INDEXED/ABSTRACTED IN: BA, CA, IM, NAR, SA, CC, CINAHL

◆

JOURNAL TITLE: British Medical Journal

MANUSCRIPT ADDRESS: The Editor
BMA House, Tavistock Square
London WC1H 9JR England

TYPES OF ARTICLES: Research, case studies

MAJOR CONTENT AREAS: Many areas listed in Appendix A including: major
health problems and diseases, medical and nursing
specialty areas, aging and aged, health sciences,
hospitals, human behavior, human sexuality,
marriage & divorce, primary care

TOPICS PREFERRED: None cited

INAPPROPRIATE TOPICS: None cited

REVIEW PROCEDURE: Editorial board and external review
REVIEW PERIOD: 4-6 weeks
MANUSCRIPT WORD LENGTH: 2000 maximum   PAGE CHARGES: No
MANUSCRIPT COPIES: 2   STYLE REQUIREMENTS: Own
PUBLICATION LAG TIME: 4 weeks   STYLE SHEET: Yes
EARLY PUBLICATION OPTION: No   REVISED THESES: No
ACCEPTANCE RATE: 10-15%   STUDENT PAPERS: No
AUTHORSHIP RESTRICTIONS: No   REPRINT POLICY: None free

SUBSCRIPTION ADDRESS: British Medical Journal
BMA House, Tavistock Square
London WC1H 9JR England

ANNUAL SUBSCRIPTION RATE: $56
FREQUENCY: Weekly   CIRCULATION: 85,000
AFFILIATION: British Medical Association
INDEXED/ABSTRACTED IN: BA, CA, IPA, IM, NAR, CINAHL, INI

43

JOURNAL TITLE: Canada's Mental Health

MANUSCRIPT ADDRESS: Department of National Health and Welfare
Health Services and Promotion Branch
Ottawa K1A 1B4 Canada
TYPES OF ARTICLES: Research, review, case studies

MAJOR CONTENT AREAS: mental health issues for all ages; groups;
child/spouse and alcoholism/drug abuse; counsel-
ing; cultural diversity; human behavior & sexuality; marriage & divorce; inservice & patient education; psychiatric nursing; research methodology
TOPICS PREFERRED: Child and family, adolescence, geriatrics,
forensic, administration, environment, evaluation
INAPPROPRIATE TOPICS: Retardation, specific program descriptives

REVIEW PROCEDURE: Editorial board, external review, blind referees		
REVIEW PERIOD: 6 months		
MANUSCRIPT WORD LENGTH: 4000-5000	**PAGE CHARGES:** No	
MANUSCRIPT COPIES: 2	**STYLE REQUIREMENTS:** APA	
PUBLICATION LAG TIME: 1 year	**STYLE SHEET:** Yes	
EARLY PUBLICATION OPTION: Yes	**REVISED THESES:** Yes	
ACCEPTANCE RATE: Not cited	**STUDENT PAPERS:** No	
AUTHORSHIP RESTRICTIONS: Yes	**REPRINT POLICY:** None free	

SUBSCRIPTION ADDRESS: Department of National Health and Welfare
Health Services and Promotion Branch
Ottawa K1A 1B4 Canada
ANNUAL SUBSCRIPTION RATE: $4
FREQUENCY: Quarterly   **CIRCULATION:** 30,000
AFFILIATION: None
INDEXED/ABSTRACTED IN: AHM, CEI, CPI, CINAHL, CC, HLI, PA, SSCI, SWRA

◆

JOURNAL TITLE: Canadian Journal of Medical Technology

MANUSCRIPT ADDRESS: P.O. Box 830
Hamilton, Ontario
Canada L8N 3N8
TYPES OF ARTICLES: Research, method assessment, instrumentation
assessment, theoretical
MAJOR CONTENT AREAS: biochemistry, biomedical research, genetics,
microbiology, research methodology

TOPICS PREFERRED: Accounts of original technical investigations,
clinical laboratory technology
INAPPROPRIATE TOPICS: Poorly disguised commercial promotions

REVIEW PROCEDURE: External review		
REVIEW PERIOD: 15-30 days		
MANUSCRIPT WORD LENGTH: 2000-4000	**PAGE CHARGES:** No	
MANUSCRIPT COPIES: 1	**STYLE REQUIREMENTS:** Own	
PUBLICATION LAG TIME: 1-12 months	**STYLE SHEET:** Yes	
EARLY PUBLICATION OPTION: Will consider	**REVISED THESES:** No	
ACCEPTANCE RATE: 30%	**STUDENT PAPERS:** Yes	
AUTHORSHIP RESTRICTIONS: No	**REPRINT POLICY:** None free	

SUBSCRIPTION ADDRESS: Canadian Journal of Medical Technology
P.O. Box 830
Hamilton, Ontario, Canada L8N 3N8
ANNUAL SUBSCRIPTION RATE: $15
FREQUENCY: Bimonthly   **CIRCULATION:** 19,500
AFFILIATION: Canadian Society of Laboratory Technologists
INDEXED/ABSTRACTED IN: BA, CA, CINAHL, IM, SCI

JOURNAL TITLE: Canadian Journal of Psychiatric Nursing

MANUSCRIPT ADDRESS: 871 Notre Dame Avenue
Winnipeg, Manitoba R3E 0M4
Canada
TYPES OF ARTICLES: Research, commentaries, case studies,
theoretical, unsolicted book reviews, review
MAJOR CONTENT AREAS: psychiatric/mental health nursing

TOPICS PREFERRED: None cited

INAPPROPRIATE TOPICS: None cited

REVIEW PROCEDURE:	Editorial board		
REVIEW PERIOD:	6 weeks		
MANUSCRIPT WORD LENGTH:	1500	**PAGE CHARGES:**	No
MANUSCRIPT COPIES:	2	**STYLE REQUIREMENTS:**	C
PUBLICATION LAG TIME:	1 year	**STYLE SHEET:**	Yes
EARLY PUBLICATION OPTION:	Yes	**REVISED THESES:**	No
ACCEPTANCE RATE:	65%	**STUDENT PAPERS:**	No
AUTHORSHIP RESTRICTIONS:	No	**REPRINT POLICY:**	2 free

SUBSCRIPTION ADDRESS: 871 Notre Dame Avenue
Winnipeg, Manitoba R3E 0M4
Canada
ANNUAL SUBSCRIPTION RATE: $10 ($8 in Canada)
FREQUENCY: Bimonthly **CIRCULATION:** 5000
AFFILIATION: Psychiatric Nurses Association of Canada
INDEXED/ABSTRACTED IN: INI, CINAHL

◆

JOURNAL TITLE: Canadian Journal of Public Health

MANUSCRIPT ADDRESS: 1335 Carling Avenue
Suite 306
Ottawa, Ontario Canada K1Z 8N8
TYPES OF ARTICLES: Research, theoretical, case studies,
commentaries, letters to the editor
MAJOR CONTENT AREAS: community/public health nursing, epidemiology,
health promotion, health policies, public health,
quality of life

TOPICS PREFERRED: None cited

INAPPROPRIATE TOPICS: None cited

REVIEW PROCEDURE:	Not cited		
REVIEW PERIOD:	Not cited		
MANUSCRIPT WORD LENGTH:	Not cited	**PAGE CHARGES:**	Not cited
MANUSCRIPT COPIES:	2	**STYLE REQUIREMENTS:**	IM, Own
PUBLICATION LAG TIME:	Not cited	**STYLE SHEET:**	Not cited
EARLY PUBLICATION OPTION:	Not cited	**REVISED THESES:**	Not cited
ACCEPTANCE RATE:	Not cited	**STUDENT PAPERS:**	Not cited
AUTHORSHIP RESTRICTIONS:	Not cited	**REPRINT POLICY:**	Not cited

SUBSCRIPTION ADDRESS: 1335 Carling Avenue
Suite 306
Ottawa, Ontario Canada K1Z 8N8
ANNUAL SUBSCRIPTION RATE: $15
FREQUENCY: Bimonthly **CIRCULATION:** 5000
AFFILIATION: Canadian Public Health Association
INDEXED/ABSTRACTED IN: BA, CINAHL, CA, IM, NAR, OA, PoIA, SSCI

JOURNAL TITLE: The Canadian Journal of Radiography, Radiotherapy and Nuclear Medicine

MANUSCRIPT ADDRESS: CSRT Office, Ste 410, 280 Metcalfe Street Ottawa Ontario Canada K2P 1R7

TYPES OF ARTICLES: Not cited

MAJOR CONTENT AREAS: Medical/surgical nursing

TOPICS PREFERRED: None cited

INAPPROPRIATE TOPICS: None cited

REVIEW PROCEDURE: External review		
REVIEW PERIOD: 60 days		
MANUSCRIPT WORD LENGTH: No limit	**PAGE CHARGES:** No	
MANUSCRIPT COPIES: 3	**STYLE REQUIREMENTS:** Not cited	
PUBLICATION LAG TIME: 4-6 months	**STYLE SHEET:** Yes	
EARLY PUBLICATION OPTION: Yes	**REVISED THESES:** Yes	
ACCEPTANCE RATE: 60%	**STUDENT PAPERS:** Yes	
AUTHORSHIP RESTRICTIONS: No	**REPRINT POLICY:** 100-200 free	

SUBSCRIPTION ADDRESS: Canadian Association of Medical Radiation Technologists, Suite 410, 280 Metcalfe Street Ottawa Ontario Canada K2P 1R7

ANNUAL SUBSCRIPTION RATE: Individuals: $12.50   Institutions: $10.00

FREQUENCY: Bimonthly   **CIRCULATION:** 8000

AFFILIATION: Canadian Assoc. of Medical Radiation Technologists

INDEXED/ABSTRACTED IN: CINAHL

JOURNAL TITLE: Canadian Nurse

MANUSCRIPT ADDRESS: Canadian Nurses Association
50 The Driveway
Ottawa   Canada K2P 1E2

TYPES OF ARTICLES: Review, case studies, commentaries

MAJOR CONTENT AREAS: accidents, adolescence, allied health personnel, alcoholism & drug abuse, anatomy & physiology, cancer, children, continuing education, cultural diversity, discharge planning, genetics, all nursing areas listed in Appendix A

TOPICS PREFERRED: Nursing related

INAPPROPRIATE TOPICS: None cited

REVIEW PROCEDURE: Editorial board and external review		
REVIEW PERIOD: 3 months		
MANUSCRIPT WORD LENGTH: 1500-3000	**PAGE CHARGES:** No	
MANUSCRIPT COPIES: 2	**STYLE REQUIREMENTS:** C	
PUBLICATION LAG TIME: 6 months	**STYLE SHEET:** Yes	
EARLY PUBLICATION OPTION: Not cited	**REVISED THESES:** No	
ACCEPTANCE RATE: 10%	**STUDENT PAPERS:** No	
AUTHORSHIP RESTRICTIONS: No	**REPRINT POLICY:** 3 free journals	

SUBSCRIPTION ADDRESS: Canadian Nurses Association
50 The Driveway
Ottawa   Canada K2P 1E2

ANNUAL SUBSCRIPTION RATE: $12

FREQUENCY: 11 times yearly   **CIRCULATION:** 97,000

AFFILIATION: Canadian Nurses Association

INDEXED/ABSTRACTED IN: INI, CINAHL, AHM, HLI, HosA, IM, CPI, IPA

JOURNAL TITLE: Cancer Clinical Trials

MANUSCRIPT ADDRESS: Luther W. Brady, M.D.
230 North Broad St.
Philadelphia PA 19102
TYPES OF ARTICLES: Research, review, case studies

MAJOR CONTENT AREAS: cancer

TOPICS PREFERRED: Evaluation and clinical trials of treatment modalities for malignancies
INAPPROPRIATE TOPICS: None cited

REVIEW PROCEDURE: Editorial board
REVIEW PERIOD: 1 month
MANUSCRIPT WORD LENGTH: 3000   PAGE CHARGES: No
MANUSCRIPT COPIES: 3   STYLE REQUIREMENTS: IM
PUBLICATION LAG TIME: 4 months   STYLE SHEET: Yes
EARLY PUBLICATION OPTION: Not cited   REVISED THESES: No
ACCEPTANCE RATE: 50%   STUDENT PAPERS: No
AUTHORSHIP RESTRICTIONS: No   REPRINT POLICY: None free

SUBSCRIPTION ADDRESS: Subscription Fulfillment Department
20th and Northampton Sts.
Easton, PA 18042
ANNUAL SUBSCRIPTION RATE: $45 ($50 Foreign)
FREQUENCY: Quarterly   CIRCULATION: 1000
AFFILIATION: None
INDEXED/ABSTRACTED IN: IM, CC

◆

JOURNAL TITLE: Cancer Detection and Prevention

MANUSCRIPT ADDRESS: Dr. Herbert Heibergs, Department of Pathology
Mt. Sinai School of Medicine
New York NY 10029
TYPES OF ARTICLES: Research, case studies

MAJOR CONTENT AREAS: biology, cancer, circulatory diseases, medicine,
pathology, stress

TOPICS PREFERRED: None cited

INAPPROPRIATE TOPICS: None cited

REVIEW PROCEDURE: Editorial board
REVIEW PERIOD: 4-6 weeks
MANUSCRIPT WORD LENGTH: Not cited   PAGE CHARGES: No
MANUSCRIPT COPIES: 3   STYLE REQUIREMENTS: AMA
PUBLICATION LAG TIME: 12 weeks   STYLE SHEET: Yes
EARLY PUBLICATION OPTION: No   REVISED THESES: No
ACCEPTANCE RATE: Not cited   STUDENT PAPERS: Not cited
AUTHORSHIP RESTRICTIONS: No   REPRINT POLICY: None free

SUBSCRIPTION ADDRESS: Marcel Dekker Journals
270 Madison Avenue
New York NY 10016
ANNUAL SUBSCRIPTION RATE: Individuals: $25   Institutions: $50
FREQUENCY: Quarterly   CIRCULATION: Not cited
AFFILIATION: Int'l. Study Group Detect. & Prevention of Cancer
INDEXED/ABSTRACTED IN: Not cited

JOURNAL TITLE: Cancer Nursing

MANUSCRIPT ADDRESS: 14 East 60th Street
New York NY 10022

TYPES OF ARTICLES: Theoretical, research, review

MAJOR CONTENT AREAS: cancer, any cancer related topic

TOPICS PREFERRED: Cancer nursing and cancer related topics

INAPPROPRIATE TOPICS: Personal experiences

REVIEW PROCEDURE: Editorial board
REVIEW PERIOD: 3-4 months
MANUSCRIPT WORD LENGTH: 1250-2500   PAGE CHARGES: No
MANUSCRIPT COPIES: 2   STYLE REQUIREMENTS: IM
PUBLICATION LAG TIME: 3-4 months   STYLE SHEET: Yes
EARLY PUBLICATION OPTION: Not cited   REVISED THESES: Yes
ACCEPTANCE RATE: 50%   STUDENT PAPERS: No
AUTHORSHIP RESTRICTIONS: No   REPRINT POLICY: None free

SUBSCRIPTION ADDRESS: Cancer Nursing
14 East 60th Street
New York   NY   10022
ANNUAL SUBSCRIPTION RATE: $20.50
FREQUENCY: Bimonthly   CIRCULATION: 10,000
AFFILIATION: None
INDEXED/ABSTRACTED IN: CINAHL, INI

◆

JOURNAL TITLE: Cardiovascular Nursing

MANUSCRIPT ADDRESS: American Heart Association
7320 Greenville Avenue
Dallas   TX   75231
TYPES OF ARTICLES: Theoretical, review, research, case studies,
commentaries, unsolicited book reviews
MAJOR CONTENT AREAS: biofeedback, family planning, human sexuality,
patient teaching, pathology, quality of life,
rehabilitation, relaxation, sleep, stress,
nursing: clinical specialties, critical care,
medical/surgical, process, research
TOPICS PREFERRED: Direct and indirect aspects of nursing care of
cardiac patients
INAPPROPRIATE TOPICS: None cited

REVIEW PROCEDURE: Editorial board
REVIEW PERIOD: 1-2 months
MANUSCRIPT WORD LENGTH: 3000-4000   PAGE CHARGES: No
MANUSCRIPT COPIES: 2   STYLE REQUIREMENTS: Own
PUBLICATION LAG TIME: 6 months   STYLE SHEET: Yes
EARLY PUBLICATION OPTION: Yes   REVISED THESES: Yes
ACCEPTANCE RATE: 50%   STUDENT PAPERS: No
AUTHORSHIP RESTRICTIONS: No   REPRINT POLICY: 25 free

SUBSCRIPTION ADDRESS: State organization of American Heart Association

ANNUAL SUBSCRIPTION RATE: Membership in AHA Council
FREQUENCY: Bimonthly ── CIRCULATION: Not cited
AFFILIATION: Council on Cardiovascular Nursing of the AHA
INDEXED/ABSTRACTED IN: INI, CINAHL

JOURNAL TITLE: CE Focus

MANUSCRIPT ADDRESS: P.O. Box 145
Pacific Palisades CA 90272

TYPES OF ARTICLES: Research, theoretical, commentaries

MAJOR CONTENT AREAS: change theory, continuing education, inservice education, teaching/learning, testing/measurement, self-directed learning; evaluation of continuing education

TOPICS PREFERRED: Experiences in developing/evaluating continuing education, issues; staff development, inservice
INAPPROPRIATE TOPICS: None cited

REVIEW PROCEDURE: Refereed, advisory board
REVIEW PERIOD: 3 months
MANUSCRIPT WORD LENGTH: Not cited
MANUSCRIPT COPIES: 2
PUBLICATION LAG TIME: 4 months
EARLY PUBLICATION OPTION: Not cited
ACCEPTANCE RATE: 75%
AUTHORSHIP RESTRICTIONS: No

PAGE CHARGES: Not cited
STYLE REQUIREMENTS: C
STYLE SHEET: Yes
REVISED THESES: Yes
STUDENT PAPERS: Yes
REPRINT POLICY: 25 free

SUBSCRIPTION ADDRESS: P.O. Box 145
Pacific Palisades CA 90272

ANNUAL SUBSCRIPTION RATE: $10
FREQUENCY: Bimonthly
AFFILIATION: None
INDEXED/ABSTRACTED IN: CINAHL

CIRCULATION: 20,000

◆

JOURNAL TITLE: Change Magazine

MANUSCRIPT ADDRESS: 4000 Abemarle Street, N.W.
Washington D.C. 20016

TYPES OF ARTICLES: Research

MAJOR CONTENT AREAS: continuing education, inservice education, nursing education, teaching/learning

TOPICS PREFERRED: Higher education

INAPPROPRIATE TOPICS: None cited

REVIEW PROCEDURE: Editorial board
REVIEW PERIOD: 6-8 weeks
MANUSCRIPT WORD LENGTH: Not cited
MANUSCRIPT COPIES: 1
PUBLICATION LAG TIME: Varies
EARLY PUBLICATION OPTION: No
ACCEPTANCE RATE: 10%
AUTHORSHIP RESTRICTIONS: No

PAGE CHARGES: No
STYLE REQUIREMENTS: Not cited
STYLE SHEET: Yes
REVISED THESES: No
STUDENT PAPERS: No
REPRINT POLICY: 10 free

SUBSCRIPTION ADDRESS: Change Magazine
4000 Abemarle Street, N.W.
Washington D.C. 20016

ANNUAL SUBSCRIPTION RATE: $18
FREQUENCY: 10 times yearly
AFFILIATION: None cited
INDEXED/ABSTRACTED IN: RGPL

CIRCULATION: 30,000

JOURNAL TITLE: Chest

MANUSCRIPT ADDRESS: Alfred Soffer, M.D.
The American College of Chest Physicians
911 Busse Highway, Park Ridge IL 60068
TYPES OF ARTICLES: Research, review, case studies, clinical investigations
MAJOR CONTENT AREAS: anesthesiology, cancer, circulatory diseases,
emergency services, epidemiology, health sciences,
medicine, pathology, pharmacology, public health,
rehabilitation, respiratory diseases

TOPICS PREFERRED: Heart and lung medicine and surgery

INAPPROPRIATE TOPICS: None cited

REVIEW PROCEDURE: Editorial board and external review
REVIEW PERIOD: 3-4 weeks
MANUSCRIPT WORD LENGTH: Not cited   PAGE CHARGES: No
MANUSCRIPT COPIES: 2   STYLE REQUIREMENTS: AMA
PUBLICATION LAG TIME: 7-9 months   STYLE SHEET: Yes
EARLY PUBLICATION OPTION: Yes   REVISED THESES: No
ACCEPTANCE RATE: 25%   STUDENT PAPERS: No
AUTHORSHIP RESTRICTIONS: No   REPRINT POLICY: None free

SUBSCRIPTION ADDRESS: The American College of Chest Physicians
911 Busse Highway
Park Ridge IL 60068
ANNUAL SUBSCRIPTION RATE: Individuals: $35   Institutions: $42
FREQUENCY: Monthly   CIRCULATION: 19,000
AFFILIATION: American College of Chest Physicians
INDEXED/ABSTRACTED IN: IM, CINAHL, BA, CA

◆

JOURNAL TITLE: Child Behavior Therapy

MANUSCRIPT ADDRESS: Cyril M. Franks
GSAPP, Psych. Bldg. Rm. 105, Busch Campus
Rutgers University, New Brunswick NJ 08903
TYPES OF ARTICLES: Research, case studies, theoretical, review,
commentaries, unsolicited book reviews
MAJOR CONTENT AREAS: Many areas listed in Appendix A, especially those
related to behavioral problems of children &
adolescents; ethics; nursing: community,
maternal/child, psychiatric/mental health;
research methodology; systems theory
TOPICS PREFERRED: Behavior therapy

INAPPROPRIATE TOPICS: None cited

REVIEW PROCEDURE: Editorial board and external review
REVIEW PERIOD: 3 months
MANUSCRIPT WORD LENGTH: No restriction   PAGE CHARGES: No
MANUSCRIPT COPIES: 2   STYLE REQUIREMENTS: APA
PUBLICATION LAG TIME: 12 months   STYLE SHEET: Yes
EARLY PUBLICATION OPTION: No   REVISED THESES: Yes
ACCEPTANCE RATE: 20%   STUDENT PAPERS: No
AUTHORSHIP RESTRICTIONS: No   REPRINT POLICY: 50 free

SUBSCRIPTION ADDRESS: The Haworth Press
28 East 22nd St.
New York NY 10010
ANNUAL SUBSCRIPTION RATE: $25
FREQUENCY: Quarterly   CIRCULATION: None cited
AFFILIATION: None
INDEXED/ABSTRACTED IN: None cited

JOURNAL TITLE: Child Care Health and Development

MANUSCRIPT ADDRESS: Editor
8 John St.
London WC1N 2E8 England

TYPES OF ARTICLES: Research, theoretical, review, case studies

MAJOR CONTENT AREAS: all aspects of the development of children, but
particularly those handicapped by physical,
intellectual, emotional and social problems;
allied health personnel, nursing:community/
public health, maternal/child, pediatric, school

TOPICS PREFERRED: Any topic of interest to the multidisciplinary
team working with normal or handicapped children

INAPPROPRIATE TOPICS: None cited

REVIEW PROCEDURE:	External review		
REVIEW PERIOD:	2-3 months		
MANUSCRIPT WORD LENGTH:	2000-4000	PAGE CHARGES:	No
MANUSCRIPT COPIES:	2	STYLE REQUIREMENTS:	Own
PUBLICATION LAG TIME:	6 months	STYLE SHEET:	Yes
EARLY PUBLICATION OPTION:	No	REVISED THESES:	Yes
ACCEPTANCE RATE:	60-70%	STUDENT PAPERS:	Yes
AUTHORSHIP RESTRICTIONS:	No	REPRINT POLICY:	50 free

SUBSCRIPTION ADDRESS: Messrs. Blackwells Scientific Publications, Ltd.
8 John St.
London WC1N 2E8 England

ANNUAL SUBSCRIPTION RATE: $52.50

FREQUENCY: Bimonthly   CIRCULATION: 600

AFFILIATION: None

INDEXED/ABSTRACTED IN: IM, INI

———◆———

JOURNAL TITLE: Child Psychiatry and Human Development

MANUSCRIPT ADDRESS: John C. Duffy, M.D., Editor
7111 44th Street
Chevy Chase MD 20015

TYPES OF ARTICLES: Research, review, theoretical, case studies

MAJOR CONTENT AREAS: abuse (child), adolescence, children, mental
health/illness, parenting, psychiatric/mental
health nursing

TOPICS PREFERRED: Child mental illness, child development

INAPPROPRIATE TOPICS: None cited

REVIEW PROCEDURE:	Editorial board		
REVIEW PERIOD:	8 weeks		
MANUSCRIPT WORD LENGTH:	4000 maximum	PAGE CHARGES:	No
MANUSCRIPT COPIES:	3	STYLE REQUIREMENTS:	IM
PUBLICATION LAG TIME:	14 months	STYLE SHEET:	No
EARLY PUBLICATION OPTION:	Yes	REVISED THESES:	No
ACCEPTANCE RATE:	20%	STUDENT PAPERS:	Yes
AUTHORSHIP RESTRICTIONS:	No	REPRINT POLICY:	None free

SUBSCRIPTION ADDRESS: Human Sciences Press
72 Fifth Avenue
New York NY 10011

ANNUAL SUBSCRIPTION RATE: $40

FREQUENCY: Quarterly   CIRCULATION: 4000

AFFILIATION: None

INDEXED/ABSTRACTED IN: IM, EM, BA, CIJE, CDA, CC, ECER, PA, SSCI

JOURNAL TITLE: Children in Contemporary Society †

MANUSCRIPT ADDRESS: P.O. Box 11173
Pittsburgh PA 15237

TYPES OF ARTICLES: Theoretical, review, commentaries

MAJOR CONTENT AREAS: adolescence, children, growth/development,
parenting

TOPICS PREFERRED: Contemporary educational, social, medical, politi-
cal & economic issues that affect young children
INAPPROPRIATE TOPICS: None cited

REVIEW PROCEDURE: Editors
REVIEW PERIOD: Not cited
MANUSCRIPT WORD LENGTH: Not cited   PAGE CHARGES: No
MANUSCRIPT COPIES: 1   STYLE REQUIREMENTS: APA
PUBLICATION LAG TIME: Not cited   STYLE SHEET: Not cited
EARLY PUBLICATION OPTION: Not cited   REVISED THESES: No
ACCEPTANCE RATE: Not cited   STUDENT PAPERS: No
AUTHORSHIP RESTRICTIONS: Not cited   REPRINT POLICY: Not cited

SUBSCRIPTION ADDRESS: Children in Contemporary Society
P.O. Box 11173
Pittsburgh PA 15237
ANNUAL SUBSCRIPTION RATE: $8
FREQUENCY: Quarterly   CIRCULATION: Not cited
AFFILIATION: Pittsburgh Assoc. Education of Young Children
INDEXED/ABSTRACTED IN: ECER, CINAHL

◆

JOURNAL TITLE: Children Today

MANUSCRIPT ADDRESS: Children's Bureau, ACYF
P.O. Box 1182
Washington DC 20013
TYPES OF ARTICLES: Articles or program experiences on specific
aspects of child care and service to families
MAJOR CONTENT AREAS: abuse, accidents, adolescence, children, counseling, crisis, cultural diversity, genetics, human
behavior, marriage & divorce, mental health/illness,
parenting, suicide, women's issues, nursing:
public health, maternal/child, pediatric, school
TOPICS PREFERRED: Programs and research relating to children, youth
and families
INAPPROPRIATE TOPICS: None cited

REVIEW PROCEDURE: Editorial board and external review
REVIEW PERIOD: 1-3 months
MANUSCRIPT WORD LENGTH: 2000-3000   PAGE CHARGES: No
MANUSCRIPT COPIES: 2   STYLE REQUIREMENTS: Own
PUBLICATION LAG TIME: 1-6 months   STYLE SHEET: Yes
EARLY PUBLICATION OPTION: No   REVISED THESES: No
ACCEPTANCE RATE: Not cited   STUDENT PAPERS: No
AUTHORSHIP RESTRICTIONS: No   REPRINT POLICY: 25 free issues

SUBSCRIPTION ADDRESS: Superintendent of Documents
U.S. Government Printing Office
Washington DC 20402
ANNUAL SUBSCRIPTION RATE: $10
FREQUENCY: Bimonthly   CIRCULATION: 14,000
AFFILIATION: Published by Children's Bureau, ACYF, HHS
INDEXED/ABSTRACTED IN: RGPL, CINAHL, CIJE, EI, ECER, HLI, BRI, IM,
IUSGP, INI

JOURNAL TITLE: Christian Nurse

MANUSCRIPT ADDRESS: P.B. 24
Nagpur, 440-001
Maharashtra, India
TYPES OF ARTICLES: Devotional, theoretical, case studies, review, research, commentaries, unsolicited book reviews
MAJOR CONTENT AREAS: Nearly all areas in Appendix A cited

TOPICS PREFERRED: All topics pertaining to health care, devotional-prayer life
INAPPROPRIATE TOPICS: None cited

REVIEW PROCEDURE: Editorial board
REVIEW PERIOD: 1 month
MANUSCRIPT WORD LENGTH: 1200-3000
MANUSCRIPT COPIES: 2
PUBLICATION LAG TIME: 2-3 months
EARLY PUBLICATION OPTION: Yes
ACCEPTANCE RATE: 60%
AUTHORSHIP RESTRICTIONS: Yes

PAGE CHARGES: Yes
STYLE REQUIREMENTS: IM
STYLE SHEET: Yes
REVISED THESES: Yes
STUDENT PAPERS: Yes
REPRINT POLICY: 15 free

SUBSCRIPTION ADDRESS: P.B. 24, Nagpur, 440-001
Maharashtra, India

ANNUAL SUBSCRIPTION RATE: $8
FREQUENCY: Bimonthly
CIRCULATION: 2000
AFFILIATION: Christian Medical Association of India
INDEXED/ABSTRACTED IN: CINAHL

◆

JOURNAL TITLE: Circulatory Shock

MANUSCRIPT ADDRESS: Dr. William Schumer, Univ. of Health Sciences
Chicago Medical School at VA Medical Center
North Chicago   IL   60064
TYPES OF ARTICLES: Research, review, unsolicited book reviews

MAJOR CONTENT AREAS: biochemistry, biomedical research, circulatory diseases, trauma nursing

TOPICS PREFERRED: Shock and trauma

INAPPROPRIATE TOPICS: None cited

REVIEW PROCEDURE: Editorial board and external review
REVIEW PERIOD: 6-8 weeks
MANUSCRIPT WORD LENGTH: 1800
MANUSCRIPT COPIES: 3
PUBLICATION LAG TIME: 4-5 months
EARLY PUBLICATION OPTION: Yes
ACCEPTANCE RATE: 60%
AUTHORSHIP RESTRICTIONS: No

PAGE CHARGES: No
STYLE REQUIREMENTS: CBE
STYLE SHEET: Yes
REVISED THESES: Yes
STUDENT PAPERS: No
REPRINT POLICY: None free

SUBSCRIPTION ADDRESS: Alan R. Liss, Inc.
150 Fifth Avenue
New York   NY   10011
ANNUAL SUBSCRIPTION RATE: $45
FREQUENCY: Quarterly
CIRCULATION: 700
AFFILIATION: The Shock Society
INDEXED/ABSTRACTED IN: IM, CC

JOURNAL TITLE: Clinical Behavior Therapy Review

MANUSCRIPT ADDRESS: Cyril M. Franks
GSAPP, Psych. Bldg. Rm. 105 Busch Campus
Rutgers University, New Brunswick NJ 08903

TYPES OF ARTICLES: Articles reviewing new developments for the practitioner. Query first.

MAJOR CONTENT AREAS: All aspects of behavior; all age groups; professionalism; research methodology; nursing: community/public health, psychiatric/mental health, school, trauma

TOPICS PREFERRED: Behavior therapy

INAPPROPRIATE TOPICS: None cited

REVIEW PROCEDURE: Editorial agreement with author
REVIEW PERIOD: 1 month
MANUSCRIPT WORD LENGTH: 12,500
MANUSCRIPT COPIES: 2
PUBLICATION LAG TIME: 6 months
EARLY PUBLICATION OPTION: No
ACCEPTANCE RATE: Not cited
AUTHORSHIP RESTRICTIONS: No

PAGE CHARGES: No
STYLE REQUIREMENTS: APA
STYLE SHEET: Yes
REVISED THESES: No
STUDENT PAPERS: No
REPRINT POLICY: 50 free

SUBSCRIPTION ADDRESS: The Haworth Press
28 East 22nd St.
New York NY 10010

ANNUAL SUBSCRIPTION RATE: $24
FREQUENCY: Quarterly
AFFILIATION: None
INDEXED/ABSTRACTED IN: None cited

CIRCULATION: None cited

◆

JOURNAL TITLE: Clinical Electroencephalography

MANUSCRIPT ADDRESS: 1427 North Astor Street
Chicago IL 60610

TYPES OF ARTICLES: Research, review, clinical research on EEG

MAJOR CONTENT AREAS: accidents, aging and aged, alcoholism and drug abuse, circulatory diseases, genetics, mental retardation, sleep, suicide

TOPICS PREFERRED: Anything connected with EEG

INAPPROPRIATE TOPICS: None cited

REVIEW PROCEDURE: Editorial board
REVIEW PERIOD: 1 month
MANUSCRIPT WORD LENGTH: 2500
MANUSCRIPT COPIES: 2
PUBLICATION LAG TIME: 3 months
EARLY PUBLICATION OPTION: No
ACCEPTANCE RATE: 80%
AUTHORSHIP RESTRICTIONS: No

PAGE CHARGES: No
STYLE REQUIREMENTS: AMA
STYLE SHEET: Yes
REVISED THESES: No
STUDENT PAPERS: No
REPRINT POLICY: None free

SUBSCRIPTION ADDRESS: 1427 North Astor Street
Chicago IL 60610

ANNUAL SUBSCRIPTION RATE: $20
FREQUENCY: Quarterly
AFFILIATION: American Medical EEG Association
INDEXED/ABSTRACTED IN: IM, CC

CIRCULATION: 2000

JOURNAL TITLE: Clinical & Experimental Hypertension

MANUSCRIPT ADDRESS: Michael J. Antonaccio, Ph.D., Editor
Squibb Institute for Medical Research, Dept. of
Pharmacology, Box 4000, Princeton NJ 08540
TYPES OF ARTICLES: Research, review, commentaries, theoretical, case
studies, unsolicited book reviews
MAJOR CONTENT AREAS: allied health personnel, anatomy & physiology,
biochemistry, biology, biomedical research, cir-
culatory diseases, epidemiology, genetics, health
sciences, life span, medicine, pharmacology,
research methodology, testing/measurement
TOPICS PREFERRED: Hypertension; circulation

INAPPROPRIATE TOPICS: None

REVIEW PROCEDURE: Editorial board and external review
REVIEW PERIOD: 4-6 weeks

MANUSCRIPT WORD LENGTH: 3000	**PAGE CHARGES:** No	
MANUSCRIPT COPIES: 2	**STYLE REQUIREMENTS:** Own	
PUBLICATION LAG TIME: 12-16 weeks	**STYLE SHEET:** Yes	
EARLY PUBLICATION OPTION: Yes	**REVISED THESES:** No	
ACCEPTANCE RATE: 60%	**STUDENT PAPERS:** No	
AUTHORSHIP RESTRICTIONS: No	**REPRINT POLICY:** 20 free	

SUBSCRIPTION ADDRESS: Marcel Dekker, Inc.
270 Madison Avenue
New York NY 10016
ANNUAL SUBSCRIPTION RATE: $90
FREQUENCY: Bimonthly   **CIRCULATION:** 400
AFFILIATION: None
INDEXED/ABSTRACTED IN: CC(LS), BD, BA, CA, EM, IPA, CINAHL

◆

JOURNAL TITLE: Clinical Otolaryngology & Allied Sciences

MANUSCRIPT ADDRESS: Editor, Dept. of Otolaryngology
University of Liverpool, Prescott St.
Liverpool L7 8XP England
TYPES OF ARTICLES: Research, review

MAJOR CONTENT AREAS: biomedical research, cancer, eating disorders,
medical/surgical nursing, medicine,
otolaryngology, patient teaching, pathology,
rehabilitation, respiratory diseases

TOPICS PREFERRED: Clinically oriented research; Otolaryngology, aud-
iology, oncology, speech pathology, plastic surgery
INAPPROPRIATE TOPICS: Endocrinology, case reports

REVIEW PROCEDURE: Editorial board
REVIEW PERIOD: 3-4 weeks

MANUSCRIPT WORD LENGTH: 3000	**PAGE CHARGES:** No	
MANUSCRIPT COPIES: 3	**STYLE REQUIREMENTS:** Own	
PUBLICATION LAG TIME: 8-12 months	**STYLE SHEET:** Yes	
EARLY PUBLICATION OPTION: Yes	**REVISED THESES:** No	
ACCEPTANCE RATE: 40%	**STUDENT PAPERS:** No	
AUTHORSHIP RESTRICTIONS: No	**REPRINT POLICY:** 25 free	

SUBSCRIPTION ADDRESS: Blackwell Scientific Publications, Ltd.
P.O. Box 88
Oxford England
ANNUAL SUBSCRIPTION RATE: $72.50
FREQUENCY: Bimonthly   **CIRCULATION:** 800
AFFILIATION: Dutch ENT, ORS-ENT, and Politzer Societies
INDEXED/ABSTRACTED IN: IM,CC

JOURNAL TITLE: Clinical Pediatrics

MANUSCRIPT ADDRESS: J.B. Lippincott Company
East Washington Square
Philadelphia PA 19105

TYPES OF ARTICLES: Review, research, case studies, commentaries, theoretical

MAJOR CONTENT AREAS: all areas related to child care, pediatric practice, behavioral and educational problems, community health situations and disorders requiring hospitalization; maternal/child, pediatric, & school nursing; research methodology

TOPICS PREFERRED: None cited

INAPPROPRIATE TOPICS: None cited

REVIEW PROCEDURE: Editorial board and external review
REVIEW PERIOD: 6-8 weeks
MANUSCRIPT WORD LENGTH: 1500-3000
MANUSCRIPT COPIES: 3
PUBLICATION LAG TIME: 6-8 months
EARLY PUBLICATION OPTION: No
ACCEPTANCE RATE: 20%
AUTHORSHIP RESTRICTIONS: No

PAGE CHARGES: No
STYLE REQUIREMENTS: CBE
STYLE SHEET: Yes
REVISED THESES: No
STUDENT PAPERS: No
REPRINT POLICY: None free

SUBSCRIPTION ADDRESS: J.B. Lippincott Company
East Washington Square
Philadelphia PA 19105
ANNUAL SUBSCRIPTION RATE: $20
FREQUENCY: Monthly
CIRCULATION: 20,000
AFFILIATION: None cited
INDEXED/ABSTRACTED IN: BA, CA, IM, INI, NAR

JOURNAL TITLE: Clinical Pharmacology and Therapeutics

MANUSCRIPT ADDRESS: P.O. Box 119
Larchmont NY 10538

TYPES OF ARTICLES: Research, theoretical, commentaries

MAJOR CONTENT AREAS: pharmacology, clinical pharmacology

TOPICS PREFERRED: Clinical pharmacology

INAPPROPRIATE TOPICS: Topics not related to clinical pharmacology

REVIEW PROCEDURE: Editorial board
REVIEW PERIOD: 3-6 months
MANUSCRIPT WORD LENGTH: No limit
MANUSCRIPT COPIES: 2
PUBLICATION LAG TIME: 4 months
EARLY PUBLICATION OPTION: No
ACCEPTANCE RATE: 30%
AUTHORSHIP RESTRICTIONS: No

PAGE CHARGES: Yes
STYLE REQUIREMENTS: Own
STYLE SHEET: No
REVISED THESES: No
STUDENT PAPERS: No
REPRINT POLICY: None free

SUBSCRIPTION ADDRESS: C.V. Mosby Company
11830 Westline Industrial Drive
St. Louis MO 63141
ANNUAL SUBSCRIPTION RATE: Individuals: $30.00   Institutions: $42.00
FREQUENCY: Monthly   CIRCULATION: 7500
AFFILIATION: Amer. Soc. for Pharmacology & Exper. Therapeutics
INDEXED/ABSTRACTED IN: BA, CA, IPA, IM, NAR

JOURNAL TITLE: Community Mental Health Journal

MANUSCRIPT ADDRESS: National Council of Community Mental Health Centers
2233 Wisconsin Avenue, Suite 322
Washington DC 20007

TYPES OF ARTICLES: Research, theoretical, review

MAJOR CONTENT AREAS: mental health/illness

TOPICS PREFERRED: Any areas relating to community mental health

INAPPROPRIATE TOPICS: None cited

REVIEW PROCEDURE: Editorial board
REVIEW PERIOD: Not cited
MANUSCRIPT WORD LENGTH: 4000-4500
MANUSCRIPT COPIES: 3
PUBLICATION LAG TIME: 4 months
EARLY PUBLICATION OPTION: No
ACCEPTANCE RATE: 5%
AUTHORSHIP RESTRICTIONS: No

PAGE CHARGES: No
STYLE REQUIREMENTS: APA
STYLE SHEET: No
REVISED THESES: Will review
STUDENT PAPERS: No
REPRINT POLICY: 1 free journal

SUBSCRIPTION ADDRESS: Human Sciences Press
72 Fifth Avenue
New York NY 10011
ANNUAL SUBSCRIPTION RATE: Individuals: $18 Institutions: $40
FREQUENCY: Quarterly CIRCULATION: 3000
AFFILIATION: Nat. Council of Community Mental Health Centers
INDEXED/ABSTRACTED IN: PA, SWRA, CSPA, CDL, MRA, HRA, HLI, CINAHL, SSCI,
CC, ASCA, SCI, AHM, SocA, SSA, MRD, SSI BA, IM,
HRA, INI

JOURNAL TITLE: Contraception

MANUSCRIPT ADDRESS: 1240 North Mission Road
Los Angeles CA 90033

TYPES OF ARTICLES: Research, case studies, review

MAJOR CONTENT AREAS: biomedical research, family planning, medicine

TOPICS PREFERRED: Relating to contraception

INAPPROPRIATE TOPICS: None cited

REVIEW PROCEDURE: External review
REVIEW PERIOD: 6 weeks
MANUSCRIPT WORD LENGTH: 2500
MANUSCRIPT COPIES: 2
PUBLICATION LAG TIME: 1 month
EARLY PUBLICATION OPTION: Yes
ACCEPTANCE RATE: 60%
AUTHORSHIP RESTRICTIONS: No

PAGE CHARGES: Yes
STYLE REQUIREMENTS: Own, IM
STYLE SHEET: Yes
REVISED THESES: No
STUDENT PAPERS: No
REPRINT POLICY: None free

SUBSCRIPTION ADDRESS: Geron-X, Inc.
P.O. Box 1108
Los Altos CA 94022
ANNUAL SUBSCRIPTION RATE: Individuals: $60 Institutions: $100
FREQUENCY: Monthly CIRCULATION: 1000
AFFILIATION: None
INDEXED/ABSTRACTED IN: IM, PSIBR, CA, CC, BA, CINAHL

JOURNAL TITLE: Critical Care Quarterly

MANUSCRIPT ADDRESS: Aspen Systems Corporation
1600 Research Boulevard
Rockville MD 20850

TYPES OF ARTICLES: Review, applied articles

MAJOR CONTENT AREAS: abuse (child/spouse, alcoholism/drug), anatomy &
physiology, cancer, chronicity, circulatory &
respiratory diseases, continuity of care, crisis
intervention/theory, nursing: critical care, clinical specialties; pain, sensory deprivation

TOPICS PREFERRED: Critical care

INAPPROPRIATE TOPICS: Many

REVIEW PROCEDURE: Editorial board and external review
REVIEW PERIOD: 1-3 months
MANUSCRIPT WORD LENGTH: 4500-6000
MANUSCRIPT COPIES: 3
PUBLICATION LAG TIME: 2-4 months
EARLY PUBLICATION OPTION: No
ACCEPTANCE RATE: 1% unsolicited
AUTHORSHIP RESTRICTIONS: No

PAGE CHARGES: No
STYLE REQUIREMENTS: C
STYLE SHEET: Yes
REVISED THESES: No
STUDENT PAPERS: No
REPRINT POLICY: None free

SUBSCRIPTION ADDRESS: Aspen Systems Corporation
16792 Oakmont Avenue
Gaithersburg MD 20877

ANNUAL SUBSCRIPTION RATE: $36
FREQUENCY: Quarterly
AFFILIATION: None
INDEXED/ABSTRACTED IN: CINAHL

CIRCULATION: 12,000

◆

JOURNAL TITLE: Critical Care Update

MANUSCRIPT ADDRESS: P.O. Box 5828
Orange CA 92667

TYPES OF ARTICLES: case studies, clinical bedside care

MAJOR CONTENT AREAS: abuse, accidents, adaptation, cancer, discharge
planning, emergency services, nursing: clinical
specialties, critical care, neurosurgical, care,
diagnosis, education, process, theory, pediatric,
trauma; pain, patient teaching, quality of life

TOPICS PREFERRED: Critical care nursing

INAPPROPRIATE TOPICS: None cited

REVIEW PROCEDURE: Editorial board
REVIEW PERIOD: 1-2 weeks
MANUSCRIPT WORD LENGTH: Not cited
MANUSCRIPT COPIES: 2
PUBLICATION LAG TIME: 3-6 months
EARLY PUBLICATION OPTION: No
ACCEPTANCE RATE: 90%
AUTHORSHIP RESTRICTIONS: No

PAGE CHARGES: No
STYLE REQUIREMENTS: Own
STYLE SHEET: Yes
REVISED THESES: Yes
STUDENT PAPERS: Yes
REPRINT POLICY: 4 free journals

SUBSCRIPTION ADDRESS: P.O. Box 5828
Orange CA 92667

ANNUAL SUBSCRIPTION RATE: Individuals: $20   Institutions: $30
FREQUENCY: Monthly   CIRCULATION: 10,000
AFFILIATION: National Critical Care Institute of Education
INDEXED/ABSTRACTED IN: CINAHL, INI

JOURNAL TITLE: Culture, Medicine and Psychiatry

MANUSCRIPT ADDRESS: c/o Arthur Kleinman
Department of Psychiatry and Behavioral Sciences
University of Washington, Seattle WA 98195
TYPES OF ARTICLES: Research, theoretical, review

MAJOR CONTENT AREAS: anthropology, communication, cultural diversity,
epidemiology, human behavior, mental health/
illness, patient teaching, primary care,
psychopathology, research methodology, stigma,
stress
TOPICS PREFERRED: Anthropology of health, cross-cultural studies of
illness and health care
INAPPROPRIATE TOPICS: None cited

REVIEW PROCEDURE: Editorial board and external review
REVIEW PERIOD: 2-4 months
MANUSCRIPT WORD LENGTH: 5000-7500   PAGE CHARGES: No
MANUSCRIPT COPIES: 4   STYLE REQUIREMENTS: AA
PUBLICATION LAG TIME: 3-6 months   STYLE SHEET: Yes
EARLY PUBLICATION OPTION: Yes   REVISED THESES: No
ACCEPTANCE RATE: 50%   STUDENT PAPERS: No
AUTHORSHIP RESTRICTIONS: No   REPRINT POLICY: 25 free

SUBSCRIPTION ADDRESS: D. Reidel Publishing Company
P.O. Box 17, 3300 AA
Dordrecht Holland
ANNUAL SUBSCRIPTION RATE: Individuals: $18   Institutions: $36
FREQUENCY: Quarterly   CIRCULATION: 500
AFFILIATION: None
INDEXED/ABSTRACTED IN: IM, SocA

◆

JOURNAL TITLE: CURATIONIS

MANUSCRIPT ADDRESS: The Editor
South African Nursing Association
Private Bag X105 PRETORIA 0001   SOUTH AFRICA
TYPES OF ARTICLES: Nursing (and allied professions) articles

MAJOR CONTENT AREAS: Many areas listed in Appendix A including: all
nursing areas, aging and aged, children, con-
tinuing education, death & dying, dependency,
health promotion, health sciences, mental health/
illness, midwifery, patient teaching, primary care
TOPICS PREFERRED: None cited

INAPPROPRIATE TOPICS: None cited

REVIEW PROCEDURE: Editorial advisory committee and panel
REVIEW PERIOD: Variable
MANUSCRIPT WORD LENGTH: 2000-4000   PAGE CHARGES: No
MANUSCRIPT COPIES: 2   STYLE REQUIREMENTS: Not cited
PUBLICATION LAG TIME: Variable   STYLE SHEET: No
EARLY PUBLICATION OPTION: No   REVISED THESES: No
ACCEPTANCE RATE: Most solicited   STUDENT PAPERS: Yes
AUTHORSHIP RESTRICTIONS: No   REPRINT POLICY: None free

SUBSCRIPTION ADDRESS: The Editor, CURATIONIS
S.A. Nursing Association, Private Bag X105
PRETORIA 0001   SOUTH AFRICA
ANNUAL SUBSCRIPTION RATE: $8
FREQUENCY: Quarterly   CIRCULATION: 2000
AFFILIATION: South African Nursing Association
INDEXED/ABSTRACTED IN: INI, CINAHL

JOURNAL TITLE: Current Microbiology

MANUSCRIPT ADDRESS: Dr. Mortimer P. Starr, Editor
Department of Bacteriology
University of California, Davis CA 95616
TYPES OF ARTICLES: Research, theoretical

MAJOR CONTENT AREAS: biochemistry, epidemiology, genetics,
immunization, microbiology, research methodology

TOPICS PREFERRED: None cited

INAPPROPRIATE TOPICS: None cited

REVIEW PROCEDURE: Editorial board and external review
REVIEW PERIOD: 2-3 weeks
MANUSCRIPT WORD LENGTH: 2500   PAGE CHARGES: No
MANUSCRIPT COPIES: 3   STYLE REQUIREMENTS: C, CBE, ASM
PUBLICATION LAG TIME: 6-10 weeks   STYLE SHEET: Yes
EARLY PUBLICATION OPTION: No   REVISED THESES: Yes
ACCEPTANCE RATE: 70%   STUDENT PAPERS: No
AUTHORSHIP RESTRICTIONS: No   REPRINT POLICY: 50 free

SUBSCRIPTION ADDRESS: Springer-Verlag, New York, Inc.
175 Fifth Avenue
New York NY 10010
ANNUAL SUBSCRIPTION RATE: Individuals: $29   Institutions: $89
FREQUENCY: Monthly   CIRCULATION: Not cited
AFFILIATION: None
INDEXED/ABSTRACTED IN: CC

◆

JOURNAL TITLE: CVP: The Journal of Cardiovascular and
Pulmonary Technology
MANUSCRIPT ADDRESS: 825 South Barrington Avenue
Los Angeles CA 90049

TYPES OF ARTICLES: Research, review, case studies, commentaries,
equipment surveys
MAJOR CONTENT AREAS: anesthesiology, cardiovascular and cardiopulmonary technology, catheterization,
stress, mechanical heart and lung operators

TOPICS PREFERRED: None cited

INAPPROPRIATE TOPICS: None cited

REVIEW PROCEDURE: Editorial board, external review, in-house review
REVIEW PERIOD: 2-3 weeks
MANUSCRIPT WORD LENGTH: 3500   PAGE CHARGES: No
MANUSCRIPT COPIES: 2   STYLE REQUIREMENTS: C
PUBLICATION LAG TIME: Varies   STYLE SHEET: Yes
EARLY PUBLICATION OPTION: Yes   REVISED THESES: Yes
ACCEPTANCE RATE: 75%   STUDENT PAPERS: Yes
AUTHORSHIP RESTRICTIONS: No   REPRINT POLICY: 1 free

SUBSCRIPTION ADDRESS: Barrington Publications
825 South Barrington Avenue
Los Angeles CA 90049
ANNUAL SUBSCRIPTION RATE: $30
FREQUENCY: Bimonthly   CIRCULATION: 20,000
AFFILIATION: None
INDEXED/ABSTRACTED IN: CINAHL

JOURNAL TITLE: Death Education

MANUSCRIPT ADDRESS: Hannelore Wass, Editor, College of Education,
Center of Gerontological Studies & Programs,
University of Florida, Gainesville FL 32611
TYPES OF ARTICLES: Theoretical, research, case studies, commentaries

MAJOR CONTENT AREAS: continuity of care, counseling, crisis, death &
dying, ethics, health policies, human behavior &
sexuality, loss/grief, nursing: critical care,
clinical specialties; pain, primary care,
quality of life, stigma, stress, suicide
TOPICS PREFERRED: None cited

INAPPROPRIATE TOPICS: None cited

REVIEW PROCEDURE: Editorial board
REVIEW PERIOD: Not cited
MANUSCRIPT WORD LENGTH: Not cited   PAGE CHARGES: No
MANUSCRIPT COPIES: 3   STYLE REQUIREMENTS: APA, Own
PUBLICATION LAG TIME: Not cited   STYLE SHEET: Yes
EARLY PUBLICATION OPTION: Not cited   REVISED THESES: Not cited
ACCEPTANCE RATE: Not cited   STUDENT PAPERS: Not cited
AUTHORSHIP RESTRICTIONS: No   REPRINT POLICY: Free journal

SUBSCRIPTION ADDRESS: Hemisphere Publishing Corporation
1025 Vermont Avenue, N.W.
Washington DC 20005
ANNUAL SUBSCRIPTION RATE: Individuals: $20   Institutions: $40
FREQUENCY: Quarterly   CIRCULATION: 850
AFFILIATION: None
INDEXED/ABSTRACTED IN: EM, CMHR, EI, RGPL, SSI, BA, CC, SCI, BD, PA,
HRA, CINAHL, CEI, CPI, SWRA

◆

JOURNAL TITLE: Developmental and Comparative Immunology

MANUSCRIPT ADDRESS: Professor Edwin L. Cooper
Dept. of Anatomy, School of Medicine
University of California, Los Angeles CA 90024
TYPES OF ARTICLES: Research, theoretical, review, unsolicited book
reviews
MAJOR CONTENT AREAS: aging and aged, anatomy and physiology, biomedical research, genetics, growth/development,
immunization, life span, microbiology, comparative
immunology, developmental immunology, evolution,
immunity
TOPICS PREFERRED: None cited

INAPPROPRIATE TOPICS: None cited

REVIEW PROCEDURE: Editorial board and external review
REVIEW PERIOD: 3-4 months
MANUSCRIPT WORD LENGTH: 300   PAGE CHARGES: No
MANUSCRIPT COPIES: 2   STYLE REQUIREMENTS: C
PUBLICATION LAG TIME: 5-6 months   STYLE SHEET: Yes
EARLY PUBLICATION OPTION: Not cited   REVISED THESES: Yes
ACCEPTANCE RATE: 70%   STUDENT PAPERS: Yes
AUTHORSHIP RESTRICTIONS: No   REPRINT POLICY: None free

SUBSCRIPTION ADDRESS: Pergamon Press, Inc.
Fairview Park
Elmsford NY 10523
ANNUAL SUBSCRIPTION RATE: Individuals: $30   Institutions: $80
FREQUENCY: Quarterly   CIRCULATION: 1020
AFFILIATION: None
INDEXED/ABSTRACTED IN: None cited

JOURNAL TITLE: Developmental Medicine and Child Neurology

MANUSCRIPT ADDRESS: 5A Netherhall Gardens
London   NW3 5RN   England

TYPES OF ARTICLES: Research, review, case studies, theoretical

MAJOR CONTENT AREAS: children, continuity of care, epidemiology, genetics, growth/development, handicapping conditions, maternal/child & pediatric nursing, medicine, mental retardation, child psychology

TOPICS PREFERRED: Child neurology, development, psychology, psychiatry, handicapping conditions in childhood
INAPPROPRIATE TOPICS: None

REVIEW PROCEDURE: Editorial board and external review		
REVIEW PERIOD: 2-3 months		
MANUSCRIPT WORD LENGTH: Varies	**PAGE CHARGES:** No	
MANUSCRIPT COPIES: 2	**STYLE REQUIREMENTS:** H	
PUBLICATION LAG TIME: 6 months	**STYLE SHEET:** Yes	
EARLY PUBLICATION OPTION: Yes	**REVISED THESES:** May submit	
ACCEPTANCE RATE: 50%	**STUDENT PAPERS:** No	
AUTHORSHIP RESTRICTIONS: No	**REPRINT POLICY:** 25 free	

SUBSCRIPTION ADDRESS: J.B. Lippincott Company
East Washington Square
Philadelphia PA 19105
ANNUAL SUBSCRIPTION RATE: $44.75
FREQUENCY: Bimonthly   **CIRCULATION:** 5500
AFFILIATION: AACPDM, British Paediatric Neurology Association
INDEXED/ABSTRACTED IN: BA, DSHA, DI, IM, MRA, PA, SCI, CINAHL

◆

JOURNAL TITLE: Diabetes Care

MANUSCRIPT ADDRESS: Jay S. Skyler, M.D.
c/o University of Miami Hospitals
1475 N.W. 12th Avenue, Miami FL 33136
TYPES OF ARTICLES: Research, review, case studies, commentaries, theoretical
MAJOR CONTENT AREAS: diabetes

TOPICS PREFERRED: Diabetes related areas

INAPPROPRIATE TOPICS: None cited

REVIEW PROCEDURE: Editorial board and external review		
REVIEW PERIOD: 6 weeks		
MANUSCRIPT WORD LENGTH: Varies	**PAGE CHARGES:** No	
MANUSCRIPT COPIES: 3	**STYLE REQUIREMENTS:** CBE	
PUBLICATION LAG TIME: 3 months	**STYLE SHEET:** Yes	
EARLY PUBLICATION OPTION: No	**REVISED THESES:** Yes	
ACCEPTANCE RATE: 35%	**STUDENT PAPERS:** No	
AUTHORSHIP RESTRICTIONS: No	**REPRINT POLICY:** None free	

SUBSCRIPTION ADDRESS: American Diabetes Association, Inc.
600 Fifth Avenue
New York NY   10020
ANNUAL SUBSCRIPTION RATE: Individuals: $20   Institutions: $30
FREQUENCY: Bimonthly   **CIRCULATION:** 7000
AFFILIATION: American Diabetes Association
INDEXED/ABSTRACTED IN: IM, CA

JOURNAL TITLE: Diabetes Dialogue

MANUSCRIPT ADDRESS: Canadian Diabetes Association
123 Edward Street, Suite 601
Toronto M5G 1E2 Canada
TYPES OF ARTICLES: Research (lay-written appeal), personal commentaries
MAJOR CONTENT AREAS: adaptation, adolescence, adulthood, body image, children, counseling, critical care nursing, genetics, handicapping conditions, health policies, human sexuality, marriage and divorce stigma
TOPICS PREFERRED: Areas relating to diabetics; personal commentaries by diabetics or relatives/friends of diabetics
INAPPROPRIATE TOPICS: None cited

REVIEW PROCEDURE: Editorial board, external review
REVIEW PERIOD: 1-2 weeks
MANUSCRIPT WORD LENGTH: 1500-2000   **PAGE CHARGES:** No
MANUSCRIPT COPIES: 1   **STYLE REQUIREMENTS:** Own
PUBLICATION LAG TIME: 8 weeks   **STYLE SHEET:** Yes
EARLY PUBLICATION OPTION: No   **REVISED THESES:** No
ACCEPTANCE RATE: 85%   **STUDENT PAPERS:** No
AUTHORSHIP RESTRICTIONS: No   **REPRINT POLICY:** 5 + free

SUBSCRIPTION ADDRESS: 123 Edward Street
Suite 601
Toronto M5G 1E2 Canada
ANNUAL SUBSCRIPTION RATE: $7 Canadian
FREQUENCY: Quarterly   **CIRCULATION:** 22,000
AFFILIATION: Canadian Diabetic Association
INDEXED/ABSTRACTED IN: None cited

JOURNAL TITLE: Diagnostic Medicine

MANUSCRIPT ADDRESS: Medical Economics Company
680 Kinderkamack Road
Oradell NJ 07649
TYPES OF ARTICLES: Review, case studies, theoretical, research

MAJOR CONTENT AREAS: aging & aged (diseases), biochemistry, circulatory diseases, epidemiology, microbiology, pathology

TOPICS PREFERRED: Pathology or lab-related subjects

INAPPROPRIATE TOPICS: Esoteric research; Inquiry required

REVIEW PROCEDURE: Editorial board
REVIEW PERIOD: 4-6 weeks
MANUSCRIPT WORD LENGTH: 2500-7500   **PAGE CHARGES:** No
MANUSCRIPT COPIES: 2   **STYLE REQUIREMENTS:** C
PUBLICATION LAG TIME: 3 months   **STYLE SHEET:** Yes
EARLY PUBLICATION OPTION: Not cited   **REVISED THESES:** Not cited
ACCEPTANCE RATE: Not cited   **STUDENT PAPERS:** Not cited
AUTHORSHIP RESTRICTIONS: No   **REPRINT POLICY:** 50 free

SUBSCRIPTION ADDRESS: Box 555
Oradell NJ 07649

ANNUAL SUBSCRIPTION RATE: $24
FREQUENCY: Bimonthly   **CIRCULATION:** 30,000
AFFILIATION: None
INDEXED/ABSTRACTED IN: CINAHL

JOURNAL TITLE: Dialysis and Transplantation

MANUSCRIPT ADDRESS: 12849 Magnolia Blvd.
North Hollywood CA 91607

TYPES OF ARTICLES: Research, theoretical, case studies,
commentaries, review

MAJOR CONTENT AREAS: adaptation, chronicity, communication, compliance, counseling, death & dying, dependency,
ethics, human behavior & sexuality, quality of
life, rehabilitation, research methodology, dialysis techniques, equipment, all health fields

TOPICS PREFERRED: Research studies, care of dialysis & transplant
patients; case studies

INAPPROPRIATE TOPICS: Poorly researched studies; topics which don't
apply to field of dialysis and transplantation

REVIEW PROCEDURE: Editorial board and peer review

REVIEW PERIOD: 2-4 weeks

MANUSCRIPT WORD LENGTH: 2000-5000	PAGE CHARGES: No	
MANUSCRIPT COPIES: 2	STYLE REQUIREMENTS: AMA, CBE	
PUBLICATION LAG TIME: 2-6 months	STYLE SHEET: Yes	
EARLY PUBLICATION OPTION: No	REVISED THESES: Will consider	
ACCEPTANCE RATE: 65%	STUDENT PAPERS: Will consider	
AUTHORSHIP RESTRICTIONS: No	REPRINT POLICY: 1-2 free journals	

SUBSCRIPTION ADDRESS: Dialysis and Transplantation
12849 Magnolia Blvd.
North Hollywood CA 91607

ANNUAL SUBSCRIPTION RATE: $25

FREQUENCY: Monthly   CIRCULATION: 9000

AFFILIATION: None

INDEXED/ABSTRACTED IN: CC, EM

◆

JOURNAL TITLE: Digestive Diseases and Sciences

MANUSCRIPT ADDRESS: Sidney F. Phillips, Editor
Mayo Clinic
Rochester MN 55901

TYPES OF ARTICLES: Research, case studies, review

MAJOR CONTENT AREAS: alcoholism & drug abuse, biomedical research,
cancer, medicine, nutrition, pathology, phar-
macology

TOPICS PREFERRED: Gastroenterology

INAPPROPRIATE TOPICS: Clinical research

REVIEW PROCEDURE: External review

REVIEW PERIOD: 2 months

MANUSCRIPT WORD LENGTH: 2500	PAGE CHARGES: No	
MANUSCRIPT COPIES: 3	STYLE REQUIREMENTS: CBE	
PUBLICATION LAG TIME: 5 months	STYLE SHEET: Yes	
EARLY PUBLICATION OPTION: No	REVISED THESES: No	
ACCEPTANCE RATE: 50%	STUDENT PAPERS: No	
AUTHORSHIP RESTRICTIONS: No	REPRINT POLICY: None free	

SUBSCRIPTION ADDRESS: Plenum Press
227 W. 17th Street
New York NY 10011

ANNUAL SUBSCRIPTION RATE: Individuals: $33   Institutions: $66

FREQUENCY: Monthly   CIRCULATION: 5000

AFFILIATION: None

INDEXED/ABSTRACTED IN: IPA, IM

JOURNAL TITLE: Dimensions in Health Service

MANUSCRIPT ADDRESS: Canadian Hospital Association, Publications Dept.
410 Laurier Avenue West
Ottawa Ontario Canada K1R 7T6

TYPES OF ARTICLES: Research, commentaries, theoretical, case studies

MAJOR CONTENT AREAS: Many areas listed in Appendix A including: all medicine and nursing areas; continuing, inservice & patient education; aging & aged, death & dying, ethics, health promotion & policies, hospitals, nurisng homes, systems theory

TOPICS PREFERRED: Administration of health care facilities

INAPPROPRIATE TOPICS: Lifestyles, stress, promotional pieces

REVIEW PROCEDURE: Editorial board
REVIEW PERIOD: 2 months
MANUSCRIPT WORD LENGTH: 1200-2000
MANUSCRIPT COPIES: 2
PUBLICATION LAG TIME: 1-12 months
EARLY PUBLICATION OPTION: No
ACCEPTANCE RATE: 75%
AUTHORSHIP RESTRICTIONS: Yes

PAGE CHARGES: No
STYLE REQUIREMENTS: C
STYLE SHEET: Yes
REVISED THESES: Yes
STUDENT PAPERS: Yes
REPRINT POLICY: Author purchase

SUBSCRIPTION ADDRESS: Canadian Hospital Association
Sales and Circulation, 410 Laurier Avenue West
Ottawa Ontario Canada K1R 7T6

ANNUAL SUBSCRIPTION RATE: $12
FREQUENCY: Monthly
CIRCULATION: 16000
AFFILIATION: The Canadian Hospital Association
INDEXED/ABSTRACTED IN: CINAHL, HAS, HLI, IPA, IM, INI

◆

JOURNAL TITLE: Diseases of the Colon and Rectum

MANUSCRIPT ADDRESS: 403 First National Bank Building
Rochester MN 55901

TYPES OF ARTICLES: Research, review, case studies

MAJOR CONTENT AREAS: epidemiology and pathology of diseases of the colon, rectum, or anus

TOPICS PREFERRED: Clinical research regarding diseases that involve anus, rectum or colon

INAPPROPRIATE TOPICS: None

REVIEW PROCEDURE: Editorial board
REVIEW PERIOD: 4-6 weeks
MANUSCRIPT WORD LENGTH: 1500-2500
MANUSCRIPT COPIES: 2
PUBLICATION LAG TIME: 4 months
EARLY PUBLICATION OPTION: Yes
ACCEPTANCE RATE: 65%
AUTHORSHIP RESTRICTIONS: No

PAGE CHARGES: No
STYLE REQUIREMENTS: CBE, IM
STYLE SHEET: Yes
REVISED THESES: No
STUDENT PAPERS: Will consider
REPRINT POLICY: Not cited

SUBSCRIPTION ADDRESS: J.B. Lippincott Company
P.O. Box 7777 - R0210
Philadelphia PA 19175

ANNUAL SUBSCRIPTION RATE: $30 (Residents: $20.00)
FREQUENCY: 8 times yearly
CIRCULATION: 3800
AFFILIATION: American Society of Colon and Rectal Surgeons
INDEXED/ABSTRACTED IN: EM, BA, CA, IM, INI

JOURNAL TITLE: Ecology of Food and Nutrition

MANUSCRIPT ADDRESS: Dr. John K. Robson, Department of Family Practice
Medical University of South Carolina
171 Ashley Avenue, Charleston SC 29403

TYPES OF ARTICLES: Research, case studies, theoretical, commentaries,
review, unsolicited book reviews

MAJOR CONTENT AREAS: anthropology, biomedical research, eating
disorders, groups, growth/development, human
behavior, inservice education, medicine,
nutrition, research methodology

TOPICS PREFERRED: Nutritional status of different ethnic groups,
the remote and immediate causation of malnutrition

INAPPROPRIATE TOPICS: Review articles of topics covered better in spe-
cialist journals

REVIEW PROCEDURE: Editorial board and external review
REVIEW PERIOD: 6-8 weeks

MANUSCRIPT WORD LENGTH: 3500	**PAGE CHARGES:** No
MANUSCRIPT COPIES: 3	**STYLE REQUIREMENTS:** CBE
PUBLICATION LAG TIME: 1-4 months	**STYLE SHEET:** Yes
EARLY PUBLICATION OPTION: No	**REVISED THESES:** Yes
ACCEPTANCE RATE: 50-60%	**STUDENT PAPERS:** Yes
AUTHORSHIP RESTRICTIONS: No	**REPRINT POLICY:** Author purchase

SUBSCRIPTION ADDRESS: Gordon and Breach Science Publishers
One Park Avenue
New York NY 10016
ANNUAL SUBSCRIPTION RATE: Individuals: $45 Institutions: $119
FREQUENCY: Quarterly   **CIRCULATION:** 4000
AFFILIATION: None
INDEXED/ABSTRACTED IN: BA, EM, CA

◆

JOURNAL TITLE: Emergency Medical Services

MANUSCRIPT ADDRESS: Joan Hart, Editor
12849 Magnolia Blvd.
North Hollywood CA 91607

TYPES OF ARTICLES: Pragmatic, research, theoretical, review, case
studies, commentaries

MAJOR CONTENT AREAS: accidents, health personnel, alcoholism/drug
abuse, children, circulatory & respiratory dis-
eases, continuing & inservice education, counseling, crisis, death & dying, emergency services,
health policies, pain, stress, suicide

TOPICS PREFERRED: Emergency medical services in general

INAPPROPRIATE TOPICS: First person and news stories

REVIEW PROCEDURE: Editorial board
REVIEW PERIOD: 6 weeks

MANUSCRIPT WORD LENGTH: 1500 and up	**PAGE CHARGES:** No
MANUSCRIPT COPIES: 2	**STYLE REQUIREMENTS:** AMA, CBE, IM
PUBLICATION LAG TIME: 2-4 months	**STYLE SHEET:** Yes
EARLY PUBLICATION OPTION: No	**REVISED THESES:** Yes
ACCEPTANCE RATE: 80%	**STUDENT PAPERS:** No
AUTHORSHIP RESTRICTIONS: No	**REPRINT POLICY:** 2 free

SUBSCRIPTION ADDRESS: Emergency Medical Services
12849 Magnolia Blvd.
North Hollywood CA 91607
ANNUAL SUBSCRIPTION RATE: $20 (EMT's & Nurses, $10.50)
FREQUENCY: Bimonthly   **CIRCULATION:** 38,000
AFFILIATION: None
INDEXED/ABSTRACTED IN: CC, IM

JOURNAL TITLE: Emergency Medicine

MANUSCRIPT ADDRESS: Fisher-Murray, Inc.
280 Madison Avenue
New York NY 10016

TYPES OF ARTICLES: Review, case studies (most articles written house staff)

MAJOR CONTENT AREAS: abuse (child/spouse), accidents, alcoholism & drug abuse, circulatory diseases, crisis intervention/ theory, death & dying, emergency services, loss/ grief, medicine, pain, pharmacology, primary care, psychopathology, respiratory diseases, suicide

TOPICS PREFERRED: Management of acute illness and injury, management of acute phase of any disorder

INAPPROPRIATE TOPICS: None cited

REVIEW PROCEDURE: Editorial board, staff review
REVIEW PERIOD: 6 weeks

MANUSCRIPT WORD LENGTH: Variable		PAGE CHARGES: No
MANUSCRIPT COPIES: 2		STYLE REQUIREMENTS: Own
PUBLICATION LAG TIME: 2-3 months		STYLE SHEET: Yes
EARLY PUBLICATION OPTION: No		REVISED THESES: No
ACCEPTANCE RATE: Not cited		STUDENT PAPERS: No
AUTHORSHIP RESTRICTIONS: No		REPRINT POLICY: 100 tear sheets

SUBSCRIPTION ADDRESS: Fisher-Murray, Inc.
280 Madison Avenue
New York NY 10016

ANNUAL SUBSCRIPTION RATE: General: $27.50 Special rates available
FREQUENCY: Twice monthly   CIRCULATION: 114,000
AFFILIATION: None cited
INDEXED/ABSTRACTED IN: CINAHL, HLI

◆

JOURNAL TITLE: EMT Journal †

MANUSCRIPT ADDRESS: P.O. Box 153
Key Colony Beach FL 33051

TYPES OF ARTICLES: Scientific teaching articles relating to pre-hospital care; theoretical, research, review

MAJOR CONTENT AREAS: abuse (child/spouse), communication, crisis intervention/theory, death & dying, health policies, human behavior, leadership, primary care, respiratory diseases, safety/first aid, prehospital trauma, emergency medical services management

TOPICS PREFERRED: Pre-hospital care (medical) and systems management

INAPPROPRIATE TOPICS: None cited

REVIEW PROCEDURE: Editorial board
REVIEW PERIOD: 3-4 weeks

MANUSCRIPT WORD LENGTH: Variable		PAGE CHARGES: No
MANUSCRIPT COPIES: 3		STYLE REQUIREMENTS: Own
PUBLICATION LAG TIME: 6 months		STYLE SHEET: Yes
EARLY PUBLICATION OPTION: Not cited		REVISED THESES: Yes
ACCEPTANCE RATE: 50%		STUDENT PAPERS: Yes
AUTHORSHIP RESTRICTIONS: No		REPRINT POLICY: None free

SUBSCRIPTION ADDRESS: National Association of EMT
Box 334
Newton Highlands MA 02161

ANNUAL SUBSCRIPTION RATE: $10 Special rates available
FREQUENCY: Bimonthly   CIRCULATION: 20,000
AFFILIATION: National Assoc. of Emergency Medical Technologists
INDEXED/ABSTRACTED IN: CINAHL

JOURNAL TITLE: Environment International

MANUSCRIPT ADDRESS: A. Alan Moghissi, Ph.D., Editor-in-Chief
P.O. Box 7166
Alexandria VA 22307

TYPES OF ARTICLES: Research, theoretical, review, unsolicited book reviews

MAJOR CONTENT AREAS: biochemistry, biology, biomedical research, health sciences, health policies, medicine, natural science, respiratory diseases

TOPICS PREFERRED: Environmental topics

INAPPROPRIATE TOPICS: None cited

REVIEW PROCEDURE: Editorial board and external review
REVIEW PERIOD: 3-5 months

MANUSCRIPT WORD LENGTH: No limit	**PAGE CHARGES:** Yes
MANUSCRIPT COPIES: 3	**STYLE REQUIREMENTS:** CBE
PUBLICATION LAG TIME: 4-6 months	**STYLE SHEET:** Yes
EARLY PUBLICATION OPTION: No	**REVISED THESES:** Yes
ACCEPTANCE RATE: 80%	**STUDENT PAPERS:** No
AUTHORSHIP RESTRICTIONS: No	**REPRINT POLICY:** 25 free

SUBSCRIPTION ADDRESS: Pergamon Press, Inc.
Fairview Park
Elmsford NY 10523

ANNUAL SUBSCRIPTION RATE: Individuals: $30   Institutions: $110
FREQUENCY: Bimonthly   **CIRCULATION:** 1100
AFFILIATION: None
INDEXED/ABSTRACTED IN: None cited

◆

JOURNAL TITLE: Ergonomics

MANUSCRIPT ADDRESS: Dr. I.D. Brown, Editor
M.R.C. Applied Psychology Unit
15 Chaucer Road, Cambridge CB1 2EF   England

TYPES OF ARTICLES: Research, theoretical, case studies

MAJOR CONTENT AREAS: accidents, anatomy & physiology, biofeedback, biorhythms, biomedical research, fatigue, natural science, pain, perception, psychology, rehabilitation, research methodology, safety/first aid, sensory deprivation, sleep, stress, testing/measurement

TOPICS PREFERRED: Ergonomics

INAPPROPRIATE TOPICS: None cited

REVIEW PROCEDURE: External review
REVIEW PERIOD: 2-3 months

MANUSCRIPT WORD LENGTH: 3000-6000	**PAGE CHARGES:** No
MANUSCRIPT COPIES: 3	**STYLE REQUIREMENTS:** Own
PUBLICATION LAG TIME: 10 months	**STYLE SHEET:** Yes
EARLY PUBLICATION OPTION: No	**REVISED THESES:** Yes
ACCEPTANCE RATE: 60%	**STUDENT PAPERS:** No
AUTHORSHIP RESTRICTIONS: No	**REPRINT POLICY:** 50 free

SUBSCRIPTION ADDRESS: Taylor & Frances Ltd.
Bankers Trust Building, P.O. 9137
Church Streek Sta., New York NY 10049

ANNUAL SUBSCRIPTION RATE: $140
FREQUENCY: Monthly   **CIRCULATION:** 2300
AFFILIATION: Ergonomics Society
INDEXED/ABSTRACTED IN: BA, CA, EI, PA, SSCI, IM

JOURNAL TITLE: Ethics in Science and Medicine

MANUSCRIPT ADDRESS: Dr. P.J. McEwan
Glengarden, Ballater
Aberdeenshire, United Kingdom, AB3 5UB
TYPES OF ARTICLES: Research, theoretical, review, commentaries, case studies, unsolicited book reviews
MAJOR CONTENT AREAS: anthropology, ethics, human behavior, human sexuality, marriage & divorce, mental health/illness, professionalism, psychology, public health, quality of life, retirement, sociology, suicide, women's issues
TOPICS PREFERRED: Social morality and professional ethics

INAPPROPRIATE TOPICS: None

REVIEW PROCEDURE: Editorial board and external review
REVIEW PERIOD: 2 months
MANUSCRIPT WORD LENGTH: 2000-5000   **PAGE CHARGES:** No
MANUSCRIPT COPIES: 2   **STYLE REQUIREMENTS:** Own
PUBLICATION LAG TIME: 2 months   **STYLE SHEET:** Yes
EARLY PUBLICATION OPTION: Yes   **REVISED THESES:** Yes
ACCEPTANCE RATE: 60%   **STUDENT PAPERS:** No
AUTHORSHIP RESTRICTIONS: No   **REPRINT POLICY:** 25 free

SUBSCRIPTION ADDRESS: Pergamon Press, Inc.
Fairview Park
Elmsford NY 10523
ANNUAL SUBSCRIPTION RATE: Individuals: $30   Institutions: $75
FREQUENCY: Quarterly   **CIRCULATION:** 1100
AFFILIATION: None
INDEXED/ABSTRACTED IN: IM, CINAHL

◆

JOURNAL TITLE: Ethos

MANUSCRIPT ADDRESS: Department of Psychiatry
University of California
Los Angeles CA 90024
TYPES OF ARTICLES: Research, theoretical

MAJOR CONTENT AREAS: anthropology, cultural diversity, human behavior, human sexuality, sociology, cross-cultural psychology

TOPICS PREFERRED: Interrelationship between the individual & social or cultural setting
INAPPROPRIATE TOPICS: None cited

REVIEW PROCEDURE: Editorial board and external review
REVIEW PERIOD: 1.5-2 months
MANUSCRIPT WORD LENGTH: Not cited   **PAGE CHARGES:** Not cited
MANUSCRIPT COPIES: 3   **STYLE REQUIREMENTS:** AA, Own
PUBLICATION LAG TIME: Not cited   **STYLE SHEET:** Yes
EARLY PUBLICATION OPTION: Not cited   **REVISED THESES:** Not cited
ACCEPTANCE RATE: 40%   **STUDENT PAPERS:** Not cited
AUTHORSHIP RESTRICTIONS: No   **REPRINT POLICY:** 25 free

SUBSCRIPTION ADDRESS: Society for Psychological Anthropology
1703 New Hampshire Avenue, N.W.
Washington DC 20009
ANNUAL SUBSCRIPTION RATE: Individuals: $20   Members: $16   Students: $12
FREQUENCY: Quarterly   **CIRCULATION:** 600
AFFILIATION: Society for Psychological Anthropology
INDEXED/ABSTRACTED IN: PA

JOURNAL TITLE: Evaluation and the Health Professions

MANUSCRIPT ADDRESS: School of Nursing, University of Maryland
655 West Lombard Street
Baltimore MD 21201

TYPES OF ARTICLES: Research, theoretical, review, unsolicited book reviews

MAJOR CONTENT AREAS: abuse (child/spouse), alcoholism and drug abuse, biomedical research, continuing education, continuity of care, epidemiology, research methodology, evaluation

TOPICS PREFERRED: Program evaluation

INAPPROPRIATE TOPICS: None cited

REVIEW PROCEDURE: Editorial board
REVIEW PERIOD: 3 months
MANUSCRIPT WORD LENGTH: 3500-7000   **PAGE CHARGES:** No
MANUSCRIPT COPIES: 3   **STYLE REQUIREMENTS:** APA
PUBLICATION LAG TIME: 3 months   **STYLE SHEET:** Yes
EARLY PUBLICATION OPTION: No   **REVISED THESES:** Yes
ACCEPTANCE RATE: 25%   **STUDENT PAPERS:** No
AUTHORSHIP RESTRICTIONS: No   **REPRINT POLICY:** 24 free

SUBSCRIPTION ADDRESS: School of Nursing, University of Maryland
655 West Lombard Street
Baltimore MD 21201

ANNUAL SUBSCRIPTION RATE: Individuals: $15   Institutions: $30
FREQUENCY: Quarterly   **CIRCULATION:** 1500-2000
AFFILIATION: None
INDEXED/ABSTRACTED IN: Not cited

◆

JOURNAL TITLE: Family and Community Health

MANUSCRIPT ADDRESS: Aspen Systems Corporation
1600 Research Boulevard
Rockville MD 20850
TYPES OF ARTICLES: Material applicable to management and practical
settings; usable, readable articles
MAJOR CONTENT AREAS: adaptation, all age groups, alcoholism and drug
abuse, body image, client teaching, community/
public health nursing, crisis intervention/theory,
cultural diversity, family planning, geriatric
nursing, health promotion, nutrition, public health
TOPICS PREFERRED: Anything related to family and community nursing;
health promotion and maintenance
INAPPROPRIATE TOPICS: Disease oriented material; treatment

REVIEW PROCEDURE: Editorial board
REVIEW PERIOD: 3 months
MANUSCRIPT WORD LENGTH: 4500-6000   PAGE CHARGES: No
MANUSCRIPT COPIES: 3   STYLE REQUIREMENTS: C, Own
PUBLICATION LAG TIME: 6 months   STYLE SHEET: Yes
EARLY PUBLICATION OPTION: No   REVISED THESES: No
ACCEPTANCE RATE: 25%   STUDENT PAPERS: No
AUTHORSHIP RESTRICTIONS: No   REPRINT POLICY: 2 free journals

SUBSCRIPTION ADDRESS: Aspen Systems Corporation
16792 Oakmont Avenue
Gaithersburg MD 20877
ANNUAL SUBSCRIPTION RATE: $42
FREQUENCY: Quarterly   CIRCULATION: 6000
AFFILIATION: None
INDEXED/ABSTRACTED IN: CINAHL

JOURNAL TITLE: Family Health †

MANUSCRIPT ADDRESS: 149 Fifth Avenue
New York NY 10010

TYPES OF ARTICLES: Research, case studies, commentaries,
theoretical, review
MAJOR CONTENT AREAS: All content areas related to health care and
prevention

TOPICS PREFERRED: Preventive medicine and sound nutrition

INAPPROPRIATE TOPICS: None cited

REVIEW PROCEDURE: Editor
REVIEW PERIOD: Not cited
MANUSCRIPT WORD LENGTH: Not cited   PAGE CHARGES: Not cited
MANUSCRIPT COPIES: Not cited   STYLE REQUIREMENTS: Own
PUBLICATION LAG TIME: Not cited   STYLE SHEET: Yes
EARLY PUBLICATION OPTION: Not cited   REVISED THESES: Not cited
ACCEPTANCE RATE: Not cited   STUDENT PAPERS: Not cited
AUTHORSHIP RESTRICTIONS: Not cited   REPRINT POLICY: Not cited

SUBSCRIPTION ADDRESS: Family Health
149 Fifth Avenue
New York NY 10010
ANNUAL SUBSCRIPTION RATE: $15
FREQUENCY: 10 times yearly   CIRCULATION: Not cited
AFFILIATION: None
INDEXED/ABSTRACTED IN: CINAHL

JOURNAL TITLE: Family Planning Perspectives

MANUSCRIPT ADDRESS: The Alan Guttmacher Institute
360 Park Avenue
New York NY 10010

TYPES OF ARTICLES: Research

MAJOR CONTENT AREAS: adolescence, biomedical research, continuity of care, ethics, family planning, genetics, health policies, human sexuality, parenting, public health

TOPICS PREFERRED: Family planning, reproductive and population research, abortion, sterilization, teenage pregnancy

INAPPROPRIATE TOPICS: None cited

REVIEW PROCEDURE: Editorial board and external review
REVIEW PERIOD: 6-8 weeks

MANUSCRIPT WORD LENGTH: 7000	PAGE CHARGES: No
MANUSCRIPT COPIES: 3	STYLE REQUIREMENTS: C
PUBLICATION LAG TIME: 3-12 months	STYLE SHEET: Yes
EARLY PUBLICATION OPTION: Yes	REVISED THESES: Yes
ACCEPTANCE RATE: 10%	STUDENT PAPERS: No
AUTHORSHIP RESTRICTIONS: No	REPRINT POLICY: 20 free

SUBSCRIPTION ADDRESS: Circulation Manager
Family Planning Perspectives
360 Park Avenue, New York NY 10010

ANNUAL SUBSCRIPTION RATE: Free with $25 membership
FREQUENCY: Bimonthly   CIRCULATION: 28000
AFFILIATION: The Alan Guttmacher Institute
INDEXED/ABSTRACTED IN: CINAHL, HRA, IM, PA, SSCI, RPR

◄►

JOURNAL TITLE: Family Process

MANUSCRIPT ADDRESS: 149 E 78th Street
New York NY 10021

TYPES OF ARTICLES: Research, theoretical, clinical

MAJOR CONTENT AREAS: counseling, crisis intervention/theory, marriage & divorce, mental health/illness, parenting, psychology, psychopathology, psych/mental health nursing, research methodology, systems theory

TOPICS PREFERRED: Family therapy, research, theory and clinical material, interdisciplinary

INAPPROPRIATE TOPICS: None cited

REVIEW PROCEDURE: Editorial board and external review
REVIEW PERIOD: 6 months

MANUSCRIPT WORD LENGTH: Not cited	PAGE CHARGES: No
MANUSCRIPT COPIES: 4	STYLE REQUIREMENTS: APA
PUBLICATION LAG TIME: 1 year	STYLE SHEET: Yes
EARLY PUBLICATION OPTION: No	REVISED THESES: Will consider
ACCEPTANCE RATE: 15%	STUDENT PAPERS: No
AUTHORSHIP RESTRICTIONS: No	REPRINT POLICY: None free

SUBSCRIPTION ADDRESS: Family Process
149 E. 78th Street
New York NY 10021

ANNUAL SUBSCRIPTION RATE: Individuals: $16   Institutions: $25
FREQUENCY: Quarterly   CIRCULATION: 7000
AFFILIATION: None
INDEXED/ABSTRACTED IN: SWRA, SPAA, PA, SocA, CINAHL, ISI, IM

JOURNAL TITLE: Fertility and Contraception

MANUSCRIPT ADDRESS: Family Planning Information Service
27-35 Mortimer Street
London WIN 7RJ England

TYPES OF ARTICLES: Research, review, theoretical, case studies

MAJOR CONTENT AREAS: biomedical research related to contraception, counseling, epidemiology, family planning, genetics, handicapping conditions, human sexuality, immunization, marriage & divorce, maternal/child nursing, medicine, mental health, nutrition, women's issues

TOPICS PREFERRED: Contraceptive methods, fertility and infertility, family planning services, abortion, menopause

INAPPROPRIATE TOPICS: Over-theoretical, statistical material

REVIEW PROCEDURE: Editor, editorial board
REVIEW PERIOD: 1 month
MANUSCRIPT WORD LENGTH: 2000
MANUSCRIPT COPIES: 1
PUBLICATION LAG TIME: 2 months
EARLY PUBLICATION OPTION: No
ACCEPTANCE RATE: 90%
AUTHORSHIP RESTRICTIONS: No

PAGE CHARGES: No
STYLE REQUIREMENTS: Own
STYLE SHEET: Yes
REVISED THESES: Yes
STUDENT PAPERS: No
REPRINT POLICY: 25 free journals

SUBSCRIPTION ADDRESS: Subscriptions Secretary
Family Planning Information Service
27-35 Mortimer St., London WIN 7RJ England

ANNUAL SUBSCRIPTION RATE: $8
FREQUENCY: Quarterly
CIRCULATION: 5200
AFFILIATION: United Kingdom Family Planning Association
INDEXED/ABSTRACTED IN: Not cited

◆

JOURNAL TITLE: Geriatric Nursing

MANUSCRIPT ADDRESS: Cynthia H. Kelly, R.N., Editor
555 W. 57th Street
New York NY 10019

TYPES OF ARTICLES: Clinical articles with direct application to care of older persons in home, hospital & community

MAJOR CONTENT AREAS: areas relevant to the older population including: accidents, adaptation, biofeedback, body image, chronicity, compliance, continuity of care, dependency, loss/grief, nutrition, pain, primary care, retirement, sensory deprivation

TOPICS PREFERRED: Programs of care with demonstrated promise for improving geriatric care/nursing practice

INAPPROPRIATE TOPICS: New journal

REVIEW PROCEDURE: Editorial board		
REVIEW PERIOD: 4 weeks		
MANUSCRIPT WORD LENGTH: 1500-2000	**PAGE CHARGES:** No	
MANUSCRIPT COPIES: 2	**STYLE REQUIREMENTS:** C, IM, T	
PUBLICATION LAG TIME: 6-12 months	**STYLE SHEET:** Yes	
EARLY PUBLICATION OPTION: Not cited	**REVISED THESES:** Yes	
ACCEPTANCE RATE: New journal	**STUDENT PAPERS:** Yes	
AUTHORSHIP RESTRICTIONS: No	**REPRINT POLICY:** 100 free	

SUBSCRIPTION ADDRESS: Subscription Fulfillment Department
American Journal of Nursing Company
555 West 57th St., New York NY 10023

ANNUAL SUBSCRIPTION RATE: $18

FREQUENCY: Bimonthly   **CIRCULATION:** 16,000

AFFILIATION: None

INDEXED/ABSTRACTED IN: INI, IM, CINAHL

◆

JOURNAL TITLE: Gerontologist

MANUSCRIPT ADDRESS: Elias S. Cohen, J.D., Editor-in-Chief
136 Farwood Rd.
Philadelphia PA 19151

TYPES OF ARTICLES: Research, education, theoretical case studies, review, commentaries, unsolicited book reviews

MAJOR CONTENT AREAS: basic & applied health sciences related to gerontology, adaptation, chronicity, death & dying, dependency, ethics, handicapping conditions, loss/grief, marriage & divorce, mental retardation, quality of life, rehabilitation, retirement

TOPICS PREFERRED: Articles particularly applicable to practitioners, planners or policy makers and administrators

INAPPROPRIATE TOPICS: None cited

REVIEW PROCEDURE: Editorial board and external review		
REVIEW PERIOD: 3-8 weeks		
MANUSCRIPT WORD LENGTH: 4500-5000	**PAGE CHARGES:** No	
MANUSCRIPT COPIES: 3	**STYLE REQUIREMENTS:** APA	
PUBLICATION LAG TIME: 3-5 months	**STYLE SHEET:** Yes	
EARLY PUBLICATION OPTION: No	**REVISED THESES:** Yes	
ACCEPTANCE RATE: 28%	**STUDENT PAPERS:** Yes	
AUTHORSHIP RESTRICTIONS: No	**REPRINT POLICY:** 2 free journals	

SUBSCRIPTION ADDRESS: Gerontological Society
1835 K St., N.W., Suite 305
Washington DC 20006

ANNUAL SUBSCRIPTION RATE: $25

FREQUENCY: Bimonthly   **CIRCULATION:** 10,000

AFFILIATION: Gerontological Society

INDEXED/ABSTRACTED IN: BA, HLI, INI, SocA, CA, IM, PA, SSI, SSCI

JOURNAL TITLE: Group and Organization Studies

MANUSCRIPT ADDRESS: University Associates, Inc.
8517 Production Avenue
P.O. Box 26240, San Diego   CA   92126
TYPES OF ARTICLES: Research, theoretical

MAJOR CONTENT AREAS: counseling, crisis intervention/theory, cultural diversity, groups, human behavior, leadership, psychology, quality of life, research methodology, sociology, stress

TOPICS PREFERRED: Leadership/management, organization, community development; intercultural communication
INAPPROPRIATE TOPICS: None cited

REVIEW PROCEDURE: Editorial board
REVIEW PERIOD: 6-10 weeks
MANUSCRIPT WORD LENGTH: 4000
MANUSCRIPT COPIES: 5
PUBLICATION LAG TIME: 3 months
EARLY PUBLICATION OPTION: No
ACCEPTANCE RATE: 25%
AUTHORSHIP RESTRICTIONS: No

PAGE CHARGES: No
STYLE REQUIREMENTS: APA
STYLE SHEET: Yes
REVISED THESES: Not cited
STUDENT PAPERS: Not cited
REPRINT POLICY: Not cited

SUBSCRIPTION ADDRESS: Order Department
8517 Production Avenue
P.O. Bos 26240, San Diego   CA   92126
ANNUAL SUBSCRIPTION RATE: Individuals: $24   Institutions: $30
FREQUENCY: Quarterly
CIRCULATION: 3000
AFFILIATION: None
INDEXED/ABSTRACTED IN: PA

◆

JOURNAL TITLE: Hastings Center Report

MANUSCRIPT ADDRESS: Institute of Society, Ethics & the Life Sciences
360 Broadway
Hastings on Hudson NY 10706
TYPES OF ARTICLES: Theoretical, case studies, commentaries, short
timely articles with "news" emphasis
MAJOR CONTENT AREAS: biomedical research, death & dying, ethics,
genetics, health policies, human behavior, mental
health/illness, mental retardation, suicide

TOPICS PREFERRED: Ethics

INAPPROPRIATE TOPICS: None cited

REVIEW PROCEDURE: Editorial board and external review
REVIEW PERIOD: 4-6 weeks
MANUSCRIPT WORD LENGTH: 3000-4000   **PAGE CHARGES:** No
MANUSCRIPT COPIES: 2   **STYLE REQUIREMENTS:** C
PUBLICATION LAG TIME: 2 months   **STYLE SHEET:** Yes
EARLY PUBLICATION OPTION: No   **REVISED THESES:** No
ACCEPTANCE RATE: 10%   **STUDENT PAPERS:** No
AUTHORSHIP RESTRICTIONS: No   **REPRINT POLICY:** 5 free

SUBSCRIPTION ADDRESS: Institute of Society, Ethics & the Life Sciences
360 Broadway
Hastings on Hudson NYI 10706
ANNUAL SUBSCRIPTION RATE: $19
FREQUENCY: Bimonthly   **CIRCULATION:** 10,000
AFFILIATION: Institute of Society, Ethics & the Life Sciences
INDEXED/ABSTRACTED IN: IM, PI, BA, CC, CINAHL

◆

JOURNAL TITLE: Health Care in Canada †

MANUSCRIPT ADDRESS: Heather Howie, Editor
1450 Don Mills Road
Don Mills Ontario Canada M3B 2X7
TYPES OF ARTICLES: Research, theoretical, review, case studies

MAJOR CONTENT AREAS: discharge planning, emergency services, family
planning, health promotion, hospitals, leadership,
nursing: assessment, audit, care, education, geriatric, homes, service administration, operating
room; pharmacology, professionalism, public health
TOPICS PREFERRED: None cited

INAPPROPRIATE TOPICS: None cited

REVIEW PROCEDURE: Editorial board
REVIEW PERIOD: 1 month
MANUSCRIPT WORD LENGTH: 1000   **PAGE CHARGES:** No
MANUSCRIPT COPIES: 2   **STYLE REQUIREMENTS:** Not cited
PUBLICATION LAG TIME: 2 months   **STYLE SHEET:** No
EARLY PUBLICATION OPTION: No   **REVISED THESES:** Yes
ACCEPTANCE RATE: 10%   **STUDENT PAPERS:** No
AUTHORSHIP RESTRICTIONS: No   **REPRINT POLICY:** 1 free

SUBSCRIPTION ADDRESS: 1450 Don Mills Road
Don Mills
Ontario Canada M3B 2X7
ANNUAL SUBSCRIPTION RATE: $21
FREQUENCY: Monthly   **CIRCULATION:** 13,000
AFFILIATION: None
INDEXED/ABSTRACTED IN: HLI, IPA, CBPI

JOURNAL TITLE: Health Care Education

MANUSCRIPT ADDRESS: Edward McCabe, Editor
Reinhardt/Keymer Publishing
60 East 42nd Street, New York NY 10017
TYPES OF ARTICLES: Research, case studies; Prefer a detailed query
letter
MAJOR CONTENT AREAS: communication, continuing education, discharge
planning, inservice education, nursing education,
patient teaching

TOPICS PREFERRED: Training and Education methods for which proof
of efficacy is available
INAPPROPRIATE TOPICS: Many

REVIEW PROCEDURE: Editorial board, the editor's judgement
REVIEW PERIOD: One week

MANUSCRIPT WORD LENGTH: 750-1500	PAGE CHARGES: No	
MANUSCRIPT COPIES: 1	STYLE REQUIREMENTS: Own	
PUBLICATION LAG TIME: 2-4 months	STYLE SHEET: Yes	
EARLY PUBLICATION OPTION: No	REVISED THESES: No	
ACCEPTANCE RATE: 20%	STUDENT PAPERS: No	
AUTHORSHIP RESTRICTIONS: No	REPRINT POLICY: 20 free journals	

SUBSCRIPTION ADDRESS: Bill Robinson, Circulation Manager
Reinhardt/Keymer Publishing Co.
60 East 42nd Street, New York NY 10017
ANNUAL SUBSCRIPTION RATE: $18
FREQUENCY: Bimonthly   CIRCULATION: 20,000
AFFILIATION: None
INDEXED/ABSTRACTED IN: CINAHL, INI

◆

JOURNAL TITLE: Health Care Management Review

MANUSCRIPT ADDRESS: Aspen Systems Corporation
1600 Research Blvd.
Rockville MD 20850
TYPES OF ARTICLES: Theoretical, commentaries, case studies, research

MAJOR CONTENT AREAS: health care administration, health promotion,
health policies, hospitals

TOPICS PREFERRED: Anything relating to health care management

INAPPROPRIATE TOPICS: None cited

REVIEW PROCEDURE: Editorial board
REVIEW PERIOD: 1-3 months

MANUSCRIPT WORD LENGTH: Up to 5000	PAGE CHARGES: No	
MANUSCRIPT COPIES: 3	STYLE REQUIREMENTS: C, APA	
PUBLICATION LAG TIME: 2-6 months	STYLE SHEET: Yes	
EARLY PUBLICATION OPTION: No	REVISED THESES: Yes	
ACCEPTANCE RATE: 40%	STUDENT PAPERS: No	
AUTHORSHIP RESTRICTIONS: No	REPRINT POLICY: 2 free journals	

SUBSCRIPTION ADDRESS: Fulfillment operations
Aspen Systems Corporation
16792 Oakmont Ave., Gaithersburg MD 20877
ANNUAL SUBSCRIPTION RATE: $44.50
FREQUENCY: Quarterly   CIRCULATION: 6000
AFFILIATION: None
INDEXED/ABSTRACTED IN: Not cited

JOURNAL TITLE: Health Education

MANUSCRIPT ADDRESS: c/o AAHPER Director of Periodicals
1900 Associate Drive
Reston VA 22091
TYPES OF ARTICLES: Research, theoretical, review, commentaries,
unsolicited book reviews
MAJOR CONTENT AREAS: abuse (child/spouse), alcoholism & drug abuse,
death & dying, handicapping conditions, nutrition,
parenting, patient teaching

TOPICS PREFERRED: Any aspect of health education

INAPPROPRIATE TOPICS: None cited

REVIEW PROCEDURE: Editorial board & external review
REVIEW PERIOD: Not cited
MANUSCRIPT WORD LENGTH: 2000-3000   PAGE CHARGES: No
MANUSCRIPT COPIES: 2   STYLE REQUIREMENTS: Own
PUBLICATION LAG TIME: Not cited   STYLE SHEET: Yes
EARLY PUBLICATION OPTION: No   REVISED THESES: Yes
ACCEPTANCE RATE: Not cited   STUDENT PAPERS: No
AUTHORSHIP RESTRICTIONS: No   REPRINT POLICY: None free

SUBSCRIPTION ADDRESS: Health Education
1900 Associate Drive
Reston VA 22091
ANNUAL SUBSCRIPTION RATE: $25
FREQUENCY: Bimonthly   CIRCULATION: 11,000
AFFILIATION: Amer. Alliance Health, Physical Ed. & Recreation
INDEXED/ABSTRACTED IN: Not cited

◆

JOURNAL TITLE: The Health Education Journal

MANUSCRIPT ADDRESS: Health Education Council
78 New Oxford Street
London WC1A 1AH England
TYPES OF ARTICLES: Research, theoretical, case studies, commentaries

MAJOR CONTENT AREAS: abuse (child/spouse/alcoholism/drug), accidents,
body image, cancer, crisis, dependency, eating
disorders, family planning, fatigue, health promotion, human behavior & sexuality, immunization,
nutrition, quality of life, relaxation, stress
TOPICS PREFERRED: All aspects of health education

INAPPROPRIATE TOPICS: Irrelevant topics

REVIEW PROCEDURE: External review
REVIEW PERIOD: 6 weeks
MANUSCRIPT WORD LENGTH: 5000   PAGE CHARGES: No
MANUSCRIPT COPIES: 1   STYLE REQUIREMENTS: H
PUBLICATION LAG TIME: 1 year maximum   STYLE SHEET: Yes
EARLY PUBLICATION OPTION: No   REVISED THESES: Yes
ACCEPTANCE RATE: 50%   STUDENT PAPERS: No
AUTHORSHIP RESTRICTIONS: No   REPRINT POLICY: 6 free

SUBSCRIPTION ADDRESS: Health Education Council
78 New Oxford Street
London WC1A 1AH England
ANNUAL SUBSCRIPTION RATE: $7.50
FREQUENCY: Quarterly   CIRCULATION: 4500
AFFILIATION: Health Education Council
INDEXED/ABSTRACTED IN: SSCI

JOURNAL TITLE: Health Policy and Education

MANUSCRIPT ADDRESS: Thomas Samph, Editor
Educational Testing Service
Princeton NY 08541
TYPES OF ARTICLES: Research, review, commentaries, theoretical, case
stduies, unsolicited book reviews
MAJOR CONTENT AREAS: health policies

TOPICS PREFERRED: Current issues in health care, health policies,
and health education
INAPPROPRIATE TOPICS: Only unfocused articles are not accepted

REVIEW PROCEDURE: Editorial board and external review
REVIEW PERIOD: 2-4 months
MANUSCRIPT WORD LENGTH: Varies   PAGE CHARGES: No
MANUSCRIPT COPIES: 3   STYLE REQUIREMENTS: Own
PUBLICATION LAG TIME: 3-6 months   STYLE SHEET: Yes
EARLY PUBLICATION OPTION: No   REVISED THESES: Will review
ACCEPTANCE RATE: 40%   STUDENT PAPERS: Yes
AUTHORSHIP RESTRICTIONS: No   REPRINT POLICY: 50 free

SUBSCRIPTION ADDRESS: Elsevier Scientific Publishing Co.
P.O. Box 211
1000 AE Amsterdam, The Netherlands
ANNUAL SUBSCRIPTION RATE: Individuals: $36.00 Institutions: $73.25
FREQUENCY: Quarterly   CIRCULATION: Not cited
AFFILIATION: None
INDEXED/ABSTRACTED IN: Not cited

◆

JOURNAL TITLE: Health Practitioner and Physician Assistant †

MANUSCRIPT ADDRESS: 515 Madison Avenue
New York NY 10022

TYPES OF ARTICLES. Review, case studies, commentaries

MAJOR CONTENT AREAS: most health practitioners, most client age
groups, & disease problems, continuing education,
continuity of care, death & dying, ethics,
hospitals, human sexuality, loss/grief, nursing
homes, nutrition, parenting, professionalism
TOPICS PREFERRED: None cited

INAPPROPRIATE TOPICS: None cited

REVIEW PROCEDURE: Editorial board
REVIEW PERIOD: 3 months
MANUSCRIPT WORD LENGTH: 2000   PAGE CHARGES: Not cited
MANUSCRIPT COPIES: 3   STYLE REQUIREMENTS: AMA
PUBLICATION LAG TIME: 6 months   STYLE SHEET: Yes
EARLY PUBLICATION OPTION: No   REVISED THESES: No
ACCEPTANCE RATE: 35%   STUDENT PAPERS: No
AUTHORSHIP RESTRICTIONS: No   REPRINT POLICY: 50 free

SUBSCRIPTION ADDRESS: Health Practitioner and Physician Assistant
515 Madison Avenue
New York NY 10022
ANNUAL SUBSCRIPTION RATE: $15
FREQUENCY: Monthly   CIRCULATION: 12,000
AFFILIATION: American Academy of Physicians Assistants
INDEXED/ABSTRACTED IN: None cited

JOURNAL TITLE: Health Services Manager

MANUSCRIPT ADDRESS: American Management Association
135 W. 50th Street
New York NY 10020

TYPES OF ARTICLES: Theoretical, commentaries, case studies,
practical articles

MAJOR CONTENT AREAS: communication, community/public health nursing,
continuing education, hospitals, inservice
education, leadership, nursing service
administration, management and administration

TOPICS PREFERRED: Administrative and management oriented articles
dealing with healthcare facilities

INAPPROPRIATE TOPICS: None cited

REVIEW PROCEDURE: Editor and editorial board
REVIEW PERIOD: 1-2 weeks
MANUSCRIPT WORD LENGTH: 2000-3000   PAGE CHARGES: No
MANUSCRIPT COPIES: 2   STYLE REQUIREMENTS: C
PUBLICATION LAG TIME: Several months   STYLE SHEET: Yes
EARLY PUBLICATION OPTION: No   REVISED THESES: No
ACCEPTANCE RATE: 35%   STUDENT PAPERS: No
AUTHORSHIP RESTRICTIONS: No   REPRINT POLICY: 100 Free

SUBSCRIPTION ADDRESS: Health Services Manager, Subscription Services
American Management Association
Box 319, Saranac Lake NY 12983
ANNUAL SUBSCRIPTION RATE: Members: $14 Nonmembers: $18
FREQUENCY: Monthly   CIRCULATION: 5000
AFFILIATION: American Management Association
INDEXED/ABSTRACTED IN: Not cited

◆

JOURNAL TITLE: Health Services Research

MANUSCRIPT ADDRESS: The Editor
840 North Lake Shore Drive
Chicago IL 60611

TYPES OF ARTICLES: Research

MAJOR CONTENT AREAS: epidemiology, health sciences, health policies,
testing/measurement

TOPICS PREFERRED: None cited

INAPPROPRIATE TOPICS: None cited

REVIEW PROCEDURE: Editorial board and external review
REVIEW PERIOD: 6-8 weeks
MANUSCRIPT WORD LENGTH: Not cited   PAGE CHARGES: No
MANUSCRIPT COPIES: 4   STYLE REQUIREMENTS: Own
PUBLICATION LAG TIME: 6 months   STYLE SHEET: Yes
EARLY PUBLICATION OPTION: No   REVISED THESES: No
ACCEPTANCE RATE: Not cited   STUDENT PAPERS: No
AUTHORSHIP RESTRICTIONS: No   REPRINT POLICY: 50 free

SUBSCRIPTION ADDRESS: Health Services Research
840 North Lake Shore Drive
Chicago IL 60611
ANNUAL SUBSCRIPTION RATE: $25
FREQUENCY: Quarterly   CIRCULATION: Not cited
AFFILIATION: None
INDEXED/ABSTRACTED IN: AHM, CC, EM, HLI, INI, MSRS, SSCI, IM

80

JOURNAL TITLE: Health and Social Service Journal

MANUSCRIPT ADDRESS: 3 Dyers Buildings
Holborn
London EC1N 2NR England

TYPES OF ARTICLES: Research, commentaries, theoretical, review

MAJOR CONTENT AREAS: most nursing specialties, health and social
problems & policies, communication, continuing &
inservice education, discharge planning, primary
care, professionalism, quality of life, research
methodology, women's issues

TOPICS PREFERRED: Hospital administration, The Health Service,
sociology, medical sociology, children

INAPPROPRIATE TOPICS: None cited

REVIEW PROCEDURE: Editorial board and external review
REVIEW PERIOD: 1 week
MANUSCRIPT WORD LENGTH: 800-900   PAGE CHARGES: Yes
MANUSCRIPT COPIES: 2   STYLE REQUIREMENTS: Not cited
PUBLICATION LAG TIME: Varies   STYLE SHEET: Yes
EARLY PUBLICATION OPTION: No   REVISED THESES: Yes
ACCEPTANCE RATE: Not cited   STUDENT PAPERS: Not cited
AUTHORSHIP RESTRICTIONS: No   REPRINT POLICY: free journal

SUBSCRIPTION ADDRESS: Subscription Department
Brunel Road, Basingstoke
Hampshire RG21 2XS England

ANNUAL SUBSCRIPTION RATE: $30
FREQUENCY: Weekly   CIRCULATION: 60,000
AFFILIATION: None cited
INDEXED/ABSTRACTED IN: HosA, HLI, CINAHL

JOURNAL TITLE: Health & Social Work

MANUSCRIPT ADDRESS: 1425 H Street, N.W.
Washington DC 20005

TYPES OF ARTICLES: Research, theoretical, review, case studies

MAJOR CONTENT AREAS: abuse, adolescence, aging & aged, substance
abuse, children, chronicity, continuity of care,
counseling, crisis, death & dying, discharge
planning, ethics, family planning, groups, handicapping conditions, health: promotion, policies

TOPICS PREFERRED: Any related to social work and health care

INAPPROPRIATE TOPICS: None cited

REVIEW PROCEDURE: Editorial board
REVIEW PERIOD: 3-4 months
MANUSCRIPT WORD LENGTH: 1500   PAGE CHARGES: No
MANUSCRIPT COPIES: 4   STYLE REQUIREMENTS: C, Own
PUBLICATION LAG TIME: 6-12 months   STYLE SHEET: Yes
EARLY PUBLICATION OPTION: No   REVISED THESES: Not cited
ACCEPTANCE RATE: Not cited   STUDENT PAPERS: No
AUTHORSHIP RESTRICTIONS: No   REPRINT POLICY: Contracted

SUBSCRIPTION ADDRESS: 49 Sheridan Avenue
Albany NY 12210

ANNUAL SUBSCRIPTION RATE: Individuals: $35 Members: $20
FREQUENCY: Quarterly   CIRCULATION: 4500
AFFILIATION: National Association of Social Workers
INDEXED/ABSTRACTED IN: SWRA, IM, CINAHL, INI

JOURNAL TITLE: Health Values: Achieving High Level Wellness

MANUSCRIPT ADDRESS: Charles B. Slack, Inc.
6900 Grove Road
Thorofare NJ 08086

TYPES OF ARTICLES: Research, theoretical, review, commentaries, unsolicited book reviews

MAJOR CONTENT AREAS: abuse (child/spouse), accidents, health promotion, health sciences, health policies, human behavior, human sexuality, life span, professionalism, public health, quality of life, health education, values clarification

TOPICS PREFERRED: Any topic which considers the body, mind, & spirit as an interrelated & interdependent whole

INAPPROPRIATE TOPICS: None cited

REVIEW PROCEDURE: Editorial board
REVIEW PERIOD: Not cited
MANUSCRIPT WORD LENGTH: 1500-2000   PAGE CHARGES: No
MANUSCRIPT COPIES: 3   STYLE REQUIREMENTS: IM
PUBLICATION LAG TIME: Not cited   STYLE SHEET: Not cited
EARLY PUBLICATION OPTION: Not cited   REVISED THESES: Not cited
ACCEPTANCE RATE: Not cited   STUDENT PAPERS: Not cited
AUTHORSHIP RESTRICTIONS: Not cited   REPRINT POLICY: Not cited

SUBSCRIPTION ADDRESS: Charles B. Slack
6900 Grove Road
Thorofare NJ 08086

ANNUAL SUBSCRIPTION RATE: $14
FREQUENCY: Bimonthly   CIRCULATION: Not cited
AFFILIATION: None
INDEXED/ABSTRACTED IN: Not cited

◆

JOURNAL TITLE: Health Visitor

MANUSCRIPT ADDRESS: Health Visitors Association
36 Eccleston Square
London SW1V 1PF England

TYPES OF ARTICLES: Research, case studies, theoretical, review, unsolicited book reviews, commentaries

MAJOR CONTENT AREAS: mental, physical & social health problems of children & adolescents, public health & school nursing, counseling, health promotion, human behavior & sexuality, loss/grief, aging & aged, marriage & divorce, parenting, professionalism

TOPICS PREFERRED: Maternal and child health, maternal child health in the field of preventive medicine

INAPPROPRIATE TOPICS: Advertising material for editorials

REVIEW PROCEDURE: Editor's decision
REVIEW PERIOD: 1 week
MANUSCRIPT WORD LENGTH: 2000-4000   PAGE CHARGES: No
MANUSCRIPT COPIES: 2   STYLE REQUIREMENTS: Not cited
PUBLICATION LAG TIME: 2-7 months   STYLE SHEET: Yes
EARLY PUBLICATION OPTION: No   REVISED THESES: Yes
ACCEPTANCE RATE: 90%   STUDENT PAPERS: Yes
AUTHORSHIP RESTRICTIONS: No   REPRINT POLICY: 25 free

SUBSCRIPTION ADDRESS: B. Edsall and Co.
36 Eccleston Square
London SW1V 1PF England

ANNUAL SUBSCRIPTION RATE: $20
FREQUENCY: Monthly   CIRCULATION: 12,000
AFFILIATION: Health Visitors Association
INDEXED/ABSTRACTED IN: CINAHL, INI

JOURNAL TITLE: Heart and Lung: The Journal of Critical Care

MANUSCRIPT ADDRESS: Sylvan L. Weinberg, M.D.
33 W. First Street
Dayton OH 45402
TYPES OF ARTICLES: Original articles, review articles, case studies

MAJOR CONTENT AREAS: critical care nursing

TOPICS PREFERRED: None cited

INAPPROPRIATE TOPICS: None cited

REVIEW PROCEDURE: Editorial Board and external review
REVIEW PERIOD: 2-3 months
MANUSCRIPT WORD LENGTH: 2500-3000   PAGE CHARGES: No
MANUSCRIPT COPIES: 3   STYLE REQUIREMENTS: CBE, IM
PUBLICATION LAG TIME: 5-6 months   STYLE SHEET: Yes
EARLY PUBLICATION OPTION: No   REVISED THESES: No
ACCEPTANCE RATE: 70%   STUDENT PAPERS: No
AUTHORSHIP RESTRICTIONS: No   REPRINT POLICY: None free

SUBSCRIPTION ADDRESS: The C.V. Mosby Company
Journal Circulation Department, 11830 Westline
Industrial Drive, St. Louis MO 63141
ANNUAL SUBSCRIPTION RATE: Individuals: $14.00   Institutions: $33.00
FREQUENCY: Bimonthly   CIRCULATION: 56,000
AFFILIATION: American Association of Critical Care Nurses
INDEXED/ABSTRACTED IN: IM, CC, CINAHL, HLI, INI

◆

JOURNAL TITLE: Holistic Health Review

MANUSCRIPT ADDRESS: Steven Markell, Editor
1030 Merced Street
Berkeley CA 94707
TYPES OF ARTICLES: Research, commentaries, theoretical, case studies
unsolicited book reviews
MAJOR CONTENT AREAS: Many areas in Appendix A including: adaptation,
aging & aged, biofeedback, body image, chronicity,
compliance, continuity of care, cultural diversity, death & dying, ethics, fatigue, nursing:
care, philosophy, public health; quality of life
TOPICS PREFERRED: Holistic health, disease prevention, health
promotion
INAPPROPRIATE TOPICS: None cited

REVIEW PROCEDURE: Editorial board & external review
REVIEW PERIOD: 3 months
MANUSCRIPT WORD LENGTH: 1500-3000   PAGE CHARGES: No
MANUSCRIPT COPIES: 3   STYLE REQUIREMENTS: APA
PUBLICATION LAG TIME: 6-9 months   STYLE SHEET: Yes
EARLY PUBLICATION OPTION: No   REVISED THESES: Yes
ACCEPTANCE RATE: 50%   STUDENT PAPERS: Yes
AUTHORSHIP RESTRICTIONS: No   REPRINT POLICY: 5 free

SUBSCRIPTION ADDRESS: Human Sciences Press
72 Fifth Avenue
New York NY 10011
ANNUAL SUBSCRIPTION RATE: Individuals: $15   Institutions: $35
FREQUENCY: Quarterly   CIRCULATION: 2000
AFFILIATION: None
INDEXED/ABSTRACTED IN: New journal

JOURNAL TITLE: Home Health Review

MANUSCRIPT ADDRESS: National Association of Home Health Agencies
205 C Street, N.E.
Washington DC 20002

TYPES OF ARTICLES: Case studies, research, review, commentaries, theoretical, unsolicited book reviews

MAJOR CONTENT AREAS: continuity of care, health promotion, midwifery, nursing: assessment, audit, care, clinical specialties, geriatric, service administration, occupational health; nursing homes, physical therapy, primary care, public health, home health care

TOPICS PREFERRED: Topics which are relevant to the continued development of home health care

INAPPROPRIATE TOPICS: Articles that are too medically technical for an audience of administrators

REVIEW PROCEDURE: Editorial board

REVIEW PERIOD: 2 months

MANUSCRIPT WORD LENGTH: 4000	PAGE CHARGES: No
MANUSCRIPT COPIES: 2	STYLE REQUIREMENTS: Own
PUBLICATION LAG TIME: 1 month	STYLE SHEET: Yes
EARLY PUBLICATION OPTION: No	REVISED THESES: Yes
ACCEPTANCE RATE: 50%	STUDENT PAPERS: No
AUTHORSHIP RESTRICTIONS: No	REPRINT POLICY: As requested

SUBSCRIPTION ADDRESS: National Association of Home Health Agencies
205 C Street, N.E.
Washington DC 20002

ANNUAL SUBSCRIPTION RATE: $20

FREQUENCY: Quarterly   CIRCULATION: 800

AFFILIATION: National Association of Home Health Agencies

INDEXED/ABSTRACTED IN: HLI

◆

JOURNAL TITLE: Hospital and Community Psychiatry

MANUSCRIPT ADDRESS: Donald W. Hammersley, M.D., Editor
The American Psychiatric Association
1700 18th Street, N.W., Washington DC 20009

TYPES OF ARTICLES: Research, case studies, evaluative studies, clinical, commentaries

MAJOR CONTENT AREAS: adolescence, aging and aged, alcoholism & drug abuse, continuity of care, counseling, crisis intervention/theory, dependency, mental health/illness, mental retardation, psychiatric/mental health nursing, stigma, stress, suicide

TOPICS PREFERRED: Program descriptions, legal and judicial issues, current topics for interdisciplinary audience

INAPPROPRIATE TOPICS: None cited

REVIEW PROCEDURE: Editorial board and external review

REVIEW PERIOD: 8 weeks

MANUSCRIPT WORD LENGTH: 1200-3000	PAGE CHARGES: No
MANUSCRIPT COPIES: 3	STYLE REQUIREMENTS: Own
PUBLICATION LAG TIME: 9-12 months	STYLE SHEET: Yes
EARLY PUBLICATION OPTION: No	REVISED THESES: Yes
ACCEPTANCE RATE: 25%	STUDENT PAPERS: No
AUTHORSHIP RESTRICTIONS: No	REPRINT POLICY: 5 free journals

SUBSCRIPTION ADDRESS: American Psychiatric Association
1700 18th Street, N.W.
Washington DC 20009

ANNUAL SUBSCRIPTION RATE: $24

FREQUENCY: Monthly   CIRCULATION: 20,000

AFFILIATION: American Psychiatric Association

INDEXED/ABSTRACTED IN: IM, CINAHL, EM, HLI, INI, PA, SSCI, BA

JOURNAL TITLE: Hospital Equipment & Supplies

MANUSCRIPT ADDRESS: Northwood House
93-99 Goswell Road
London EC1V 7QA England
TYPES OF ARTICLES: Reviews, research, theoretical, commentaries,
unsolicited book reviews
MAJOR CONTENT AREAS: biomedical research & personnel, nursing: geriatric, maternal/child, medical/surgical, service
administration, operating room, trauma; nutrition,
physics, research methodology, safety/first aid,
systems theory, teaching/learning
TOPICS PREFERRED: New research on equipment, supplies and clinical
systems to be developed or marketed in England
INAPPROPRIATE TOPICS: None cited

REVIEW PROCEDURE: Editorial board
REVIEW PERIOD: 1-2 weeks
MANUSCRIPT WORD LENGTH: 1000-1500   PAGE CHARGES: No
MANUSCRIPT COPIES: 1   STYLE REQUIREMENTS: Own
PUBLICATION LAG TIME: 6 weeks   STYLE SHEET: Yes
EARLY PUBLICATION OPTION: Not cited   REVISED THESES: Yes
ACCEPTANCE RATE: 90%   STUDENT PAPERS: No
AUTHORSHIP RESTRICTIONS: No   REPRINT POLICY: 12 free

SUBSCRIPTION ADDRESS: Circulation Manager
23-29 Emerald Street
London WC1N 3QJ England
ANNUAL SUBSCRIPTION RATE: $30
FREQUENCY: Monthly   CIRCULATION: 10,200
AFFILIATION: None
INDEXED/ABSTRACTED IN: Not cited

◆

JOURNAL TITLE: Hospital Formulary

MANUSCRIPT ADDRESS: Arthur G. Lipman, Editor
Department of Pharmacy Practice
University of Utah, Salt Lake City UT 84112
TYPES OF ARTICLES: Research, review, case studies

MAJOR CONTENT AREAS: most health problems & health sciences;
hospitals, compliance, primary care, emergency
services, nursing: clinical specialties, critical care, geriatric, medical/surgical,
neurological, theory, trauma; research methodology
TOPICS PREFERRED: Drugs, drug therapy, patient compliance, health
policy
INAPPROPRIATE TOPICS: Incomplete or biased reviews

REVIEW PROCEDURE: Editorial board (refereed)
REVIEW PERIOD: 3 months
MANUSCRIPT WORD LENGTH: 2000-3000   PAGE CHARGES: No
MANUSCRIPT COPIES: 3   STYLE REQUIREMENTS: IM
PUBLICATION LAG TIME: 4-6 months   STYLE SHEET: Yes
EARLY PUBLICATION OPTION: No   REVISED THESES: Yes
ACCEPTANCE RATE: 30-40%   STUDENT PAPERS: No
AUTHORSHIP RESTRICTIONS: Yes   REPRINT POLICY: Not cited

SUBSCRIPTION ADDRESS: Circulation Department
1 East First Street
Duluth MN 55802
ANNUAL SUBSCRIPTION RATE: $15
FREQUENCY: Monthly   CIRCULATION: 30,000
AFFILIATION: None
INDEXED/ABSTRACTED IN: CINAHL

JOURNAL TITLE: Hospital Forum

MANUSCRIPT ADDRESS: Association of Western Hospitals
830 Market Street
San Francisco CA 94102
TYPES OF ARTICLES: Theoretical, commentaries

MAJOR CONTENT AREAS: health policies, hospitals

TOPICS PREFERRED: Hospital administration; practical information
for hospital administrators and managers
INAPPROPRIATE TOPICS: Articles promoting a product

REVIEW PROCEDURE: Editor reviews
REVIEW PERIOD: 6 months
MANUSCRIPT WORD LENGTH: 2000-3000   PAGE CHARGES: No
MANUSCRIPT COPIES: 1   STYLE REQUIREMENTS: WT
PUBLICATION LAG TIME: 1-3 months   STYLE SHEET: No
EARLY PUBLICATION OPTION: Not cited   REVISED THESES: No
ACCEPTANCE RATE: Not cited   STUDENT PAPERS: Yes
AUTHORSHIP RESTRICTIONS: No   REPRINT POLICY: 3 free

SUBSCRIPTION ADDRESS: Association of Western Hospitals
830 Market Street
San Francisco CA 94102
ANNUAL SUBSCRIPTION RATE: $20
FREQUENCY: 7 times yearly   CIRCULATION: 10,000
AFFILIATION: Association of Western Hospitals
INDEXED/ABSTRACTED IN: CINAHL, AHM, EM, HLI, IPA

◆

JOURNAL TITLE: Hospital and Health Services Administration

MANUSCRIPT ADDRESS: Stuart A. Wesbury, Jr., FACHA, Executive Editor
840 North Lake Shore Drive
Chicago IL 60611
TYPES OF ARTICLES: Theoretical, research, commentaries (with
documentation), unsolicited book reviews
MAJOR CONTENT AREAS: communication, continuing education, health
policies, hospitals, human behavior, leadership,
nursing service administration, professionalism,
systems theory

TOPICS PREFERRED: The art and science of management/administration
for hospitals & health service facilities
INAPPROPRIATE TOPICS: "How to" and success stores from PR firms

REVIEW PROCEDURE: Editorial board
REVIEW PERIOD: 6-8 weeks
MANUSCRIPT WORD LENGTH: 3000-4200   PAGE CHARGES: No
MANUSCRIPT COPIES: 4   STYLE REQUIREMENTS: C
PUBLICATION LAG TIME: 12-18 months   STYLE SHEET: Yes
EARLY PUBLICATION OPTION: Yes   REVISED THESES: Will consider
ACCEPTANCE RATE: 35%   STUDENT PAPERS: No
AUTHORSHIP RESTRICTIONS: No   REPRINT POLICY: 6 free

SUBSCRIPTION ADDRESS: 840 North Lake Shore Drive
Chicago IL 60611

ANNUAL SUBSCRIPTION RATE: $12.50
FREQUENCY: Quarterly   CIRCULATION: 15,000
AFFILIATION: American College of Hospital Adminsitrators
INDEXED/ABSTRACTED IN: HLI, IPA, CINAHL

JOURNAL TITLE: Hospital Pharmacy

MANUSCRIPT ADDRESS: Neil M. Davis, Editor
1143 Wright Drive
Huntingdon Valley PA 19006
TYPES OF ARTICLES: Practical articles on running a hospital pharmacy, case studies, review, theoretical, research
MAJOR CONTENT AREAS: accidents, communication, inservice education

TOPICS PREFERRED: Medication errors, medication systems, medication administration records
INAPPROPRIATE TOPICS: None cited

REVIEW PROCEDURE: External review and peer review
REVIEW PERIOD: 8 weeks
MANUSCRIPT WORD LENGTH: 1000-2000
MANUSCRIPT COPIES: 3
PUBLICATION LAG TIME: 6 months
EARLY PUBLICATION OPTION: No
ACCEPTANCE RATE: 30%
AUTHORSHIP RESTRICTIONS: No

PAGE CHARGES: No
STYLE REQUIREMENTS: AMA, CBE
STYLE SHEET: No
REVISED THESES: Yes
STUDENT PAPERS: No
REPRINT POLICY: 25 free

SUBSCRIPTION ADDRESS: J.B. Lippincott Company
East Washington Square
Philadelphia PA 19105
ANNUAL SUBSCRIPTION RATE: Individuals: $16 Institutions: $16
FREQUENCY: Monthly
CIRCULATION: 20,000
AFFILIATION: None
INDEXED/ABSTRACTED IN: IPA

◆

JOURNAL TITLE: Hospital Practice

MANUSCRIPT ADDRESS: HP Publishing Co., Inc.
575 Lexington Avenue
New York NY 10022
TYPES OF ARTICLES: Research, theoretical, case studies, commentaries

MAJOR CONTENT AREAS: biochemistry, biomedical research, hospitals, medicine, microbiology, pathology, psychopathology

TOPICS PREFERRED: None cited

INAPPROPRIATE TOPICS: None cited

REVIEW PROCEDURE: Not cited
REVIEW PERIOD: Not cited
MANUSCRIPT WORD LENGTH: Not cited
MANUSCRIPT COPIES: Not cited
PUBLICATION LAG TIME: Not cited
EARLY PUBLICATION OPTION: Not cited
ACCEPTANCE RATE: Not cited
AUTHORSHIP RESTRICTIONS: Not cited

PAGE CHARGES: Not cited
STYLE REQUIREMENTS: Not cited
STYLE SHEET: Not cited
REVISED THESES: Not cited
STUDENT PAPERS: Not cited
REPRINT POLICY: Not cited

SUBSCRIPTION ADDRESS: HP Publishing Co., Inc.
575 Lexington Avenue
New York NY 10022
ANNUAL SUBSCRIPTION RATE: Individuals: $20 Students: $15
FREQUENCY: Monthly
CIRCULATION: 185,000
AFFILIATION: None
INDEXED/ABSTRACTED IN: IM, CINAHL, BA, HLI

JOURNAL TITLE: Hospital Progress

MANUSCRIPT ADDRESS: The Catholic Hospital Association
4455 Woodson Road
St. Louis MO 63134

TYPES OF ARTICLES: Research, case studies, commentaries

MAJOR CONTENT AREAS: death & dying, genetics, health policies,
hospitals, quality of life

TOPICS PREFERRED: Hospital organization, government, legal

INAPPROPRIATE TOPICS: Clinical topics

REVIEW PROCEDURE: Editorial board and external review
REVIEW PERIOD: 6 months
MANUSCRIPT WORD LENGTH: 1500-2000   **PAGE CHARGES:** No
MANUSCRIPT COPIES: 2   **STYLE REQUIREMENTS:** C
PUBLICATION LAG TIME: 3 months   **STYLE SHEET:** Yes
EARLY PUBLICATION OPTION: No   **REVISED THESES:** Yes
ACCEPTANCE RATE: 20%   **STUDENT PAPERS:** No
AUTHORSHIP RESTRICTIONS: No   **REPRINT POLICY:** 100 free

SUBSCRIPTION ADDRESS: The Catholic Hospital Association
4455 Woodson Rd.
St. Louis MO 63134
ANNUAL SUBSCRIPTION RATE: $20
FREQUENCY: Monthly   **CIRCULATION:** 14,000
AFFILIATION: Catholic Hospital Association
INDEXED/ABSTRACTED IN: HLI, IM, CINAHL, AHM, IPA, MSRS, CPLI, INI

◆

JOURNAL TITLE: Hospital Topics

MANUSCRIPT ADDRESS: 3807 Bond Place
Sarasota FL 33582

TYPES OF ARTICLES: Short illustrated "how to do it" articles and new
techniques, products and systems
MAJOR CONTENT AREAS: communication, continuing education, continuity of
care, epidemiology, hospitals, leadership,
medicine, microbiology, nursing: assessment, care,
clinical specialties, education, medical/surgical,
process, service administration, operating room
TOPICS PREFERRED: Materials & nursing management, pharmacy, OR, cen-
ral service, infection control, nursing education
INAPPROPRIATE TOPICS: Construction and food articles

REVIEW PROCEDURE: Consultants
REVIEW PERIOD: 7-10 days
MANUSCRIPT WORD LENGTH: 3000   **PAGE CHARGES:** No
MANUSCRIPT COPIES: 1   **STYLE REQUIREMENTS:** AMA
PUBLICATION LAG TIME: 2-4 months   **STYLE SHEET:** Yes
EARLY PUBLICATION OPTION: Yes   **REVISED THESES:** No
ACCEPTANCE RATE: 70%   **STUDENT PAPERS:** No
AUTHORSHIP RESTRICTIONS: No   **REPRINT POLICY:** 10 free journals

SUBSCRIPTION ADDRESS: Hospital Topics
3807 Bond Place
Sarasota FL 33582
ANNUAL SUBSCRIPTION RATE: $25
FREQUENCY: Bimonthly   **CIRCULATION:** 16,000
AFFILIATION: None cited
INDEXED/ABSTRACTED IN: HLI, IM, CINAHL, IPA, INI

JOURNAL TITLE: Hospitals

MANUSCRIPT ADDRESS: American Hospital Association
840 N. Lakeshore Drive
Chicago IL 60611

TYPES OF ARTICLES: Research, theoretical, review, case studies

MAJOR CONTENT AREAS: communication, continuing education, continuity of care, discharge planning, emergency services, health promotion, hospitals, leadership, nursing: assessment, audit, care, education, philosophy, administration; nursing homes, patient teaching

TOPICS PREFERRED: Current issues in hospital nursing service administration

INAPPROPRIATE TOPICS: Clinical articles

REVIEW PROCEDURE: Editorial board and external review
REVIEW PERIOD: 4-6 weeks

MANUSCRIPT WORD LENGTH: 2500-3000	PAGE CHARGES: No
MANUSCRIPT COPIES: 2	STYLE REQUIREMENTS: C
PUBLICATION LAG TIME: 3-6 months	STYLE SHEET: Yes
EARLY PUBLICATION OPTION: No	REVISED THESES: Yes
ACCEPTANCE RATE: 30%	STUDENT PAPERS: No
AUTHORSHIP RESTRICTIONS: No	REPRINT POLICY: None free

SUBSCRIPTION ADDRESS: American Hospital Association
840 N. Lake Shore Drive
Chicago IL 60611

ANNUAL SUBSCRIPTION RATE: $30

FREQUENCY: Biweekly	CIRCULATION: 80,000

AFFILIATION: American Hospital Association

INDEXED/ABSTRACTED IN: HLI, CINAHL, CA, IPA, INI, IM

◆

JOURNAL TITLE: Human Biology

MANUSCRIPT ADDRESS: Dr. Gabriel W. Lasker, Editor-in-Chief
Dept. of Anatomy, Wayne State University
540 East Canfield, Detroit MI 48201

TYPES OF ARTICLES: Research

MAJOR CONTENT AREAS: adaptation, anthropology, genetics, growth/development

TOPICS PREFERRED: Biology of human populations

INAPPROPRIATE TOPICS: Further small studies by the same methods with no original hypotheses or ideas

REVIEW PROCEDURE: External review (primarily Human Biology Council)
REVIEW PERIOD: 5 weeks

MANUSCRIPT WORD LENGTH: 6000	PAGE CHARGES: Extra costs
MANUSCRIPT COPIES: 3	STYLE REQUIREMENTS: CBE, Own
PUBLICATION LAG TIME: 6 months	STYLE SHEET: No
EARLY PUBLICATION OPTION: No	REVISED THESES: Some
ACCEPTANCE RATE: 40%	STUDENT PAPERS: No
AUTHORSHIP RESTRICTIONS: No	REPRINT POLICY: 25 free

SUBSCRIPTION ADDRESS: Wayne State University Press
Wayne State University
Detroit MI 48201

ANNUAL SUBSCRIPTION RATE: Individuals: $17   Institutions: $23

FREQUENCY: Quarterly	CIRCULATION: 1800

AFFILIATION: Human Biology Council

INDEXED/ABSTRACTED IN: BA, CC, AA, EM, CA, IM, NAR, PA, BAI, DA

JOURNAL TITLE: Human Organization

MANUSCRIPT ADDRESS: Department of Sociology & Anthropology
University of Rhode Island
Kingston RI 02881

TYPES OF ARTICLES: Research, case studies, commentaries

MAJOR CONTENT AREAS: aging and aged, alcoholism & drug abuse,
anthropology, communication, cultural diversity,
ethics, research methodology, sociology,
testing/measurement, women's issues

TOPICS PREFERRED: Applied social science

INAPPROPRIATE TOPICS: None cited

REVIEW PROCEDURE: External review
REVIEW PERIOD: 6-8 weeks
MANUSCRIPT WORD LENGTH: 3000-7000   PAGE CHARGES: No
MANUSCRIPT COPIES: 4   STYLE REQUIREMENTS: C
PUBLICATION LAG TIME: 6-12 months   STYLE SHEET: Yes
EARLY PUBLICATION OPTION: No   REVISED THESES: No
ACCEPTANCE RATE: 15%   STUDENT PAPERS: No
AUTHORSHIP RESTRICTIONS: No   REPRINT POLICY: None free

SUBSCRIPTION ADDRESS: American Anthropological Association
1703 New Hampshire Avenue, N.W.
Washington DC 20009
ANNUAL SUBSCRIPTION RATE: Individuals: $17   Institutions: $25
FREQUENCY: Quarterly   CIRCULATION: 4000
AFFILIATION: Society for Applied Anthropology
INDEXED/ABSTRACTED IN: SSI, SSCI, AA

◆

JOURNAL TITLE: Image

MANUSCRIPT ADDRESS: Sigma Theta Tau
1100 W. Michigan St.
Indianapolis IN 46223
TYPES OF ARTICLES: Research, theoretical

MAJOR CONTENT AREAS: leadership, nursing education, nursing philosophy, nursing theory, research methodology
women's issues

TOPICS PREFERRED: None cited

INAPPROPRIATE TOPICS: None cited

REVIEW PROCEDURE: Editorial board and external review
REVIEW PERIOD: 3-6 months
MANUSCRIPT WORD LENGTH: 2000-4000   PAGE CHARGES: No
MANUSCRIPT COPIES: 3   STYLE REQUIREMENTS: APA, C
PUBLICATION LAG TIME: 3-6 months   STYLE SHEET: Yes
EARLY PUBLICATION OPTION: No   REVISED THESES: No
ACCEPTANCE RATE: Not cited   STUDENT PAPERS: Yes
AUTHORSHIP RESTRICTIONS: No   REPRINT POLICY: 25 free

SUBSCRIPTION ADDRESS: Sigma Theta Tau
Nursing Building
1100 West Michigan St., Indianapolis IN 46223
ANNUAL SUBSCRIPTION RATE: $5
FREQUENCY: 3 times yearly   CIRCULATION: 30,000
AFFILIATION: Sigma Theta Tau
INDEXED/ABSTRACTED IN: CINAHL, INI

◆

JOURNAL TITLE: Imprint

MANUSCRIPT ADDRESS: National Student Nurses' Association
10 Columbus Circle
New York NY 10019
TYPES OF ARTICLES: Theoretical, case studies, commentaries

MAJOR CONTENT AREAS: biorhythms, communication, counseling, death &
dying, ethics, health promotion & policies,
marriage/divorce, nursing: care, clinical specialties, education, history; primary care, professionalism, stress, suicide, teaching/learning
TOPICS PREFERRED: Student experiences

INAPPROPRIATE TOPICS: Term papers

REVIEW PROCEDURE: Editorial board
REVIEW PERIOD: 3 months
MANUSCRIPT WORD LENGTH: 1500-2000   PAGE CHARGES: No
MANUSCRIPT COPIES: 2   STYLE REQUIREMENTS: C
PUBLICATION LAG TIME: 6-24 months   STYLE SHEET: Yes
EARLY PUBLICATION OPTION: No   REVISED THESES: No
ACCEPTANCE RATE: 20%   STUDENT PAPERS: Yes
AUTHORSHIP RESTRICTIONS: No   REPRINT POLICY: 3 free

SUBSCRIPTION ADDRESS: National Student Nurses' Association
10 Columbus Circle
New York NY 10019
ANNUAL SUBSCRIPTION RATE: $8
FREQUENCY: 5 times yearly   CIRCULATION: 35,000
AFFILIATION: National Student Nurses' Association
INDEXED/ABSTRACTED IN: CINAHL, INI

JOURNAL TITLE: Infant Behavior and Development

MANUSCRIPT ADDRESS: Lewis P. Lipsitt Child Study Center
Brown University, Box 1836
Providence RI 02912

TYPES OF ARTICLES: Research

MAJOR CONTENT AREAS: child abuse, adaptation, crisis intervention/
theory, death & dying, dependency, eating dis-
orders, handicapping conditions, mental retardation, nursing process, nutrition, pain, parenting, perception, rehabilitation, sleep, stress

TOPICS PREFERRED: Normal and abnormal infancy

INAPPROPRIATE TOPICS: None

REVIEW PROCEDURE:	Editorial board		
REVIEW PERIOD:	2-3 months		
MANUSCRIPT WORD LENGTH:	2400-3000	PAGE CHARGES:	No
MANUSCRIPT COPIES:	3	STYLE REQUIREMENTS:	APA
PUBLICATION LAG TIME:	5 months	STYLE SHEET:	Yes
EARLY PUBLICATION OPTION:	No	REVISED THESES:	Yes
ACCEPTANCE RATE:	50%	STUDENT PAPERS:	No
AUTHORSHIP RESTRICTIONS:	No	REPRINT POLICY:	None free

SUBSCRIPTION ADDRESS: Ablex Inc.
355 Chestnut St.
Norwood NJ 07648

ANNUAL SUBSCRIPTION RATE: Individuals: $25   Institutions: $49
FREQUENCY: Quarterly   CIRCULATION: 800
AFFILIATION: None
INDEXED/ABSTRACTED IN: CDA

JOURNAL TITLE: Infertility

MANUSCRIPT ADDRESS: Dr. Wayne H. Decker, Editor
New York Fertility Research Foundation
1430 Second Ave., New York NY 10021

TYPES OF ARTICLES: Clinical research, case studies, review, research

MAJOR CONTENT AREAS: genetics, human sexuality, human reproduction and
infertility

TOPICS PREFERRED: As cited in content areas

INAPPROPRIATE TOPICS: None cited

REVIEW PROCEDURE:	Editorial board		
REVIEW PERIOD:	2 months		
MANUSCRIPT WORD LENGTH:	1680	PAGE CHARGES:	No
MANUSCRIPT COPIES:	2	STYLE REQUIREMENTS:	Own
PUBLICATION LAG TIME:	3 months	STYLE SHEET:	Yes
EARLY PUBLICATION OPTION:	No	REVISED THESES:	Yes
ACCEPTANCE RATE:	90%	STUDENT PAPERS:	No
AUTHORSHIP RESTRICTIONS:	No	REPRINT POLICY:	20 free

SUBSCRIPTION ADDRESS: Marcel Dekker Journals
P.O. Box 11305
Church Street Station, New York NY 10249

ANNUAL SUBSCRIPTION RATE: Individuals: $20   Institutions: $40
FREQUENCY: Quarterly   CIRCULATION: Not cited
AFFILIATION: None
INDEXED/ABSTRACTED IN: CA, CC

JOURNAL TITLE: Inflammation

MANUSCRIPT ADDRESS: Gerald Weissman, M.D., Editor-in-Chief
Department of Medicine, New York University School
of Medicine, 550 First Avenue, New York NY 10016
TYPES OF ARTICLES: Research, review

MAJOR CONTENT AREAS: biochemistry, biology, circulatory diseases,
medicine, microbiology, pain, pathology,
pharmacology

TOPICS PREFERRED: Inflammation

INAPPROPRIATE TOPICS: None cited

REVIEW PROCEDURE: Editorial board and external review
REVIEW PERIOD: 1 month
MANUSCRIPT WORD LENGTH: 8000   PAGE CHARGES: No
MANUSCRIPT COPIES: 2   STYLE REQUIREMENTS: CBE
PUBLICATION LAG TIME: 6 months   STYLE SHEET: Yes
EARLY PUBLICATION OPTION: No   REVISED THESES: No
ACCEPTANCE RATE: 50%   STUDENT PAPERS: No
AUTHORSHIP RESTRICTIONS: No   REPRINT POLICY: None free

SUBSCRIPTION ADDRESS: Department of Medicine
New York University School of Medicine
550 First Avenue, New York NY 10016
ANNUAL SUBSCRIPTION RATE: $40
FREQUENCY: Quarterly   CIRCULATION: 800
AFFILIATION: International Inflammation Research Society
INDEXED/ABSTRACTED IN: None cited

◆

JOURNAL TITLE: Inquiry

MANUSCRIPT ADDRESS: Marilyn H. Cutler
Blue Cross Association
676 North St. Clair St., Chicago IL 60611
TYPES OF ARTICLES: Research, theoretical, commentaries

MAJOR CONTENT AREAS: allied health personnel, continuity of care,
discharge planning, epidemiology, ethics, groups,
health promotion & policies, hospitals, nursing:
audit, community health, service administration;
nursing homes, public health, sociology
TOPICS PREFERRED: Health care organization, provision, & financing;
third-party reimbursement systems
INAPPROPRIATE TOPICS: Reviews of the literature

REVIEW PROCEDURE: Editorial board and external review
REVIEW PERIOD: 8-16 weeks
MANUSCRIPT WORD LENGTH: 5000-7500   PAGE CHARGES: No
MANUSCRIPT COPIES: 4   STYLE REQUIREMENTS: AMA
PUBLICATION LAG TIME: 3-12 months   STYLE SHEET: No
EARLY PUBLICATION OPTION: No   REVISED THESES: No
ACCEPTANCE RATE: 30%   STUDENT PAPERS: No
AUTHORSHIP RESTRICTIONS: No   REPRINT POLICY: 10 free

SUBSCRIPTION ADDRESS: Inquiry
P.O. Box 527
Glenview IL 60025
ANNUAL SUBSCRIPTION RATE: Individuals: $15   Institutions: $20
FREQUENCY: Quarterly   CIRCULATION: 3200
AFFILIATION: None
INDEXED/ABSTRACTED IN: PAIS, HLI, IM, EM, HosA, MCR, HRA, JEL, INI

JOURNAL TITLE: International Journal of the Addictions

MANUSCRIPT ADDRESS: Dr. Stanley Ernstein
113/41 East Talpiot
Jerusalem   Israel
TYPES OF ARTICLES: Research, theoretical, case studies

MAJOR CONTENT AREAS: alcoholism and drug abuse, human behavior,
pharmacology, sociology

TOPICS PREFERRED: None cited

INAPPROPRIATE TOPICS: None cited

REVIEW PROCEDURE: Editorial board
REVIEW PERIOD: 4-6 weeks

MANUSCRIPT WORD LENGTH: Not cited	**PAGE CHARGES:** No	
MANUSCRIPT COPIES: 3	**STYLE REQUIREMENTS:** APA	
PUBLICATION LAG TIME: 6 months	**STYLE SHEET:** Yes	
EARLY PUBLICATION OPTION: No	**REVISED THESES:** Yes	
ACCEPTANCE RATE: 40%	**STUDENT PAPERS:** No	
AUTHORSHIP RESTRICTIONS: No	**REPRINT POLICY:** 20 free	

SUBSCRIPTION ADDRESS: Marcel Dekker Journals
270 Madison Avenue
New York NY 10016
ANNUAL SUBSCRIPTION RATE: Individuals: $50   Institutions: $100
FREQUENCY: 8 times yearly   **CIRCULATION:** Not cited
AFFILIATION: None cited
INDEXED/ABSTRACTED IN: CC, IM, EM, PA, BA, CA, SSCI

JOURNAL TITLE: International Journal of Aging & Human Development

MANUSCRIPT ADDRESS: Dr. Robert J. Kastenbaum, Editor
Deptartment of Psychology, College 1
Columbia Point Campus, Dorchester MA 02125
TYPES OF ARTICLES: Research, theoretical, case studies

MAJOR CONTENT AREAS: aging and aged, growth/development, human
behavior, human sexuality, quality of life

TOPICS PREFERRED: Psychology & social studies of aging & aged

INAPPROPRIATE TOPICS: None cited

REVIEW PROCEDURE: Editorial board
REVIEW PERIOD: Not cited

MANUSCRIPT WORD LENGTH: Not cited	**PAGE CHARGES:** Not cited	
MANUSCRIPT COPIES: 3	**STYLE REQUIREMENTS:** Own	
PUBLICATION LAG TIME: Not cited	**STYLE SHEET:** Yes	
EARLY PUBLICATION OPTION: Not cited	**REVISED THESES:** Not cited	
ACCEPTANCE RATE: Not cited	**STUDENT PAPERS:** Not cited	
AUTHORSHIP RESTRICTIONS: Not cited	**REPRINT POLICY:** 20 free	

SUBSCRIPTION ADDRESS: Baywood Publishing Co.
120 Marine St., P.O. Box D
Farmingdale NY 11735
ANNUAL SUBSCRIPTION RATE: Individuals: $27   Institutions: $45
FREQUENCY: Quarterly   **CIRCULATION:** Not cited
AFFILIATION: None
INDEXED/ABSTRACTED IN: IM, PA, SSCI, ACSR

JOURNAL TITLE: International Journal of Epidemiology

MANUSCRIPT ADDRESS: Professor A.E. Bennett
St. George's Hospital Medical School
Cranmer Terrace, London SW17 ORE England
TYPES OF ARTICLES: Research, theoretical, review

MAJOR CONTENT AREAS: epidemiology, public health, research methodology
evaluation of medical care

TOPICS PREFERRED: None cited

INAPPROPRIATE TOPICS: None cited

REVIEW PROCEDURE: External review
REVIEW PERIOD: 2-3 months
MANUSCRIPT WORD LENGTH: 1500   **PAGE CHARGES:** No
MANUSCRIPT COPIES: 3   **STYLE REQUIREMENTS:** Own
PUBLICATION LAG TIME: 3-6 months   **STYLE SHEET:** Yes
EARLY PUBLICATION OPTION: No   **REVISED THESES:** No
ACCEPTANCE RATE: 40%   **STUDENT PAPERS:** No
AUTHORSHIP RESTRICTIONS: No   **REPRINT POLICY:** 50 free

SUBSCRIPTION ADDRESS: Oxford Journals
Oxford University Press
Press Road, Neasden, London NW10 ODD
ANNUAL SUBSCRIPTION RATE: $45
FREQUENCY: Quarterly   **CIRCULATION:** 2500
AFFILIATION: International Epidemiological Association
INDEXED/ABSTRACTED IN: IM, CC, BA, EM, SSCI, INI

◆

JOURNAL TITLE: International Journal of Family Therapy

MANUSCRIPT ADDRESS: Dr. Gerald Zuk, Editor, Dept. of Psychiatry
Medical College of Georgia
Augusta GA 30912
TYPES OF ARTICLES: Research, theoretical, case studies, review,
commentaries
MAJOR CONTENT AREAS: most age groups, health professionals, and
psychosocial health problems listed in Appendix A;
counseling interventions; continuing & inservice
education; nursing: maternal/child, psychiatric/
mental health; family planning; parenting
TOPICS PREFERRED: Family therapy

INAPPROPRIATE TOPICS: None cited

REVIEW PROCEDURE: Editorial board
REVIEW PERIOD: 8 weeks
MANUSCRIPT WORD LENGTH: 4000   **PAGE CHARGES:** No
MANUSCRIPT COPIES: 3   **STYLE REQUIREMENTS:** APA
PUBLICATION LAG TIME: 12 months   **STYLE SHEET:** Yes
EARLY PUBLICATION OPTION: No   **REVISED THESES:** Yes
ACCEPTANCE RATE: 25%   **STUDENT PAPERS:** No
AUTHORSHIP RESTRICTIONS: No   **REPRINT POLICY:** None free

SUBSCRIPTION ADDRESS: Human Sciences Press
72 Fifth Avenue
New York NY 10011
ANNUAL SUBSCRIPTION RATE: Individuals: $16   Institutions: $36
FREQUENCY: Quarterly   **CIRCULATION:** Not cited
AFFILIATION: None
INDEXED/ABSTRACTED IN: Not cited

JOURNAL TITLE: International Journal of Health Education

MANUSCRIPT ADDRESS: 3 Rue Voillier
1207 Geneva Switzerland

TYPES OF ARTICLES: Case studies, practical experiments

MAJOR CONTENT AREAS: change theory, communication, family planning, health promotion, human behavior, nutrition, primary care, public health, research methodology

TOPICS PREFERRED: Any topics which have implications for health education

INAPPROPRIATE TOPICS: None cited

REVIEW PROCEDURE: Editorial board		
REVIEW PERIOD: 6 months		
MANUSCRIPT WORD LENGTH: 5000-7000	**PAGE CHARGES:** No	
MANUSCRIPT COPIES: 3	**STYLE REQUIREMENTS:** Own	
PUBLICATION LAG TIME: 1-6 months	**STYLE SHEET:** No (in journal)	
EARLY PUBLICATION OPTION: Not cited	**REVISED THESES:** No	
ACCEPTANCE RATE: 50%	**STUDENT PAPERS:** No	
AUTHORSHIP RESTRICTIONS: No	**REPRINT POLICY:** 1 free journal	

SUBSCRIPTION ADDRESS: International Journal of Health Education
3 Rue Voillier
1207 Geneva Switzerland

ANNUAL SUBSCRIPTION RATE: $13.50

FREQUENCY: Quarterly   **CIRCULATION:** 8000

AFFILIATION: International Union for Health Education

INDEXED/ABSTRACTED IN: CC, BA, SSCI

◆

JOURNAL TITLE: International Journal of Health Services

MANUSCRIPT ADDRESS: Dr. Vicente Navarro, Editor-in-Chief, The Johns Hopkins Univ., School of Hygiene & Public Health, 615 North Wolfe St., Baltimore MD 21205

TYPES OF ARTICLES: Research, theoretical, review

MAJOR CONTENT AREAS: ethics, health sciences, health policies, hospitals, mental health/illness, professionalism, psychology, public health, quality of life, sociology, women's issues

TOPICS PREFERRED: None cited

INAPPROPRIATE TOPICS: None cited

REVIEW PROCEDURE: Editorial board		
REVIEW PERIOD: Not cited		
MANUSCRIPT WORD LENGTH: 5000-7500	**PAGE CHARGES:** Not cited	
MANUSCRIPT COPIES: 3	**STYLE REQUIREMENTS:** IM	
PUBLICATION LAG TIME: Not cited	**STYLE SHEET:** Yes	
EARLY PUBLICATION OPTION: No	**REVISED THESES:** No	
ACCEPTANCE RATE: Not cited	**STUDENT PAPERS:** No	
AUTHORSHIP RESTRICTIONS: No	**REPRINT POLICY:** Not cited	

SUBSCRIPTION ADDRESS: Baywood Publishing Co., Inc.
120 Marine Street, P.O. Box D
Farmingdale NY 11735

ANNUAL SUBSCRIPTION RATE: Individuals: $25   Institutions: $55

FREQUENCY: Quarterly   **CIRCULATION:** Not cited

AFFILIATION: None cited

INDEXED/ABSTRACTED IN: AHM, EM, HLI, IM, MCR, MSRS

JOURNAL TITLE: International Journal of Nursing Studies

MANUSCRIPT ADDRESS: Dr. Rosemary Crow, Director, Nursing Practice &
Research Unit, Watford Rd., Harrow,
Middlesex HA1 3UJ England

TYPES OF ARTICLES: Research, commentaries

MAJOR CONTENT AREAS: new ideas based on scientific study in any area
related to nursing

TOPICS PREFERRED: Developments in any aspect of nursing in any
country

INAPPROPRIATE TOPICS: None cited

REVIEW PROCEDURE: Specialists review when appropriate
REVIEW PERIOD: 6 weeks max.

MANUSCRIPT WORD LENGTH: 4000-5000	PAGE CHARGES:	No
MANUSCRIPT COPIES: 2	STYLE REQUIREMENTS:	Own
PUBLICATION LAG TIME: 4-6 months	STYLE SHEET:	Yes
EARLY PUBLICATION OPTION: Not usually	REVISED THESES:	Yes
ACCEPTANCE RATE: 90%	STUDENT PAPERS:	May submit
AUTHORSHIP RESTRICTIONS: No	REPRINT POLICY:	25 free

SUBSCRIPTION ADDRESS: Pergamon Press, Inc.
Fairview Park
Elmsford NY 10523

ANNUAL SUBSCRIPTION RATE: Individuals: $30   Institutions: $65
FREQUENCY: Quarterly   CIRCULATION: 1150
AFFILIATION: None
INDEXED/ABSTRACTED IN: CINAHL, IM, SSCI, INI

◆

JOURNAL TITLE: International Journal of Obesity

MANUSCRIPT ADDRESS: Dr. George A. Bray
Univ. of Calif., Harbor General Hospital
1000 West Carson St., Torrance CA 90509

TYPES OF ARTICLES: Research, theoretical, review, commentaries, case
studies, unsolicited book reviews

MAJOR CONTENT AREAS: eating disorders, nutrition, obesity

TOPICS PREFERRED: None cited

INAPPROPRIATE TOPICS: None cited

REVIEW PROCEDURE: Editorial board and external review
REVIEW PERIOD: 4-6 weeks

MANUSCRIPT WORD LENGTH: 4000	PAGE CHARGES:	No
MANUSCRIPT COPIES: 2	STYLE REQUIREMENTS:	IM, Own
PUBLICATION LAG TIME: 3-6 months	STYLE SHEET:	Yes
EARLY PUBLICATION OPTION: No	REVISED THESES:	No
ACCEPTANCE RATE: Not cited	STUDENT PAPERS:	No
AUTHORSHIP RESTRICTIONS: No	REPRINT POLICY:	None free

SUBSCRIPTION ADDRESS: John Libbey and Company, Ltd.
80-84 Bondway
London SW8 1SF England

ANNUAL SUBSCRIPTION RATE: Individuals: $42   Institutions: $68
FREQUENCY: Quarterly   CIRCULATION: 500
AFFILIATION: Association for the Study of Obesity
INDEXED/ABSTRACTED IN: IM, CC(CP)

JOURNAL TITLE: International Journal of Social Psychiatry

MANUSCRIPT ADDRESS: Dr. Joshua Bierer
140 Harley St.
London W1 1AH England
TYPES OF ARTICLES: Research, theoretical, case studies, commentaries

MAJOR CONTENT AREAS: social psychiatry

TOPICS PREFERRED: The state of psychiatric care and treatment &
social welfare in particular countries
INAPPROPRIATE TOPICS: None cited

REVIEW PROCEDURE: Editorial board
REVIEW PERIOD: Not cited
MANUSCRIPT WORD LENGTH: Not cited   PAGE CHARGES: Yes
MANUSCRIPT COPIES: 4   STYLE REQUIREMENTS: Own
PUBLICATION LAG TIME: 12-18 months   STYLE SHEET: Not cited
EARLY PUBLICATION OPTION: Not cited   REVISED THESES: Not cited
ACCEPTANCE RATE: Not cited   STUDENT PAPERS: Not cited
AUTHORSHIP RESTRICTIONS: Not cited   REPRINT POLICY: Not cited

SUBSCRIPTION ADDRESS: Avenue Publishing Company
18 Park Avenue
London NW11 7SJ England
ANNUAL SUBSCRIPTION RATE: Individuals: $30 Institutions: $50
FREQUENCY: Quarterly   CIRCULATION: 2000
AFFILIATION: None cited
INDEXED/ABSTRACTED IN: IM, PA, SSCI, SSI, CINAHL

◆

JOURNAL TITLE: International Nursing Review

MANUSCRIPT ADDRESS: The Editor
P.O. Box 42
CH-1211 Geneva 20 Switzerland
TYPES OF ARTICLES: Commentaries, theoretical, review, research

MAJOR CONTENT AREAS: Many areas in Appendix A including: nursing:
assessment, audit, care, clinical specialties,
public health, critical care, diagnosis,
education, history, philosophy, process, research,
science, service administration, theory
TOPICS PREFERRED: Topics relating to programmes and achievements of
professional nurses' associations
INAPPROPRIATE TOPICS: None cited

REVIEW PROCEDURE: None cited
REVIEW PERIOD: 1-2 months
MANUSCRIPT WORD LENGTH: 2000-3000   PAGE CHARGES: No
MANUSCRIPT COPIES: 1   STYLE REQUIREMENTS: Own
PUBLICATION LAG TIME: 1 year   STYLE SHEET: Yes
EARLY PUBLICATION OPTION: Not cited   REVISED THESES: Yes
ACCEPTANCE RATE: 40%   STUDENT PAPERS: Yes
AUTHORSHIP RESTRICTIONS: No   REPRINT POLICY: 50 free

SUBSCRIPTION ADDRESS: International Nursing Review
c/o Imprimeriers Reunies S.A., 33,av. de la Gare,
Ch-1001 Lausanne Switzerland
ANNUAL SUBSCRIPTION RATE: $20
FREQUENCY: Bimonthly   CIRCULATION: 3500
AFFILIATION: International Council of Nurses
INDEXED/ABSTRACTED IN: INI, HLI, CINAHL, IM, SSCI

JOURNAL TITLE: International Quarterly of Community Health
Education

MANUSCRIPT ADDRESS: Division of Public Health, Arnold House
University of Massachusetts
Amherst MA 01003

TYPES OF ARTICLES: Research, case studies, review, theoretical,
unsolicited book reviews, commentaries

MAJOR CONTENT AREAS: allied health personnel, change theory,
communication, continuing education, family
planning, health promotion, health sciences,
health policies, human behavior, public health,
research methodology, prevention in health care

TOPICS PREFERRED: Community health education, application of social
& behavioral sciences to health problems

INAPPROPRIATE TOPICS: None cited

REVIEW PROCEDURE: Editorial board, external review, peer review
REVIEW PERIOD: 2 months
MANUSCRIPT WORD LENGTH: 4000-5000	**PAGE CHARGES:** No
MANUSCRIPT COPIES: 3	**STYLE REQUIREMENTS:** Own
PUBLICATION LAG TIME: 6 months	**STYLE SHEET:** Yes
EARLY PUBLICATION OPTION: No	**REVISED THESES:** No
ACCEPTANCE RATE: 30%	**STUDENT PAPERS:** No
AUTHORSHIP RESTRICTIONS: No	**REPRINT POLICY:** 20 free

SUBSCRIPTION ADDRESS: Baywood Publishing Co., Inc.
120 Marine St., P.O. Box 609
Farmingdale NY 11735
ANNUAL SUBSCRIPTION RATE: Individuals: $15   Institutions: $25
FREQUENCY: Quarterly   **CIRCULATION:** 500
AFFILIATION: None
INDEXED/ABSTRACTED IN: New journal

JOURNAL TITLE: International Review of Natural Family Planning

MANUSCRIPT ADDRESS: c/o Human Life Center
Saint John's University
Collegeville MN 56321

TYPES OF ARTICLES: Research, theoretical, practical articles

MAJOR CONTENT AREAS: biorhythms, body image, communication, counseling, crisis, ethics, growth/development, human
behavior & sexuality, marriage & divorce, midwifery, parenting, patient teaching, public health
nursing, psychology, quality of life, women's issues

TOPICS PREFERRED: Fertility & infertility, menstrual cycle, human
reproduction, integrated sexuality

INAPPROPRIATE TOPICS: None cited

REVIEW PROCEDURE: Editorial board
REVIEW PERIOD: 3-4 weeks
MANUSCRIPT WORD LENGTH: 500-2000	**PAGE CHARGES:** No
MANUSCRIPT COPIES: 2	**STYLE REQUIREMENTS:** C
PUBLICATION LAG TIME: 1-3 months	**STYLE SHEET:** Yes
EARLY PUBLICATION OPTION: No	**REVISED THESES:** Yes
ACCEPTANCE RATE: 50%	**STUDENT PAPERS:** No
AUTHORSHIP RESTRICTIONS: No	**REPRINT POLICY:** 10 free

SUBSCRIPTION ADDRESS: Mrs. Judy England
The Human Life Center
St. John's University, Collegeville MN 56321
ANNUAL SUBSCRIPTION RATE: $13
FREQUENCY: Quarterly   **CIRCULATION:** 1500
AFFILIATION: Human Life Center
INDEXED/ABSTRACTED IN: None cited

JOURNAL TITLE: Issues in Comprehensive Pediatric Nursing

MANUSCRIPT ADDRESS: Hemisphere Publishers, Inc.
14 West 44th St., Suite 613
New York NY 10036
TYPES OF ARTICLES: Relationship of theory and research to clinical
practice, research, theoretical
MAJOR CONTENT AREAS: Most areas listed in Appendix A including: all
nursing areas, abuse (child/spouse), adolescence,
children, cultural diversity, death & dying,
growth/development, health promotion, human
behavior & sexuality, parenting, public health
TOPICS PREFERRED: Any topic relating to nursing care of children
and their families
INAPPROPRIATE TOPICS: Articles prior to 1980 were all solicited; unso-
licited manuscripts now accepted
REVIEW PROCEDURE: Editorial board
REVIEW PERIOD: 4-6 weeks
MANUSCRIPT WORD LENGTH: 4500-6000   PAGE CHARGES: No
MANUSCRIPT COPIES: 2   STYLE REQUIREMENTS: APA
PUBLICATION LAG TIME: 6-9 months   STYLE SHEET: Yes
EARLY PUBLICATION OPTION: Possibly   REVISED THESES: No
ACCEPTANCE RATE: 40-50%   STUDENT PAPERS: Yes
AUTHORSHIP RESTRICTIONS: No   REPRINT POLICY: 20 free

SUBSCRIPTION ADDRESS: Hemisphere Publishers, Inc.
14 West 44th St.
New York NY 10036
ANNUAL SUBSCRIPTION RATE: Individuals: $17 Institutions: $34
FREQUENCY: Bimonthly   CIRCULATION: 4500
AFFILIATION: None
INDEXED/ABSTRACTED IN: CINAHL, INI

JOURNAL TITLE: Issues in Health Care of Women

MANUSCRIPT ADDRESS: Carole A. McKenzie, Editor, Graduate
Maternal-Newborn Nursing, Medical Univ. of
South Carolina, Charleston SC 29401
TYPES OF ARTICLES: Articles related to recent developments in Ob-Gyn
nursing, theoretical, research, case studies
MAJOR CONTENT AREAS: Many areas listed in Appendix A including:
nursing: assessment, audit, care, community/public
health, diagnosis, maternal/child, process,
research, theory, office; family planning, human
behavior & sexuality, parenting, quality of life
TOPICS PREFERRED: Women's issues, maternity nursing, women's health
care
INAPPROPRIATE TOPICS: Articles prior to 1980 were all solicited; unso-
licited manuscripts now accepted
REVIEW PROCEDURE: Editorial board
REVIEW PERIOD: 4-6 weeks
MANUSCRIPT WORD LENGTH: 4000-6500   PAGE CHARGES: No
MANUSCRIPT COPIES: 2   STYLE REQUIREMENTS: APA
PUBLICATION LAG TIME: 6-9 months   STYLE SHEET: Yes
EARLY PUBLICATION OPTION: Possibly   REVISED THESES: No
ACCEPTANCE RATE: 40-50%   STUDENT PAPERS: Yes
AUTHORSHIP RESTRICTIONS: No   REPRINT POLICY: 20 free journals

SUBSCRIPTION ADDRESS: Hemisphere Publishers, Inc.
14 West 44th Street, Suite 613
New York NY 10036
ANNUAL SUBSCRIPTION RATE: Individuals: $20 Institutions: $40
FREQUENCY: Bimonthly   CIRCULATION: 2500
AFFILIATION: None
INDEXED/ABSTRACTED IN: Several pending, new journal

JOURNAL TITLE: Issues in Mental Health Nursing

MANUSCRIPT ADDRESS: Barbara Flynn Sideleau
15 Deepdene Road
Trumbull CT 06611

TYPES OF ARTICLES: Research, theoretical

MAJOR CONTENT AREAS: Most areas listed in Appendix A including:
nursing: assessment, audit, care, clinical
specialties, community/public health, diagnosis,
geriatric, neurological, office, philosophy, process, research, theory, psychiatric/mental health

TOPICS PREFERRED: None cited

INAPPROPRIATE TOPICS: Articles prior to 1980 were all solicited; unsolicited manuscripts now accepted

REVIEW PROCEDURE: Editorial board

REVIEW PERIOD: 6-8 weeks

MANUSCRIPT WORD LENGTH: 6000-8000

MANUSCRIPT COPIES: 2

PUBLICATION LAG TIME: 6-12 months

EARLY PUBLICATION OPTION: Possibly

ACCEPTANCE RATE: 30-40%

AUTHORSHIP RESTRICTIONS: No

PAGE CHARGES: No

STYLE REQUIREMENTS: APA

STYLE SHEET: Yes

REVISED THESES: No

STUDENT PAPERS: Yes

REPRINT POLICY: 20 free

SUBSCRIPTION ADDRESS: Hemisphere Publishers, Inc.
15 Deepdene Road
Trumbull CT 06611

ANNUAL SUBSCRIPTION RATE: Individuals: $20   Institutions: $40

FREQUENCY: Quarterly   CIRCULATION: 2500

AFFILIATION: None

INDEXED/ABSTRACTED IN: Several pending, new journal

JOURNAL TITLE: JAMA: Journal of the American Medical Association

MANUSCRIPT ADDRESS: Editor
535 N. Dearborn
Chicago IL 60610

TYPES OF ARTICLES: Research, commentaries, case studies, review, unsolicited book reviews, theoretical

MAJOR CONTENT AREAS: biomedical research, cancer, circulatory & respiratory diseases, emergency services, epidemiology, ethics, genetics, health: policies, promotion, sciences; immunization, medicine, pathology, pharmacology, primary care, public health

TOPICS PREFERRED: As listed under major content areas

INAPPROPRIATE TOPICS: Single case studies on a variety of topics

REVIEW PROCEDURE: Editorial Board, external review, editors
REVIEW PERIOD: 6 weeks
MANUSCRIPT WORD LENGTH: 1500
MANUSCRIPT COPIES: 2
PUBLICATION LAG TIME: 3 months
EARLY PUBLICATION OPTION: Yes
ACCEPTANCE RATE: 30%
AUTHORSHIP RESTRICTIONS: No

PAGE CHARGES: No
STYLE REQUIREMENTS: AMA
STYLE SHEET: Yes
REVISED THESES: No
STUDENT PAPERS: Yes
REPRINT POLICY: None free

SUBSCRIPTION ADDRESS: Circulation Department
535 N. Dearborn
Chicago IL 60610

ANNUAL SUBSCRIPTION RATE: $36
FREQUENCY: Weekly
CIRCULATION: 230,000
AFFILIATION: American Medical Association
INDEXED/ABSTRACTED IN: IM, BA, CA, EM, INI, NAR, PAIS, PA, CINAHL

◆

JOURNAL TITLE: JEN: Journal of Emergency Nursing

MANUSCRIPT ADDRESS: 666 N. Lake Shore Drive
Suite 1729
Chicago IL 60611

TYPES OF ARTICLES: Clinical, research, case studies, unsolicited book reviews, review, theoretical

MAJOR CONTENT AREAS: abuse (child/spouse), accidents, biomedical research, crisis, emergency services, mental health, nursing: assessment, clinical specialties, critical care, neurological, research, mental health, trauma; pharmacology, respiratory diseases, suicide

TOPICS PREFERRED: Emergency nursing, trauma

INAPPROPRIATE TOPICS: None Cited

REVIEW PROCEDURE: Editorial board
REVIEW PERIOD: 3 months
MANUSCRIPT WORD LENGTH: 3000
MANUSCRIPT COPIES: 2
PUBLICATION LAG TIME: 1 year
EARLY PUBLICATION OPTION: Not cited
ACCEPTANCE RATE: 70%
AUTHORSHIP RESTRICTIONS: No

PAGE CHARGES: Not cited
STYLE REQUIREMENTS: AMA
STYLE SHEET: Yes
REVISED THESES: Yes
STUDENT PAPERS: Yes
REPRINT POLICY: 3 free journals

SUBSCRIPTION ADDRESS: 666 N. Lake Shore Drive
Suite 1729
Chicago IL 60611

ANNUAL SUBSCRIPTION RATE: $15
FREQUENCY: Bimonthly
CIRCULATION: 14,000
AFFILIATION: Emergency Department Nurses' Association
INDEXED/ABSTRACTED IN: CINAHL, INI

JOURNAL TITLE: JOGN Nursing: Journal of Obstetric, Gynecologic
and Neonatal Nursing
MANUSCRIPT ADDRESS: Mark Hobbs, Editor
600 Maryland Avenue, Suite 200
Washington DC 20024
TYPES OF ARTICLES: Research, case studies, theoretical, clinical
studies, commentaries, review of literature
MAJOR CONTENT AREAS: Many areas listed in Appendix A including:
nursing: assessment, audit, care, clinical
specialties, diagnosis, maternal/child, office,
philosophy, research, theory; body image, family
planning, human sexuality, midwifery, parenting
TOPICS PREFERRED: Topics related to obstetrical-gynecological
nursing
INAPPROPRIATE TOPICS: None cited

REVIEW PROCEDURE: Editorial board
REVIEW PERIOD: 6 months
MANUSCRIPT WORD LENGTH: Not cited   PAGE CHARGES: No
MANUSCRIPT COPIES: 3   STYLE REQUIREMENTS: AMA
PUBLICATION LAG TIME: 6-12 months   STYLE SHEET: Yes
EARLY PUBLICATION OPTION: No   REVISED THESES: Yes
ACCEPTANCE RATE: 55%   STUDENT PAPERS: No
AUTHORSHIP RESTRICTIONS: No   REPRINT POLICY: 10 free

SUBSCRIPTION ADDRESS: Harper & Row Publishers
2350 Virginia Avenue
Hagerstown MD 21740
ANNUAL SUBSCRIPTION RATE: $17.50
FREQUENCY: Bimonthly   CIRCULATION: 24,000
AFFILIATION: Nurses' Assoc. of Amer. Coll. of Obst. & Gynecol.
INDEXED/ABSTRACTED IN: INI, CINAHL, IM

◆

JOURNAL TITLE: Journal of Advanced Nursing

MANUSCRIPT ADDRESS: 8 John Street
London WC1N 2ES England

TYPES OF ARTICLES: Research, theoretical, philosophical,
commentaries, review, case studies
MAJOR CONTENT AREAS: All nursing areas listed in appendix A, midwifery,
patient teaching, primary care, professionalism

TOPICS PREFERRED: Topics which focus on nursing and emphasize the
dynamics of the role of the nurse
INAPPROPRIATE TOPICS: None cited

REVIEW PROCEDURE: Editorial board and editor
REVIEW PERIOD: 4-6 weeks
MANUSCRIPT WORD LENGTH: 5000   PAGE CHARGES: No
MANUSCRIPT COPIES: 2   STYLE REQUIREMENTS: Own
PUBLICATION LAG TIME: 6 months   STYLE SHEET: Yes
EARLY PUBLICATION OPTION: No   REVISED THESES: Yes
ACCEPTANCE RATE: 45%   STUDENT PAPERS: Yes
AUTHORSHIP RESTRICTIONS: No   REPRINT POLICY: 50 free

SUBSCRIPTION ADDRESS: Blackwell Scientific Publications
P.O. Box 88
Oxford, England
ANNUAL SUBSCRIPTION RATE: $48.50
FREQUENCY: Bimonthly   CIRCULATION: Not cited
AFFILIATION: None
INDEXED/ABSTRACTED IN: INI, IM CINAHL

JOURNAL TITLE: Journal of Affective Disorders

MANUSCRIPT ADDRESS: Elsevier North Holland
52 Vanderbilt Avenue
New York NY 10017
TYPES OF ARTICLES: Research, review, case studies

MAJOR CONTENT AREAS: biology, biomedical research, counseling,
epidemiology, genetics, health sciences, human
behavior, loss/grief, mental health/illness,
pharmacology, psychopathology, research
methodology, sociology, suicide
TOPICS PREFERRED: Articles on depression mania, anxiety states and
schizoaffective disorders
INAPPROPRIATE TOPICS: Theoretical articles

REVIEW PROCEDURE: Editorial board and external review
REVIEW PERIOD: 4-6 weeks
MANUSCRIPT WORD LENGTH: New journal
MANUSCRIPT COPIES: 3
PUBLICATION LAG TIME: 3-4 months
EARLY PUBLICATION OPTION: No
ACCEPTANCE RATE: 80%
AUTHORSHIP RESTRICTIONS: No

PAGE CHARGES: No
STYLE REQUIREMENTS: H
STYLE SHEET: Yes
REVISED THESES: No
STUDENT PAPERS: No
REPRINT POLICY: Not cited

SUBSCRIPTION ADDRESS: Journal Information Center
Elsevier's Science Division
52 Vanderbilt Avenue, New York NY 10017
ANNUAL SUBSCRIPTION RATE: $75.50
FREQUENCY: Quarterly
AFFILIATION: No
INDEXED/ABSTRACTED IN: New journal

CIRCULATION: New journal

◆

JOURNAL TITLE: Journal of Allied Health

MANUSCRIPT ADDRESS: John E. Burke, Editor
School of Allied Medical Professions, Ohio State
University, 1583 Perry St., Columbus OH 43210
TYPES OF ARTICLES: Research, case studies, theoretical, review,
unsolicited book reviews
MAJOR CONTENT AREAS: Many areas listed in Appendix A including: health
sciences & policies, continuing, inservice and
patient education, continuity of care,
professionalism, quality of life, women's issues,
minorities in allied health professions
TOPICS PREFERRED: Articles with an interdisciplinary allied health
focus
INAPPROPRIATE TOPICS: Articles which are discipline specific & do not
have interdisciplinary allied health implications
REVIEW PROCEDURE: Editorial board
REVIEW PERIOD: 6-8 weeks
MANUSCRIPT WORD LENGTH: 2500-3000
MANUSCRIPT COPIES: 3
PUBLICATION LAG TIME: Depends on topic
EARLY PUBLICATION OPTION: Not cited
ACCEPTANCE RATE: 50%
AUTHORSHIP RESTRICTIONS: No

PAGE CHARGES: Yes
STYLE REQUIREMENTS: APA, AMA
STYLE SHEET: Yes
REVISED THESES: May submit
STUDENT PAPERS: May submit
REPRINT POLICY: 6 free

SUBSCRIPTION ADDRESS: American Society of Allied Health Professions
One Dupont Circle, Suite 300
Washington DC 20036
ANNUAL SUBSCRIPTION RATE: Non-members: $45 Members: $35
FREQUENCY: Quarterly
AFFILIATION: American Society of Allied Health Professions
INDEXED/ABSTRACTED IN: CINAHL

CIRCULATION: 2000

104

JOURNAL TITLE: Journal of Ambulatory Care Management

MANUSCRIPT ADDRESS: Aspen Systems Corporation
1600 Research Blvd.
Rockville MD 20850

TYPES OF ARTICLES: Case studies, theoretical, research, review, commentaries, unsolicited book reviews

MAJOR CONTENT AREAS: continuity of care, discharge planning, health promotion, health policies, hospitals, primary care

TOPICS PREFERRED: "How to" articles; improvements of ambulatory care management

INAPPROPRIATE TOPICS: Research papers as opposed to articles

REVIEW PROCEDURE: Editorial board
REVIEW PERIOD: 4-6 weeks

MANUSCRIPT WORD LENGTH: 6000	PAGE CHARGES: Not cited	
MANUSCRIPT COPIES: 3	STYLE REQUIREMENTS: C	
PUBLICATION LAG TIME: 3-7 months	STYLE SHEET: Yes	
EARLY PUBLICATION OPTION: No	REVISED THESES: Yes	
ACCEPTANCE RATE: Not cited	STUDENT PAPERS: No	
AUTHORSHIP RESTRICTIONS: No	REPRINT POLICY: 2 free journals	

SUBSCRIPTION ADDRESS: Subscription Fulfillment
Aspen Systems Corporation
16792 Oakmont Ave., Gaithersburg MD 20877

ANNUAL SUBSCRIPTION RATE: $29.75
FREQUENCY: Quarterly   CIRCULATION: 4000
AFFILIATION: None
INDEXED/ABSTRACTED IN: Not cited

JOURNAL TITLE: Journal of the American Association of Nephrology Nurses and Technicians

MANUSCRIPT ADDRESS: North Woodbury Road, Box 56
Pitmann NJ 08071

TYPES OF ARTICLES: Research, theoretical, review

MAJOR CONTENT AREAS: adaptation, aging & aged, chronicity, human behavior, medical/surgical nursing, nursing assessment, nursing care, nursing process, nursing research, nursing science, patient teaching, primary care, quality of life, teaching/learning

TOPICS PREFERRED: Nephrology nursing

INAPPROPRIATE TOPICS: None cited

REVIEW PROCEDURE: Editorial board
REVIEW PERIOD: 4 months

MANUSCRIPT WORD LENGTH: 3000	PAGE CHARGES: Yes	
MANUSCRIPT COPIES: 4	STYLE REQUIREMENTS: C	
PUBLICATION LAG TIME: 1 year	STYLE SHEET: Yes	
EARLY PUBLICATION OPTION: No	REVISED THESES: No	
ACCEPTANCE RATE: 42%	STUDENT PAPERS: Yes	
AUTHORSHIP RESTRICTIONS: No	REPRINT POLICY: 1 free	

SUBSCRIPTION ADDRESS: AANNT Journal
North Woodbury Road, Box 56
Pitmann NJ 08071

ANNUAL SUBSCRIPTION RATE: $15
FREQUENCY: Quarterly   CIRCULATION: 4000
AFFILIATION: American Assoc. of Nephrology Nurses & Technicians
INDEXED/ABSTRACTED IN: INI, CINAHL

JOURNAL TITLE: Journal of the American College Health Association

MANUSCRIPT ADDRESS: 152 Rollins Drive
Rockville MD 20852

TYPES OF ARTICLES: Research, review, case studies, commentaries, unsolicited book reviews
MAJOR CONTENT AREAS: community/public health nursing, continuing education, dependency, emergency services, family planning, health promotion, human sexuality, immunization, medicine, nursing education, psychiatric/mental health nursing, suicide
TOPICS PREFERRED: Topics relating to health & health services in college and university communities
INAPPROPRIATE TOPICS: None cited

REVIEW PROCEDURE: Editorial board and external review
REVIEW PERIOD: 3-4 months
MANUSCRIPT WORD LENGTH: Not cited	**PAGE CHARGES:** Not cited	
MANUSCRIPT COPIES: 3	**STYLE REQUIREMENTS:** IM, Own	
PUBLICATION LAG TIME: 2-4 months	**STYLE SHEET:** Yes	
EARLY PUBLICATION OPTION: No	**REVISED THESES:** Yes	
ACCEPTANCE RATE: Not cited	**STUDENT PAPERS:** Yes	
AUTHORSHIP RESTRICTIONS: Not cited	**REPRINT POLICY:** Not cited	

SUBSCRIPTION ADDRESS: American College Health Association
152 Rollins Drive
Rockville MD 20852
ANNUAL SUBSCRIPTION RATE: $25.50 (non-members)
FREQUENCY: Bimonthly   **CIRCULATION:** 1700
AFFILIATION: American College Health Association
INDEXED/ABSTRACTED IN: CA, IM, PA, CINAHL, INI

JOURNAL TITLE: Journal of the American Dietetic Association

MANUSCRIPT ADDRESS: 430 N. Michigan Avenue
Chicago IL 60611

TYPES OF ARTICLES: Research, review, commentaries

MAJOR CONTENT AREAS: eating disorders, growth/development, human behavior, nutrition, teaching/learning

TOPICS PREFERRED: None cited

INAPPROPRIATE TOPICS: None cited

REVIEW PROCEDURE: Editorial board
REVIEW PERIOD: Varies
MANUSCRIPT WORD LENGTH: 1800-2000	**PAGE CHARGES:** No	
MANUSCRIPT COPIES: 4	**STYLE REQUIREMENTS:** IM, C	
PUBLICATION LAG TIME: 6-8 months	**STYLE SHEET:** No	
EARLY PUBLICATION OPTION: No	**REVISED THESES:** Yes	
ACCEPTANCE RATE: Not cited	**STUDENT PAPERS:** No	
AUTHORSHIP RESTRICTIONS: No	**REPRINT POLICY:** 25 free	

SUBSCRIPTION ADDRESS: Journal of the American Dietetic Association
430 N. Michigan Avenue
Chicago IL 60611
ANNUAL SUBSCRIPTION RATE: $24
FREQUENCY: Monthly   **CIRCULATION:** 45,000
AFFILIATION: American Dietetic Association
INDEXED/ABSTRACTED IN: CC, IM, BA, BAI, CA, HLI, INI, NAR, PA, CINAHL

JOURNAL TITLE: Journal of the American Geriatrics Society

MANUSCRIPT ADDRESS: Dr. Charles Elyght, Editor
10 Columbus Circle
New York NY 10019
TYPES OF ARTICLES: Research, theoretical, case studies

MAJOR CONTENT AREAS: clinical medicine aspects of: aging & aged,
biology, biomedical research, geriatric nursing,
pharmacology, respiratory diseases, retirement

TOPICS PREFERRED: Clinical medical geriatrics

INAPPROPRIATE TOPICS: None cited

REVIEW PROCEDURE: Editorial board
REVIEW PERIOD: promptly
MANUSCRIPT WORD LENGTH: Not cited
MANUSCRIPT COPIES: 2
PUBLICATION LAG TIME: 6-7 months
EARLY PUBLICATION OPTION: No
ACCEPTANCE RATE: 50%
AUTHORSHIP RESTRICTIONS: No

PAGE CHARGES: No
STYLE REQUIREMENTS: CBE
STYLE SHEET: Yes
REVISED THESES: No
STUDENT PAPERS: No
REPRINT POLICY: None free

SUBSCRIPTION ADDRESS: Journal of the American Geriatrics Society
10 Columbus Circle
New York Ny 10019
ANNUAL SUBSCRIPTION RATE: $25
FREQUENCY: Monthly
CIRCULATION: 10,000
AFFILIATION: American Geriatrics Society
INDEXED/ABSTRACTED IN: BA, CA, HLI, IM, INI, NAR, PA, SSCI, CINAHL

◆

JOURNAL TITLE: Journal of the American Medical Technologists

MANUSCRIPT ADDRESS: 710 Higgins Road
Park Ridge IL 60068

TYPES OF ARTICLES: Research, theoretical, commentaries, features in
allied health areas
MAJOR CONTENT AREAS: allied health personnel, biochemistry,
microbiology, areas related to medical laboratory

TOPICS PREFERRED: Topics related to medical laboratory

INAPPROPRIATE TOPICS: None cited

REVIEW PROCEDURE: Editorial board
REVIEW PERIOD: 2 weeks
MANUSCRIPT WORD LENGTH: 1000-2000
MANUSCRIPT COPIES: 2
PUBLICATION LAG TIME: 3-6 months
EARLY PUBLICATION OPTION: Yes
ACCEPTANCE RATE: 90%
AUTHORSHIP RESTRICTIONS: No

PAGE CHARGES: No
STYLE REQUIREMENTS: CBE
STYLE SHEET: Yes
REVISED THESES: Yes
STUDENT PAPERS: No
REPRINT POLICY: 50 free

SUBSCRIPTION ADDRESS: Journal of the American Medical Technologists
710 Higgins Rd.
Park Ridge IL 60068
ANNUAL SUBSCRIPTION RATE: $7
FREQUENCY: Bimonthly
CIRCULATION: 17,000
AFFILIATION: American Medical Technologists
INDEXED/ABSTRACTED IN: CINAHL

JOURNAL TITLE: Journal of Applied Behavioral Science

MANUSCRIPT ADDRESS: Manuscript Editor
P.O. Box 9155, Rosslyn Station
Arlington VA 22209

TYPES OF ARTICLES: Applied research, theoretical, case studies,
research, review

MAJOR CONTENT AREAS: crisis intervention/theory, growth/development,
health policies, human behavior, psychology,
research methodology, sociology, systems theory,
teaching/learning

TOPICS PREFERRED: Planned change in organizations and small groups

INAPPROPRIATE TOPICS: None cited

REVIEW PROCEDURE: Editorial board and external review
REVIEW PERIOD: 2-10 weeks
MANUSCRIPT WORD LENGTH: 1500-6000   **PAGE CHARGES:** No
MANUSCRIPT COPIES: 4   **STYLE REQUIREMENTS:** APA
PUBLICATION LAG TIME: 12-18 months   **STYLE SHEET:** Yes
EARLY PUBLICATION OPTION: No   **REVISED THESES:** Yes
ACCEPTANCE RATE: 10%   **STUDENT PAPERS:** No
AUTHORSHIP RESTRICTIONS: No   **REPRINT POLICY:** 3 free journals

SUBSCRIPTION ADDRESS: Subscription Administrator
P.O. Box 9155, Rosslyn Station
Arlington VA 22209

ANNUAL SUBSCRIPTION RATE: $23
FREQUENCY: Quarterly   **CIRCULATION:** 5000
AFFILIATION: NTL Institute
INDEXED/ABSTRACTED IN: EAA, SocA, PA, EI, SSCI, SSI

JOURNAL TITLE: Journal of Applied Nutrition

MANUSCRIPT ADDRESS: The Editor
P.O. Box 386
La Habra CA 90631

TYPES OF ARTICLES: Research, review

MAJOR CONTENT AREAS: aging & aged, biochemistry, biomedical research,
continuing education, eating disorders, health
sciences, nutrition, public health, quality of
life

TOPICS PREFERRED: All phases of nutrition

INAPPROPRIATE TOPICS: None cited

REVIEW PROCEDURE: Editorial board
REVIEW PERIOD: 2 months
MANUSCRIPT WORD LENGTH: Varies   **PAGE CHARGES:** No
MANUSCRIPT COPIES: 3   **STYLE REQUIREMENTS:** AMA
PUBLICATION LAG TIME: 6 months   **STYLE SHEET:** Yes
EARLY PUBLICATION OPTION: No   **REVISED THESES:** Yes
ACCEPTANCE RATE: 70%   **STUDENT PAPERS:** Yes
AUTHORSHIP RESTRICTIONS: No   **REPRINT POLICY:** None free

SUBSCRIPTION ADDRESS: I.C.A.N.
Box 386
La Habra CA 90631

ANNUAL SUBSCRIPTION RATE: $10
FREQUENCY: 2 times yearly   **CIRCULATION:** 2500
AFFILIATION: International College of Applied Nutrition
INDEXED/ABSTRACTED IN: NAR, BAI, CA, EM, IM, BA

JOURNAL TITLE: Journal of Audiovisual Media in Medicine

MANUSCRIPT ADDRESS: Department of Medical Illustration
University of Aberdeen Medical Bldg.
Aberdeen AB9 2ZD Scotland

TYPES OF ARTICLES: Research, review

MAJOR CONTENT AREAS: communication, instructional technology, nursing education, teaching/learning

TOPICS PREFERRED: The use of all types of audiovisual media in health science education

INAPPROPRIATE TOPICS: None cited

REVIEW PROCEDURE: Editorial board, external review
REVIEW PERIOD: 2 months
MANUSCRIPT WORD LENGTH: 2000
MANUSCRIPT COPIES: 2
PUBLICATION LAG TIME: 4 months
EARLY PUBLICATION OPTION: No
ACCEPTANCE RATE: 70%
AUTHORSHIP RESTRICTIONS: No
PAGE CHARGES: No
STYLE REQUIREMENTS: Own
STYLE SHEET: Yes
REVISED THESES: No
STUDENT PAPERS: No
REPRINT POLICY: 50 free

SUBSCRIPTION ADDRESS: Update Publications, Ltd.
33/34 Alfred Place
London WC1E 7DP England

ANNUAL SUBSCRIPTION RATE: $27
FREQUENCY: Quarterly
CIRCULATION: 1500
AFFILIATION: Institute of Medical and Biological Illustration
INDEXED/ABSTRACTED IN: CC, BA, CA, IM

◆

JOURNAL TITLE: Journal of the Autonomic Nervous System

MANUSCRIPT ADDRESS: Downstate Medical Center, SUNY
Physiology, Box 31, 450 Clarkson Avenue
Brooklyn New York NY 11203

TYPES OF ARTICLES: Research, review, theoretical, case studies, commentaries, unsolicited book reviews

MAJOR CONTENT AREAS: adaptation, biofeedback, biorhythms, chronicity, circulatory & respiratory diseases, death & dying, fatigue, genetics, human behavior & sexuality, mental health/illness, pain, perception, sensory deprivation, sleep, stress

TOPICS PREFERRED: Autonomic nervous system-structure, function, development, chemistry, pharmacology

INAPPROPRIATE TOPICS: Articles with no relevance to autonomic system

REVIEW PROCEDURE: Editorial board and external review
REVIEW PERIOD: 1-2 months
MANUSCRIPT WORD LENGTH: 2500
MANUSCRIPT COPIES: 3
PUBLICATION LAG TIME: 3-4 months
EARLY PUBLICATION OPTION: Yes
ACCEPTANCE RATE: 60%
AUTHORSHIP RESTRICTIONS: No
PAGE CHARGES: No
STYLE REQUIREMENTS: Own
STYLE SHEET: Yes
REVISED THESES: No
STUDENT PAPERS: No
REPRINT POLICY: 20 free

SUBSCRIPTION ADDRESS: Elsevier/North Holland Biomedical Press
P.O. Box 211
1000 AE Amsterdam The Netherlands

ANNUAL SUBSCRIPTION RATE: $75.50
FREQUENCY: Quarterly
CIRCULATION: Not established
AFFILIATION: None
INDEXED/ABSTRACTED IN: None (new journal)

JOURNAL TITLE: Journal of Behavioral Medicine

MANUSCRIPT ADDRESS: Department of Psychiatry and Behavioral Sciences
University of Texas Medical Branch
Galveston TX 77550
TYPES OF ARTICLES: Research, review, theoretical, case studies

MAJOR CONTENT AREAS: adaptation, aging and aged, alcoholism & drug
abuse, biofeedback, body image, compliance,
death & dying, eating disorders, health promotion,
human behavior & sexuality, loss/grief,
pain, rehabilitation, relaxation, stress
TOPICS PREFERRED: Topics in biomedical and/or behavioral science
field addressing issues of physical health/illness
INAPPROPRIATE TOPICS: None

REVIEW PROCEDURE: Editorial board and external review
REVIEW PERIOD: 1-12 weeks
MANUSCRIPT WORD LENGTH: 5000-6000   PAGE CHARGES: No
MANUSCRIPT COPIES: 3   STYLE REQUIREMENTS: CBE
PUBLICATION LAG TIME: 3 months   STYLE SHEET: No (in journal)
EARLY PUBLICATION OPTION: No   REVISED THESES: Yes
ACCEPTANCE RATE: 20%   STUDENT PAPERS: No
AUTHORSHIP RESTRICTIONS: No   REPRINT POLICY: None free

SUBSCRIPTION ADDRESS: Plenum Publishing Corporation
227 West 17th Street
New York NY 10011
ANNUAL SUBSCRIPTION RATE: Individuals: $18   Institutions: $36
FREQUENCY: Quarterly   CIRCULATION: 1000
AFFILIATION: None
INDEXED/ABSTRACTED IN: PA, IM, SCI, SSCI, BA

◆

JOURNAL TITLE: Journal of Biochemical and Biophysical Methods

MANUSCRIPT ADDRESS: Dr. C.F. Chignell, National Institute of
Environmental Health Sciences, P.O. Box 12233
Research Triangle Park, New York NY 27709
TYPES OF ARTICLES: Research, review

MAJOR CONTENT AREAS: biochemistry, biology, biomedical research,
physics, research methodology

TOPICS PREFERRED: New methodology developed for application to
biochemistry and biophysics
INAPPROPRIATE TOPICS: Papers describing trivial modifications of
methods
REVIEW PROCEDURE: Editorial board and external review
REVIEW PERIOD: 6 weeks
MANUSCRIPT WORD LENGTH: 7000   PAGE CHARGES: No
MANUSCRIPT COPIES: 4   STYLE REQUIREMENTS: Own
PUBLICATION LAG TIME: 4-6 months   STYLE SHEET: Yes
EARLY PUBLICATION OPTION: No   REVISED THESES: No
ACCEPTANCE RATE: 60%   STUDENT PAPERS: No
AUTHORSHIP RESTRICTIONS: No   REPRINT POLICY: 50 free

SUBSCRIPTION ADDRESS: Elsevier/North Holland Biomedical Press
Journal Division
P.O. Box 211, 1000 AE Amsterdam, The Netherlands
ANNUAL SUBSCRIPTION RATE: $78
FREQUENCY: Bimonthly   CIRCULATION: New journal
AFFILIATION: No
INDEXED/ABSTRACTED IN: CC(LS)

JOURNAL TITLE: Journal of Chronic Disease

MANUSCRIPT ADDRESS: Department of Medicine, Northwestern University Medical School, 303 East Chicago Avenue Chicago IL 60611

TYPES OF ARTICLES: Research, review, theoretical, case studies

MAJOR CONTENT AREAS: natural history of: chronic disease, early diagnosis, treatment, impact of chronically ill on the community, long-term medical and nursing care, rehabilitation, and preventive medicine; epidemiological and biostatistical studies

TOPICS PREFERRED: As cited in content areas

INAPPROPRIATE TOPICS: None cited

REVIEW PROCEDURE: Editorial board and external review
REVIEW PERIOD: 3-4 months

MANUSCRIPT WORD LENGTH: 4000	**PAGE CHARGES:** Yes	
MANUSCRIPT COPIES: 2	**STYLE REQUIREMENTS:** IM	
PUBLICATION LAG TIME: 4-6 months	**STYLE SHEET:** No	
EARLY PUBLICATION OPTION: No	**REVISED THESES:** No	
ACCEPTANCE RATE: 35%	**STUDENT PAPERS:** No	
AUTHORSHIP RESTRICTIONS: No	**REPRINT POLICY:** 100 free	

SUBSCRIPTION ADDRESS: Subscription Fulfillment Manager Pergamon Press, Ltd., Headington Hill Hall Oxford OX3 0BW England

ANNUAL SUBSCRIPTION RATE: Individuals: $30   Institutions: $95
FREQUENCY: Monthly   **CIRCULATION:** 3000
AFFILIATION: None
INDEXED/ABSTRACTED IN: CC(LS), BA, EM, CA, HLI, IM, INI, NAR, PA

◆

JOURNAL TITLE: Journal of Clinical Engineering

MANUSCRIPT ADDRESS: Quest Publishing 1351 Titan Way Brea CA 92621

TYPES OF ARTICLES: Practical articles on new medical device developments, review

MAJOR CONTENT AREAS: allied health personnel, biomedical research, continuing education, hospitals, instructional technology, nursing: clinical specialties, critical care, education, neurological; physical therapy, research methodology, testing/measurement

TOPICS PREFERRED: Practical technology, regulation & biomedical technology, biomedical technology development

INAPPROPRIATE TOPICS: Abstract, theory-oriented topics

REVIEW PROCEDURE: External review
REVIEW PERIOD: 2 months

MANUSCRIPT WORD LENGTH: 3000	**PAGE CHARGES:** No	
MANUSCRIPT COPIES: 1	**STYLE REQUIREMENTS:** Own	
PUBLICATION LAG TIME: 4 months	**STYLE SHEET:** Yes	
EARLY PUBLICATION OPTION: No	**REVISED THESES:** Yes	
ACCEPTANCE RATE: Not cited	**STUDENT PAPERS:** No	
AUTHORSHIP RESTRICTIONS: No	**REPRINT POLICY:** 100 free	

SUBSCRIPTION ADDRESS: Quest Publishing 1351 Titan Way Brea CA 92621

ANNUAL SUBSCRIPTION RATE: $30
FREQUENCY: Quarterly   **CIRCULATION:** 4000
AFFILIATION: None
INDEXED/ABSTRACTED IN: BEA, BA, EM

JOURNAL TITLE: Journal of Clinical Psychology

MANUSCRIPT ADDRESS: Vladimir Pishkin
c/o V.A. Hospital
921 N.E. 13th Street, Oklahoma City OK 73104
TYPES OF ARTICLES: Research

MAJOR CONTENT AREAS: alcoholism & drug abuse, body image, eating disorders, epidemiology, human behavior, development, &
sexuality, marriage/divorce, mental health, mental
retardation, pain, parenting, psychology, psychopathology, sensory deprivation, stress, suicide
TOPICS PREFERRED: None cited

INAPPROPRIATE TOPICS: None cited

REVIEW PROCEDURE: Editorial board and external review
REVIEW PERIOD: 4 months
MANUSCRIPT WORD LENGTH: 750-1000   PAGE CHARGES: Yes
MANUSCRIPT COPIES: 3   STYLE REQUIREMENTS: APA
PUBLICATION LAG TIME: 9-12 months   STYLE SHEET: Yes
EARLY PUBLICATION OPTION: No   REVISED THESES: Not cited
ACCEPTANCE RATE: 40%   STUDENT PAPERS: Not cited
AUTHORSHIP RESTRICTIONS: No   REPRINT POLICY: None free

SUBSCRIPTION ADDRESS: Clinical Psychology Publishing Co.
4 Conant Square
Brandon VT 05733
ANNUAL SUBSCRIPTION RATE: Individuals: $20   Institutions: $25
FREQUENCY: Quarterly   CIRCULATION: 2700
AFFILIATION: None
INDEXED/ABSTRACTED IN: PA, BA, CA, HLI, INI, SSCI, IM

◆

JOURNAL TITLE: Journal of Community Health

MANUSCRIPT ADDRESS: Robert Kane, Editor
The Rand Corporation
1700 Main St., Santa Monica CA 90406
TYPES OF ARTICLES: Research, review, theoretical, case studies,
commentaries
MAJOR CONTENT AREAS: aging & aged, communication, compliance, discharge planning, emergency services, epidemiology,
ethics, health promotion & policies, hospitals,
human behavior, nursing audit, pain, public
health, quality of life, research methodology
TOPICS PREFERRED: None cited

INAPPROPRIATE TOPICS: Health education and definition of wellness

REVIEW PROCEDURE: Editorial board and external review
REVIEW PERIOD: 3 months
MANUSCRIPT WORD LENGTH: 2500   PAGE CHARGES: No
MANUSCRIPT COPIES: 3   STYLE REQUIREMENTS: AMA, IM, Own
PUBLICATION LAG TIME: 9 months   STYLE SHEET: Yes
EARLY PUBLICATION OPTION: No   REVISED THESES: Yes
ACCEPTANCE RATE: 25%   STUDENT PAPERS: Yes
AUTHORSHIP RESTRICTIONS: No   REPRINT POLICY: None free

SUBSCRIPTION ADDRESS: Human Sciences Press
72 5th Avenue
New York NY 10011
ANNUAL SUBSCRIPTION RATE: Individuals: $25   Institutions: $40
FREQUENCY: Quarterly   CIRCULATION: 1400
AFFILIATION: Association of Teachers of Preventive Medicine
INDEXED/ABSTRACTED IN: IM, CINAHL

JOURNAL TITLE: Journal of Continuing Education in Cardiology

MANUSCRIPT ADDRESS: Editorial Offices, Medical Digest, Inc.
445 Central
Northfield IL 60093
TYPES OF ARTICLES: Review

MAJOR CONTENT AREAS: Most age groups, major disease categories, &
behavioral concepts; abuse (child/spouse/alcohol-
ism/drug), accidents, death & dying, family
planning, genetics, growth/development, human
behavior & sexuality, nutrition, patient teaching
TOPICS PREFERRED: Diagnosis, treatment of diseases of interest to
specialty physicians
INAPPROPRIATE TOPICS: Case reports, anecdotal material

REVIEW PROCEDURE: Editorial board and external review		
REVIEW PERIOD: 2 weeks		
MANUSCRIPT WORD LENGTH: 5000-6000	**PAGE CHARGES:** No	
MANUSCRIPT COPIES: 1	**STYLE REQUIREMENTS:** AMA, IM	
PUBLICATION LAG TIME: 6 months	**STYLE SHEET:** Yes	
EARLY PUBLICATION OPTION: No	**REVISED THESES:** No	
ACCEPTANCE RATE: Not cited	**STUDENT PAPERS:** No	
AUTHORSHIP RESTRICTIONS: Generally M.D.'s	**REPRINT POLICY:** 100 free	

SUBSCRIPTION ADDRESS: Medical Digest Inc., Subscriptions
445 Central
Northfield IL 60093
ANNUAL SUBSCRIPTION RATE: $27.50
FREQUENCY: Monthly   **CIRCULATION:** Not cited
AFFILIATION: None
INDEXED/ABSTRACTED IN: None

JOURNAL TITLE: The Journal of Continuing Education in Nursing

MANUSCRIPT ADDRESS: Charles B. Slack, Inc.
6900 Grove Road
Thorofare NJ 08086
TYPES OF ARTICLES: Research, theoretical, case studies,
unsolicited book reviews
MAJOR CONTENT AREAS: continuing education, inservice education,
nursing education, teaching/learning,
testing/measurement

TOPICS PREFERRED: Continuing education

INAPPROPRIATE TOPICS: None cited

REVIEW PROCEDURE: Editorial board		
REVIEW PERIOD: 1-3 months		
MANUSCRIPT WORD LENGTH: Varies	**PAGE CHARGES:** No	
MANUSCRIPT COPIES: 2	**STYLE REQUIREMENTS:** AMA	
PUBLICATION LAG TIME: 6 months	**STYLE SHEET:** Yes	
EARLY PUBLICATION OPTION: Yes	**REVISED THESES:** Yes	
ACCEPTANCE RATE: 60%	**STUDENT PAPERS:** No	
AUTHORSHIP RESTRICTIONS: No	**REPRINT POLICY:** 5 free journals	

SUBSCRIPTION ADDRESS: Charles B. Slack, Inc.
6900 Grove Road
Thorofare NJ 08086
ANNUAL SUBSCRIPTION RATE: $22
FREQUENCY: Bimonthly   **CIRCULATION:** 4000
AFFILIATION: None
INDEXED/ABSTRACTED IN: CINAHL, INI

JOURNAL TITLE: Journal of Dialysis

MANUSCRIPT ADDRESS: Rogosin Kidney Center, Room D208
525 E. 68th Street
New York NY 10021
TYPES OF ARTICLES: Research, theoretical, review, commentaries, case studies
MAJOR CONTENT AREAS: biomedical research, medicine

TOPICS PREFERRED: Articles dealing with hemodialysis, peritoneal dialysis and dialysis technology
INAPPROPRIATE TOPICS: None cited

REVIEW PROCEDURE: Editorial board
REVIEW PERIOD: 1-2 months
MANUSCRIPT WORD LENGTH: 3700
MANUSCRIPT COPIES: 1
PUBLICATION LAG TIME: 4 months
EARLY PUBLICATION OPTION: No
ACCEPTANCE RATE: 75-80%
AUTHORSHIP RESTRICTIONS: No

PAGE CHARGES: No
STYLE REQUIREMENTS: CBE
STYLE SHEET: Yes
REVISED THESES: No
STUDENT PAPERS: No
REPRINT POLICY: Not cited

SUBSCRIPTION ADDRESS: Marcel Dekker Journals
P.O. Box 11305, Church Street Station
New York NY 10249
ANNUAL SUBSCRIPTION RATE: Individuals: $30   Institutions: $60
FREQUENCY: Quarterly   CIRCULATION: Not cited
AFFILIATION: None
INDEXED/ABSTRACTED IN: BA, EM, IM, SCI, CC(CP), CINAHL, INI

◆

JOURNAL TITLE: Journal of Enterostomal Therapy

MANUSCRIPT ADDRESS: Editor
2506 Gross Point Rd.
Evanston IL 60201
TYPES OF ARTICLES: Case studies, research, theoretical, review, commentaries, unsolicited book reviews
MAJOR CONTENT AREAS: body image, cancer, clinical nurse specialties, counseling, loss/grief, nursing research, nutrition, rehabilitation

TOPICS PREFERRED: Care of persons with ostomies, and draining wounds
INAPPROPRIATE TOPICS: None cited

REVIEW PROCEDURE: Editorial board
REVIEW PERIOD: 2-3 months
MANUSCRIPT WORD LENGTH: 1000-2000
MANUSCRIPT COPIES: 2
PUBLICATION LAG TIME: 2-6 months
EARLY PUBLICATION OPTION: No
ACCEPTANCE RATE: 80%
AUTHORSHIP RESTRICTIONS: No

PAGE CHARGES: No
STYLE REQUIREMENTS: C
STYLE SHEET: Yes
REVISED THESES: Yes
STUDENT PAPERS: Yes
REPRINT POLICY: 2 free

SUBSCRIPTION ADDRESS: ET Journal
2506 Gross Point Road
Evanston IL 60201
ANNUAL SUBSCRIPTION RATE: $20
FREQUENCY: Bimonthly   CIRCULATION: 1750
AFFILIATION: International Association for Enterostomal Therapy
INDEXED/ABSTRACTED IN: CINAHL

JOURNAL TITLE: Journal of Epidemiology & Community Health

MANUSCRIPT ADDRESS: Welsh National School of Medicine
Department of Medical Statistics
Heath Park, Cardiff CF4 4XN
TYPES OF ARTICLES: Research

MAJOR CONTENT AREAS: distribution and behavior of disease in human
populations, effects of environment or social
conditions on disease evolution, health
assessment, epidemiology, community/public health

TOPICS PREFERRED: Problems of public health & their solution

INAPPROPRIATE TOPICS: None cited

REVIEW PROCEDURE: Editorial board
REVIEW PERIOD: Not cited
MANUSCRIPT WORD LENGTH: Not cited   **PAGE CHARGES:** Not cited
MANUSCRIPT COPIES: Not cited   **STYLE REQUIREMENTS:** Own, IM
PUBLICATION LAG TIME: Not cited   **STYLE SHEET:** Not cited
EARLY PUBLICATION OPTION: Not cited   **REVISED THESES:** Not cited
ACCEPTANCE RATE: Not cited   **STUDENT PAPERS:** Not cited
AUTHORSHIP RESTRICTIONS: Not cited   **REPRINT POLICY:** 25 free

SUBSCRIPTION ADDRESS: British Medical Journal
1172 Commonwealth Avenue
Boston MA 02134
ANNUAL SUBSCRIPTION RATE: $42
FREQUENCY: Not cited   **CIRCULATION:** Not cited
AFFILIATION: Not cited
INDEXED/ABSTRACTED IN: CINAHL

JOURNAL TITLE: Journal of Geriatric Psychiatry

MANUSCRIPT ADDRESS: The Editors
9 Elba Street
Brookline MA 02146
TYPES OF ARTICLES: Case studies, research, theoretical, review,
unsolicited book reviews, commentaries
MAJOR CONTENT AREAS: aging & aged, chronicity, counseling, crisis,
death, human behavior, life span, loss/grief,
nursing: care, education, geriatric, psychiatric;
pathology, pharmacology, psychology, psychopathology, retirement, sleep, substance abuse, suicide
TOPICS PREFERRED: Normal & pathological aging, geriatric & mental
health issues in nursing, nursing homes
INAPPROPRIATE TOPICS: None cited

REVIEW PROCEDURE: Editorial board
REVIEW PERIOD: 1-3 months
MANUSCRIPT WORD LENGTH: 4500   **PAGE CHARGES:** No
MANUSCRIPT COPIES: 4   **STYLE REQUIREMENTS:** Own, APA
PUBLICATION LAG TIME: 6-12 months   **STYLE SHEET:** Yes
EARLY PUBLICATION OPTION: No   **REVISED THESES:** Yes
ACCEPTANCE RATE: 33%   **STUDENT PAPERS:** No
AUTHORSHIP RESTRICTIONS: No   **REPRINT POLICY:** None free

SUBSCRIPTION ADDRESS: International Universities Press, Inc.
315 Fifth Avenue
New York NY 10016
ANNUAL SUBSCRIPTION RATE: Individuals: $20.00 Institutions: $32.50
FREQUENCY: Semi-annually   **CIRCULATION:** 900
AFFILIATION: Boston Society for Gerontologic Psychiatry
INDEXED/ABSTRACTED IN: IM, PA, SSCI, INI

JOURNAL TITLE: Journal of Gerontological Nursing

MANUSCRIPT ADDRESS: Charles B. Slack
6900 Grove Road
Thorofare NJ 08086
TYPES OF ARTICLES: Research, theoretical, review, case studies

MAJOR CONTENT AREAS: aging & aged, death & dying, geriatric nursing, loss/grief, nursing care, nursing homes, retirement

TOPICS PREFERRED: Any age-related nursing article

INAPPROPRIATE TOPICS: None cited

REVIEW PROCEDURE: Editorial board
REVIEW PERIOD: 1-3 months
MANUSCRIPT WORD LENGTH: Varies   PAGE CHARGES: No
MANUSCRIPT COPIES: 2   STYLE REQUIREMENTS: AMA
PUBLICATION LAG TIME: 6-8 months   STYLE SHEET: Yes
EARLY PUBLICATION OPTION: Yes   REVISED THESES: Yes
ACCEPTANCE RATE: 50%   STUDENT PAPERS: No
AUTHORSHIP RESTRICTIONS: No   REPRINT POLICY: 2 free journals

SUBSCRIPTION ADDRESS: Charles B. Slack
6900 Grove Road
Thorofare NJ 08086
ANNUAL SUBSCRIPTION RATE: $20
FREQUENCY: Bimonthly   CIRCULATION: 8000
AFFILIATION: None
INDEXED/ABSTRACTED IN: CINAHL, INI

JOURNAL TITLE: Journal of Gerontology

MANUSCRIPT ADDRESS: Martha Storandt, Ph.D.
Department of Psychology, Box 1125
Washington University, St. Louis MO 63130
TYPES OF ARTICLES: Research, theoretical, review

MAJOR CONTENT AREAS: adaptation, biofeedback, biomedical research, body image, communication, crisis, death & dying, geriatric nursing, loss/grief, nursing research, public health, quality of life, retirement, sleep, stress, suicide; areas of gerontology, geriatrics
TOPICS PREFERRED: Research in aging, experimentation in biology, clinical medicine, psychological & social sciences
INAPPROPRIATE TOPICS: Case studies, anecdotes, non-research

REVIEW PROCEDURE: External review
REVIEW PERIOD: 3 weeks-2 months
MANUSCRIPT WORD LENGTH: 5000   PAGE CHARGES: No
MANUSCRIPT COPIES: 4   STYLE REQUIREMENTS: APA, CBE
PUBLICATION LAG TIME: 6-9 months   STYLE SHEET: Yes
EARLY PUBLICATION OPTION: Yes   REVISED THESES: Yes
ACCEPTANCE RATE: 25%   STUDENT PAPERS: No
AUTHORSHIP RESTRICTIONS: No   REPRINT POLICY: None free

SUBSCRIPTION ADDRESS: Gerontological Society
1835 K St., N.W.
Washington DC 20006
ANNUAL SUBSCRIPTION RATE: $35
FREQUENCY: Bimonthly   CIRCULATION: 7000
AFFILIATION: Gerontology Society
INDEXED/ABSTRACTED IN: EM, IM, BA, CA, HLI, NAR, PAIS, PA, SSCI, SSI

JOURNAL TITLE: Journal of Health & Human Resources Administration

MANUSCRIPT ADDRESS: Jack Rabin, Editor
Graduate Program for Administrators, Rider College
P.O. Box 6400, Lawrenceville NJ 08648

TYPES OF ARTICLES: Research, theoretical, review, case studies, commentaries, unsolicited book reviews

MAJOR CONTENT AREAS: continuity of care, ethics, health promotion, sciences, policies; nursing: assessment, audit, care, community/public health, education, history, homes, philosophy, process, service administration; public health, women's issues

TOPICS PREFERRED: Administrative issues

INAPPROPRIATE TOPICS: Scientific studies

REVIEW PROCEDURE: Editorial board
REVIEW PERIOD: 2 months
MANUSCRIPT WORD LENGTH: 6000
MANUSCRIPT COPIES: 3
PUBLICATION LAG TIME: 3-6 months
EARLY PUBLICATION OPTION: No
ACCEPTANCE RATE: 30%
AUTHORSHIP RESTRICTIONS: No

PAGE CHARGES: No
STYLE REQUIREMENTS: Own
STYLE SHEET: Yes
REVISED THESES: Yes
STUDENT PAPERS: Yes
REPRINT POLICY: 2 free journals

SUBSCRIPTION ADDRESS: Southern Public Administration Education Foundation, P.O. Box 4434
Montgomery AL 36101
ANNUAL SUBSCRIPTION RATE: $21
FREQUENCY: Quarterly
AFFILIATION: None
INDEXED/ABSTRACTED IN: Not cited

CIRCULATION: 1000

◆

JOURNAL TITLE: Journal of Health, Politics, Policy and the Law

MANUSCRIPT ADDRESS: Professor T.R. Marmor, Editor
JHPPL, Box 15-A, Yale Station
New Haven CT 06520

TYPES OF ARTICLES: Research, theoretical, review, case studies, commentaries

MAJOR CONTENT AREAS: community/public health nursing, ethics, health policies, hospitals, leadership, mental health/illness, nursing philosophy, nursing research, nursing service administration, professionalism, public health, women's issues

TOPICS PREFERRED: Health and mental health policy

INAPPROPRIATE TOPICS: Not applicable

REVIEW PROCEDURE: Editorial board, external review
REVIEW PERIOD: 6-8 weeks
MANUSCRIPT WORD LENGTH: 4000-5000
MANUSCRIPT COPIES: 3
PUBLICATION LAG TIME: 6-9 months
EARLY PUBLICATION OPTION: Yes
ACCEPTANCE RATE: 25-30%
AUTHORSHIP RESTRICTIONS: No

PAGE CHARGES: No
STYLE REQUIREMENTS: C, T
STYLE SHEET: Yes
REVISED THESES: No
STUDENT PAPERS: No
REPRINT POLICY: Author purchase

SUBSCRIPTION ADDRESS: Journal of Health, Politics, Policy and the Law
P.O. Box 2421
Durham NC 27705
ANNUAL SUBSCRIPTION RATE: Individuals: $32   Institutions: $48
FREQUENCY: Quarterly
AFFILIATION: None
INDEXED/ABSTRACTED IN: CINAHL, INI

CIRCULATION: 2000

JOURNAL TITLE: Journal of Health and Social Behavior

MANUSCRIPT ADDRESS: Leonard I. Pearlin, Ph.D., Editor
Human Development & Aging Program, Univ. of Calif.
745 Parnassus Ave., San Francisco CA 94143

TYPES OF ARTICLES: Research, theoretical, review

MAJOR CONTENT AREAS: sociology

TOPICS PREFERRED: None cited

INAPPROPRIATE TOPICS: None cited

REVIEW PROCEDURE: Editorial board and external review
REVIEW PERIOD: 8-9 weeks

MANUSCRIPT WORD LENGTH:	Not cited	PAGE CHARGES:	Yes
MANUSCRIPT COPIES:	4	STYLE REQUIREMENTS:	APA
PUBLICATION LAG TIME:	Not cited	STYLE SHEET:	Yes
EARLY PUBLICATION OPTION:	No	REVISED THESES:	Not cited
ACCEPTANCE RATE:	Not cited	STUDENT PAPERS:	Not cited
AUTHORSHIP RESTRICTIONS:	No	REPRINT POLICY:	Author purchase

SUBSCRIPTION ADDRESS: American Sociological Association
1722 N St., N.W.
Washington DC 20036

ANNUAL SUBSCRIPTION RATE: Individuals: $14 Institutions: $19
FREQUENCY: Quarterly   CIRCULATION: 5000
AFFILIATION: American Sociological Association
INDEXED/ABSTRACTED IN: BA, HLI, INI, PA, SSCI, SSI, CINAHL

◆

JOURNAL TITLE: Journal of the History of Medicine & Allied
Sciences

MANUSCRIPT ADDRESS: Dr. Leonard Wilson, Editor
510 Diehl Hall, University of Minnesota
Minneapolis MN 55455

TYPES OF ARTICLES: Research

MAJOR CONTENT AREAS: history of medicine and biological sciences

TOPICS PREFERRED: History of medicine and related subjects

INAPPROPRIATE TOPICS: None cited

REVIEW PROCEDURE: Editorial board and external review
REVIEW PERIOD: 3 months

MANUSCRIPT WORD LENGTH:	6000-8000	PAGE CHARGES:	No
MANUSCRIPT COPIES:	2	STYLE REQUIREMENTS:	Own
PUBLICATION LAG TIME:	6 months	STYLE SHEET:	Yes
EARLY PUBLICATION OPTION:	No	REVISED THESES:	No
ACCEPTANCE RATE:	25%	STUDENT PAPERS:	No
AUTHORSHIP RESTRICTIONS:	No	REPRINT POLICY:	None free

SUBSCRIPTION ADDRESS: Journal of the History of Medicine
333 Cedar Street
New Haven CT 06510

ANNUAL SUBSCRIPTION RATE: Individuals: $25 Institutions: $35
FREQUENCY: Quarterly   CIRCULATION: 900
AFFILIATION: None
INDEXED/ABSTRACTED IN: SCI, CC, CWHM, BA, CA, IM, CINAHL

JOURNAL TITLE: Journal of Histotechnology

MANUSCRIPT ADDRESS: Sarah L. Lindmark, Managing Editor
Mayo Publications, P.O. Box 247
Downer's Grove   IL   60515
TYPES OF ARTICLES: Research, theoretical, review, commentaries,
unsolicited book reviews, case studies
MAJOR CONTENT AREAS: biomedical research, communication, health:
promotion, sciences, policies; medicine, nursing:
education, research, science, service administration, clinical nurse specialties, community/public
health; teaching/learning
TOPICS PREFERRED: Histology, histochemistry, pathology, toxicology,
biology, physiology, management, administration
INAPPROPRIATE TOPICS: None cited

REVIEW PROCEDURE: Editorial board
REVIEW PERIOD: 5-6 weeks
MANUSCRIPT WORD LENGTH: 500-1000   PAGE CHARGES: Yes
MANUSCRIPT COPIES: 3   STYLE REQUIREMENTS: CBE, IM
PUBLICATION LAG TIME: 3 months   STYLE SHEET: Yes
EARLY PUBLICATION OPTION: Yes   REVISED THESES: Yes
ACCEPTANCE RATE: 80%   STUDENT PAPERS: Yes
AUTHORSHIP RESTRICTIONS: No   REPRINT POLICY: 3 free journals

SUBSCRIPTION ADDRESS: National Society for Histotechnology
P.O. Box 36
Lanham   MD   20706
ANNUAL SUBSCRIPTION RATE: $12 (free to members)
FREQUENCY: Quarterly   CIRCULATION: 3500
AFFILIATION: National Society for Histotechnology
INDEXED/ABSTRACTED IN: EM, BA

◆

JOURNAL TITLE: Journal of Human Nutrition

MANUSCRIPT ADDRESS: John Libbey & Company Ltd.
80-84 Bondway
London SW8 1SF   England
TYPES OF ARTICLES: Research, theoretical, review, commentaries, case
studies, unsolicited book reviews
MAJOR CONTENT AREAS: eating disorders, nutrition

TOPICS PREFERRED: None cited

INAPPROPRIATE TOPICS: None cited

REVIEW PROCEDURE: Editorial board and external review
REVIEW PERIOD: 6-8 weeks
MANUSCRIPT WORD LENGTH: 3500   PAGE CHARGES: No
MANUSCRIPT COPIES: 2   STYLE REQUIREMENTS: IM, Own
PUBLICATION LAG TIME: 4 months   STYLE SHEET: Yes
EARLY PUBLICATION OPTION: No   REVISED THESES: No
ACCEPTANCE RATE: Not cited   STUDENT PAPERS: No
AUTHORSHIP RESTRICTIONS: No   REPRINT POLICY: None free

SUBSCRIPTION ADDRESS: John Libbey & Company Ltd.
80-84 Bondway
London SW8 1SF   England
ANNUAL SUBSCRIPTION RATE: Individuals: $30   Institutions: $53
FREQUENCY: Bimonthly   CIRCULATION: 3000
AFFILIATION: British Dietetic Association
INDEXED/ABSTRACTED IN: CC(CP), IM

JOURNAL TITLE: Journal of Human Stress

MANUSCRIPT ADDRESS: Opinion Publications, Inc.
R.R. 1, Box 396
Shelburne Falls MA 01370

TYPES OF ARTICLES: Research, case studies, review

MAJOR CONTENT AREAS: physical disorders, environmental stress, emotional stress

TOPICS PREFERRED: Effects of environmental and emotional stress on the development & course of physical disorders

INAPPROPRIATE TOPICS: None cited

REVIEW PROCEDURE: Editorial board
REVIEW PERIOD: 2 months
MANUSCRIPT WORD LENGTH: 3500
MANUSCRIPT COPIES: 3
PUBLICATION LAG TIME: Not cited
EARLY PUBLICATION OPTION: Not cited
ACCEPTANCE RATE: Not cited
AUTHORSHIP RESTRICTIONS: No

PAGE CHARGES: Not cited
STYLE REQUIREMENTS: Own
STYLE SHEET: Yes
REVISED THESES: No
STUDENT PAPERS: No
REPRINT POLICY: 10 free journals

SUBSCRIPTION ADDRESS: Opinion Publications, Inc.
R.R. 1, Box 396
Shelburne Falls MA 01370

ANNUAL SUBSCRIPTION RATE: Individuals: $33 Institutions: $43
FREQUENCY: Quarterly **CIRCULATION:** 31,500
AFFILIATION: None
INDEXED/ABSTRACTED IN: BA, CC, EM, IM, PA, SSCI, CINAHL

◆

JOURNAL TITLE: Journal of Laboratory and Clinical Medicine

MANUSCRIPT ADDRESS: Charles E. Mengel, M.D., Editor
Department of Medicine, N-424, Univ. of Missouri
Health Sciences Center, Columbia MO 65212

TYPES OF ARTICLES: Research

MAJOR CONTENT AREAS: medicine

TOPICS PREFERRED: None cited

INAPPROPRIATE TOPICS: None cited

REVIEW PROCEDURE: Editorial board, external review
REVIEW PERIOD: 2-3 months
MANUSCRIPT WORD LENGTH: 2500-3000
MANUSCRIPT COPIES: 3
PUBLICATION LAG TIME: 3-4 months
EARLY PUBLICATION OPTION: No
ACCEPTANCE RATE: 37%
AUTHORSHIP RESTRICTIONS: No

PAGE CHARGES: Yes
STYLE REQUIREMENTS: CBE, IM
STYLE SHEET: Yes
REVISED THESES: No
STUDENT PAPERS: No
REPRINT POLICY: None free

SUBSCRIPTION ADDRESS: The C.V. Mosby Company, Circulation Department
11830 Westline Industrial Drive
St. Louis MO 63141

ANNUAL SUBSCRIPTION RATE: Individuals: $41 Institutions: $62
FREQUENCY: Monthly **CIRCULATION:** 6400
AFFILIATION: Central Society for Clinical Research
INDEXED/ABSTRACTED IN: IM, CC, CINAHL, BA, CA, NAR

JOURNAL TITLE: The Journal of Long-Term Care Administration

MANUSCRIPT ADDRESS: Assistant Managing Editor
Bethesda   MD   20814

TYPES OF ARTICLES: Research, commentaries, case studies, theoretical, review, unsolicited book reviews
MAJOR CONTENT AREAS: communication, crisis, education, ethics, growth/development, health promotion & policies, leadership, nursing: education, geriatric, history, psychiatric; nursing homes, nutrition, physical therapy, public health, rehabilitation
TOPICS PREFERRED: Articles on innovations in the long-term care health field, administrative aspects
INAPPROPRIATE TOPICS: Speeches, long and very technical student papers

REVIEW PROCEDURE: Editorial board
REVIEW PERIOD: 2-3 months
MANUSCRIPT WORD LENGTH: 3000
MANUSCRIPT COPIES: 3
PUBLICATION LAG TIME: 3-12 months
EARLY PUBLICATION OPTION: Not cited
ACCEPTANCE RATE: 90%
AUTHORSHIP RESTRICTIONS: No

PAGE CHARGES: No
STYLE REQUIREMENTS: C
STYLE SHEET: Yes
REVISED THESES: No
STUDENT PAPERS: No
REPRINT POLICY: 2 free journals

SUBSCRIPTION ADDRESS: Journal Subscription Department
American College of Nursing Home Administrators
4650 East-West Highway, Washington   DC   20014
ANNUAL SUBSCRIPTION RATE: $30
FREQUENCY: Quarterly
CIRCULATION: 6600
AFFILIATION: American College of Nursing Home Administrators
INDEXED/ABSTRACTED IN: HLI, AHM, CINAHL, IPA, MCR

◆

JOURNAL TITLE: Journal of Marriage and the Family

MANUSCRIPT ADDRESS: Felix M. Berardo, Editor
Department of Sociology, University of Florida
Gainesville   FL   32611
TYPES OF ARTICLES: Research, theoretical

MAJOR CONTENT AREAS: abuse, communication, crisis, death, & dying, family planning, groups, human behavior & sexuality, life span, loss/grief, marriage & divorce, parenting, psychology, quality of life, research methodology, retirement, sociology, women's issues
TOPICS PREFERRED: Research or theory in which marital or family variables are central focus
INAPPROPRIATE TOPICS: Deviance (e.g. drug abuse, crime), fertility/population dynamics
REVIEW PROCEDURE: Editorial board
REVIEW PERIOD: 2-3 months
MANUSCRIPT WORD LENGTH: 5000
MANUSCRIPT COPIES: 3
PUBLICATION LAG TIME: 3-6 months
EARLY PUBLICATION OPTION: No
ACCEPTANCE RATE: 13-17%
AUTHORSHIP RESTRICTIONS: No

PAGE CHARGES: Yes
STYLE REQUIREMENTS: APA
STYLE SHEET: Yes
REVISED THESES: Yes
STUDENT PAPERS: No
REPRINT POLICY: None free

SUBSCRIPTION ADDRESS: National Council on Family Relations
1219 University Avenue Southeast
Minneapolis   MN   55414
ANNUAL SUBSCRIPTION RATE: Individuals: $20   Institutions: $30
FREQUENCY: Quarterly   **CIRCULATION:** 11,000
AFFILIATION: National Council on Family Relations
INDEXED/ABSTRACTED IN: SSI, CC, SWRA, BRI, ECER, PA, SSCI, PCCA, SocA

JOURNAL TITLE: Journal of Maternal and Child Health

MANUSCRIPT ADDRESS: Barker Publications, Ltd.
Church View, Lancaster Park
Richmond Surrey TW10 6A G England
TYPES OF ARTICLES: Theoretical, research, commentaries, case studies

MAJOR CONTENT AREAS: abuse (child/spouse), adolescence, children,
family planning, handicapping conditions, human
sexuality, marriage & divorce, midwifery, nursing:
public health, maternal/child, occupational,
pediatric; parenting, primary care, women's issues
TOPICS PREFERRED: None cited

INAPPROPRIATE TOPICS: None cited

REVIEW PROCEDURE: Editorial board
REVIEW PERIOD: Not cited
MANUSCRIPT WORD LENGTH: 1700   PAGE CHARGES: Not cited
MANUSCRIPT COPIES: 2   STYLE REQUIREMENTS: Own
PUBLICATION LAG TIME: 4-6 months   STYLE SHEET: Yes
EARLY PUBLICATION OPTION: No   REVISED THESES: No
ACCEPTANCE RATE: 90%   STUDENT PAPERS: No
AUTHORSHIP RESTRICTIONS: No   REPRINT POLICY: 10 free journals

SUBSCRIPTION ADDRESS: Barker Publications, Ltd.
Church View, Lancaster Park
Richmond Surrey TW10 6A G England
ANNUAL SUBSCRIPTION RATE: $44
FREQUENCY: Monthly   CIRCULATION: 22,500
AFFILIATION: None
INDEXED/ABSTRACTED IN: Not cited

◆

JOURNAL TITLE: Journal of Medical Ethics

MANUSCRIPT ADDRESS: Tavistock House North
Tavistock Square
London WC1H 9LG England
TYPES OF ARTICLES: Research, case studies, theoretical

MAJOR CONTENT AREAS: abuse (child/spouse), aging and aged, alcoholism &
drug abuse, cancer, compliance, death & dying,
dependency, ethics, health promotion, human
sexuality, loss/grief, nursing philosophy, pain,
professionalism
TOPICS PREFERRED: Ethics

INAPPROPRIATE TOPICS: None cited

REVIEW PROCEDURE: External review
REVIEW PERIOD: 3 Months
MANUSCRIPT WORD LENGTH: 3000-5000   PAGE CHARGES: No
MANUSCRIPT COPIES: 2   STYLE REQUIREMENTS: Own
PUBLICATION LAG TIME: 3 Months   STYLE SHEET: Yes
EARLY PUBLICATION OPTION: No   REVISED THESES: No
ACCEPTANCE RATE: 30%   STUDENT PAPERS: No
AUTHORSHIP RESTRICTIONS: No   REPRINT POLICY: 4 free journals

SUBSCRIPTION ADDRESS: Professional & Scientific Publications
1172 Commonwealth Avenue
Boston MA 02134
ANNUAL SUBSCRIPTION RATE: $40
FREQUENCY: Quarterly   CIRCULATION: 1000
AFFILIATION: Society for Study of Medical Ethics
INDEXED/ABSTRACTED IN: IM

JOURNAL TITLE: Journal of Medicine & Philosophy

MANUSCRIPT ADDRESS: Dr. H. Tristram Engelhardt, Jr., Associate Editor
The Kennedy Institute of Ethics
Georgetown University, Washington DC 20057
TYPES OF ARTICLES: Research, theoretical

MAJOR CONTENT AREAS: ethics, health promotion, health sciences
medicine, quality of life

TOPICS PREFERRED: Philosophical dimensions of medical research and
practice
INAPPROPRIATE TOPICS: None cited

REVIEW PROCEDURE: Editorial board		
REVIEW PERIOD: Not cited		
MANUSCRIPT WORD LENGTH: 5000-10,000	**PAGE CHARGES:** No	
MANUSCRIPT COPIES: 1	**STYLE REQUIREMENTS:** C, Own	
PUBLICATION LAG TIME: Not cited	**STYLE SHEET:** Yes	
EARLY PUBLICATION OPTION: No	**REVISED THESES:** No	
ACCEPTANCE RATE: Not cited	**STUDENT PAPERS:** No	
AUTHORSHIP RESTRICTIONS: No	**REPRINT POLICY:** 25 free	

SUBSCRIPTION ADDRESS: D. Reidel Publishing Company
P.O. Box 17, 3300AA
Dordecht, Holland
ANNUAL SUBSCRIPTION RATE: Individuals: $18   Institutions: $30
FREQUENCY: Quarterly   **CIRCULATION:** New journal
AFFILIATION: Society for Health & Human Values
INDEXED/ABSTRACTED IN: New journal

◆

JOURNAL TITLE: Journal of the National Cancer Institute

MANUSCRIPT ADDRESS: Blair Building, Room 2A01
8300 Colesville Road
Silver Spring MD 20910
TYPES OF ARTICLES: Research, theoretical, review, case studies,
letters to the editor, guest editorials
MAJOR CONTENT AREAS: biochemistry, biology, biomedical research,
epidemiology, genetics, microbiology, pathology,
research methodology; all as related to cancer
research

TOPICS PREFERRED: Cancer: cause, treatment, prevention,
carcinogenesis
INAPPROPRIATE TOPICS: None cited

REVIEW PROCEDURE: 3 external reviewers and editorial board		
REVIEW PERIOD: 1 1/2-2 months		
MANUSCRIPT WORD LENGTH: No limitations	**PAGE CHARGES:** No	
MANUSCRIPT COPIES: 3	**STYLE REQUIREMENTS:** CBE, IM, GPO	
PUBLICATION LAG TIME: 4 months	**STYLE SHEET:** Yes	
EARLY PUBLICATION OPTION: No	**REVISED THESES:** Will review	
ACCEPTANCE RATE: 50%	**STUDENT PAPERS:** No	
AUTHORSHIP RESTRICTIONS: No	**REPRINT POLICY:** 100 free	

SUBSCRIPTION ADDRESS: Subscriptions
Government Printing Office
Washington DC 20402
ANNUAL SUBSCRIPTION RATE: $55
FREQUENCY: Monthly   **CIRCULATION:** 4400
AFFILIATION: None
INDEXED/ABSTRACTED IN: CC, IM

JOURNAL TITLE: Journal of Nervous and Mental Disease

MANUSCRIPT ADDRESS: Journal of Nervous and Mental Disease
University of Maryland School of Medicine
660 West Redwood Street, HHT, Baltimore MD 21201
TYPES OF ARTICLES: Research, review, case studies

MAJOR CONTENT AREAS: human behavior, mental health/illness, psychology

TOPICS PREFERRED: Articles in the fields of psychiatry, psychology and human behavior
INAPPROPRIATE TOPICS: None cited

REVIEW PROCEDURE: Editorial board and external review
REVIEW PERIOD: 2 months
MANUSCRIPT WORD LENGTH: 1250-6000   **PAGE CHARGES:** No
MANUSCRIPT COPIES: 2   **STYLE REQUIREMENTS:** IM, Own
PUBLICATION LAG TIME: 6-8 months   **STYLE SHEET:** Yes
EARLY PUBLICATION OPTION: Sometimes   **REVISED THESES:** Yes
ACCEPTANCE RATE: 27%   **STUDENT PAPERS:** No
AUTHORSHIP RESTRICTIONS: No   **REPRINT POLICY:** Author purchase

SUBSCRIPTION ADDRESS: Subscription Department
The Williams & Wilkins Company
428 East Preston St., Baltimore MD 21202
ANNUAL SUBSCRIPTION RATE: Individuals: $50 Institutions: $70
FREQUENCY: Monthly   **CIRCULATION:** 2200
AFFILIATION: None
INDEXED/ABSTRACTED IN: BA, EM, ISI, CA, IPA, IM, INI, PA, SSCI, CINAHL

JOURNAL TITLE: Journal of Neurosurgical Nursing

MANUSCRIPT ADDRESS: Barbara Krojewski, R.N., CNRN, Editor
Crozer Chester Medical Center, Neurosurgical Dept.
15th & Upland, Chester PA 19013
TYPES OF ARTICLES: Research, case studies, unsolicited book reviews, review
MAJOR CONTENT AREAS: accidents, cancer, communication, death & dying, leadership, nursing: assessment, care, critical care, occupational, OR, pediatric, research; pain, physical therapy, primary care, rehabilitation, sensory deprivation, suicide
TOPICS PREFERRED: Nursing papers in neurosurgery, any new neurological ideas
INAPPROPRIATE TOPICS: None to present

REVIEW PROCEDURE: Editorial board
REVIEW PERIOD: 1-2 months
MANUSCRIPT WORD LENGTH: Varies   **PAGE CHARGES:** No
MANUSCRIPT COPIES: 2   **STYLE REQUIREMENTS:** IM
PUBLICATION LAG TIME: 3 months   **STYLE SHEET:** Yes
EARLY PUBLICATION OPTION: No   **REVISED THESES:** Yes
ACCEPTANCE RATE: 99%   **STUDENT PAPERS:** No
AUTHORSHIP RESTRICTIONS: No   **REPRINT POLICY:** None free

SUBSCRIPTION ADDRESS: American Association of Neurosurgical Nurses
625 North Michigan Avenue, Suite 1519
Chicago IL 60611
ANNUAL SUBSCRIPTION RATE: Individuals: $27 Institutions: $30
FREQUENCY: Bimonthly   **CIRCULATION:** 1500
AFFILIATION: American Association of Neurosurgical Nurses
INDEXED/ABSTRACTED IN: CINAHL, INI

JOURNAL TITLE: Journal of Nurse-Midwifery †

MANUSCRIPT ADDRESS: The American College of Nurse-Midwives
Suite 1120, 1522 K. Street, N.W.
Washington DC 20005
TYPES OF ARTICLES: Theoretical, research, review, case studies, commentaries, unsolicited book reviews
MAJOR CONTENT AREAS: family planning, genetics, human sexuality, maternal/child nursing, midwifery, parenting, well-woman gynecology

TOPICS PREFERRED: Child birth, parenting, midwifery

INAPPROPRIATE TOPICS: None cited

REVIEW PROCEDURE: Editorial board		
REVIEW PERIOD: 3 months		
MANUSCRIPT WORD LENGTH: 3000-4000	**PAGE CHARGES:** No	
MANUSCRIPT COPIES: 2	**STYLE REQUIREMENTS:** AMA	
PUBLICATION LAG TIME: 6-9 months	**STYLE SHEET:** Yes	
EARLY PUBLICATION OPTION: Not cited	**REVISED THESES:** Yes	
ACCEPTANCE RATE: 50%	**STUDENT PAPERS:** No	
AUTHORSHIP RESTRICTIONS: No	**REPRINT POLICY:** 1 free journal	

SUBSCRIPTION ADDRESS: Elsevier-North Holland, Inc.
52 Vanderbilt Avenue
New York NYI 10017
ANNUAL SUBSCRIPTION RATE: Individuals: $19   Institutions: $38
FREQUENCY: Bimonthly   **CIRCULATION:** 4500
AFFILIATION: American College of Nurse-Midwives
INDEXED/ABSTRACTED IN: INI, CINAHL

◆

JOURNAL TITLE: The Journal of Nursing Administration

MANUSCRIPT ADDRESS: Editorial Director
12 Lakeside Park, 607 North Avenue
Wakefield MA 01880
TYPES OF ARTICLES: Practical, case studies, theoretical, research, review, commentaries, unsolicited book reviews
MAJOR CONTENT AREAS: change theory, communication, continuing & inservice education, ethics, groups, health policies, hospitals, human behavior, leadership, nursing: audit, care, diagnosis, philosophy, research, administration, theory; professionalism, systems theory
TOPICS PREFERRED: Topics pertinent to the information needs of top nursing administrators
INAPPROPRIATE TOPICS: Topics not addressing nursing administrators, or those with little new information; poorly developed

REVIEW PROCEDURE: Editorial board		
REVIEW PERIOD: 60 days		
MANUSCRIPT WORD LENGTH: 4000-5000	**PAGE CHARGES:** No	
MANUSCRIPT COPIES: 3	**STYLE REQUIREMENTS:** C	
PUBLICATION LAG TIME: 6-9 months	**STYLE SHEET:** Yes	
EARLY PUBLICATION OPTION: No	**REVISED THESES:** Occasionally	
ACCEPTANCE RATE: 40%	**STUDENT PAPERS:** No	
AUTHORSHIP RESTRICTIONS: No	**REPRINT POLICY:** 500 free	

SUBSCRIPTION ADDRESS: Circulation Department
12 Lakeside Park
607 North Avenue, Wakefield MA 01880
ANNUAL SUBSCRIPTION RATE: $22.95 (Group rates available)
FREQUENCY: Monthly   **CIRCULATION:** 17,000
AFFILIATION: None
INDEXED/ABSTRACTED IN: INI, CINAHL, HLI, IM

JOURNAL TITLE: Journal of Nursing Care

MANUSCRIPT ADDRESS: Gerald C. Melson, R.N., M.A., Editor
265 Post Road West
Westport CT 06880
TYPES OF ARTICLES: Research, theoretical, case studies, clinical

MAJOR CONTENT AREAS: Most areas listed in Appendix A including clinical and educational articles relating to specific patients and/or disorders, nurse's role, chronicity, dying, ethics, professionalism, quality of life, rehabilitation
TOPICS PREFERRED: Issues involving LPN/LVN, bedside nursing

INAPPROPRIATE TOPICS: None cited

REVIEW PROCEDURE: Editor		
REVIEW PERIOD: 2 weeks		
MANUSCRIPT WORD LENGTH: 1200-2000	**PAGE CHARGES:** No	
MANUSCRIPT COPIES: 1	**STYLE REQUIREMENTS:** Own	
PUBLICATION LAG TIME: 4 months	**STYLE SHEET:** Yes	
EARLY PUBLICATION OPTION: No	**REVISED THESES:** Yes	
ACCEPTANCE RATE: 50%	**STUDENT PAPERS:** Yes	
AUTHORSHIP RESTRICTIONS: No	**REPRINT POLICY:** 3 free	

SUBSCRIPTION ADDRESS: Subscription Department
265 Post Road West
Westport CT 06880
ANNUAL SUBSCRIPTION RATE: $12
FREQUENCY: Monthly   **CIRCULATION:** 45,000
AFFILIATION: National Federation of Licensed Practical Nurses
INDEXED/ABSTRACTED IN: CINAHL, HLI, INI

JOURNAL TITLE: Journal of Nursing Education

MANUSCRIPT ADDRESS: Margaret Carnine, R.N., Executive Editor
Charles B. Slack, Inc., 6900 Grove Rd.
Thorofare NJ 08086
TYPES OF ARTICLES: Research, theoretical, case studies

MAJOR CONTENT AREAS: All subjects pertaining to nursing education

TOPICS PREFERRED: None cited

INAPPROPRIATE TOPICS: None cited

REVIEW PROCEDURE: Editorial board		
REVIEW PERIOD: 6 weeks		
MANUSCRIPT WORD LENGTH: 3000	**PAGE CHARGES:** No	
MANUSCRIPT COPIES: 2	**STYLE REQUIREMENTS:** AMA	
PUBLICATION LAG TIME: 1 year	**STYLE SHEET:** Yes	
EARLY PUBLICATION OPTION: Yes	**REVISED THESES:** No	
ACCEPTANCE RATE: Not cited	**STUDENT PAPERS:** Yes	
AUTHORSHIP RESTRICTIONS: No	**REPRINT POLICY:** None free	

SUBSCRIPTION ADDRESS: Charles B. Slack, Inc.
6900 Grove Road
Thorofare NJ 08086
ANNUAL SUBSCRIPTION RATE: $18
FREQUENCY: 9 times yearly   **CIRCULATION:** 4000
AFFILIATION: None
INDEXED/ABSTRACTED IN: CINAHL, HLI, IM, INI

JOURNAL TITLE: Journal of Nutrition

MANUSCRIPT ADDRESS: Dr. James S. Dinning, Editor
Institute of Food and Agricultural Sciences
University of Florida, Gainesville FL 32611
TYPES OF ARTICLES: Research articles; invited papers: biographies, editorial papers
MAJOR CONTENT AREAS: biochemistry, nutrition, pathology, research methodology, others if nutrition related

TOPICS PREFERRED: Experimental nutrition

INAPPROPRIATE TOPICS: None cited

REVIEW PROCEDURE: Editorial board and external review
REVIEW PERIOD: 6 weeks
MANUSCRIPT WORD LENGTH: 3000   **PAGE CHARGES:** No
MANUSCRIPT COPIES: 3   **STYLE REQUIREMENTS:** CBE
PUBLICATION LAG TIME: 3-4 months   **STYLE SHEET:** Yes
EARLY PUBLICATION OPTION: No   **REVISED THESES:** Yes
ACCEPTANCE RATE: 70%   **STUDENT PAPERS:** No
AUTHORSHIP RESTRICTIONS: No   **REPRINT POLICY:** None free

SUBSCRIPTION ADDRESS: The Journal of Nutrition
Subscription Department
9650 Rockville Pike, Bethesda MD 20014
ANNUAL SUBSCRIPTION RATE: $42 (non-members)
FREQUENCY: Monthly   **CIRCULATION:** 5000
AFFILIATION: American Institute of Nutrition
INDEXED/ABSTRACTED IN: BA, NAR, IM, CA, BAI

◆

JOURNAL TITLE: Journal of Nutrition Education

MANUSCRIPT ADDRESS: Susan M. Oace, Editor
Department of Nutritional Sciences
University of California, Berkeley CA 94704
TYPES OF ARTICLES: Research

MAJOR CONTENT AREAS: nutrition education

TOPICS PREFERRED: None cited

INAPPROPRIATE TOPICS: None cited

REVIEW PROCEDURE: Editorial board and external review
REVIEW PERIOD: 3-6 months
MANUSCRIPT WORD LENGTH: 4600-5000   **PAGE CHARGES:** Yes
MANUSCRIPT COPIES: 5   **STYLE REQUIREMENTS:** C
PUBLICATION LAG TIME: 1-3 months   **STYLE SHEET:** Yes
EARLY PUBLICATION OPTION: No   **REVISED THESES:** No
ACCEPTANCE RATE: 20-25%   **STUDENT PAPERS:** No
AUTHORSHIP RESTRICTIONS: No   **REPRINT POLICY:** 1 free

SUBSCRIPTION ADDRESS: Subscriptions Department
1736 Franklin Street
Oakland CA 94612
ANNUAL SUBSCRIPTION RATE: Individuals: $25   Institutions: $30
FREQUENCY: Quarterly   **CIRCULATION:** 7500
AFFILIATION: Society for Nutrition Education
INDEXED/ABSTRACTED IN: EI, CC

127

JOURNAL TITLE: Journal of the Parenteral Drug Association

MANUSCRIPT ADDRESS: School of Pharmacy
University of Wisconsin
Madison WI 53706
TYPES OF ARTICLES: Research, review, case studies, theoretical, commentaries, unsolicited book reviews
MAJOR CONTENT AREAS: biology, biomedical research, body image, medicine, microbiology, pain, pathology, pharmacology, research methodology

TOPICS PREFERRED: Sterilization, parenteral drugs (therapeutics, pathology, etc.), new drug delivery systems
INAPPROPRIATE TOPICS: None cited

REVIEW PROCEDURE: External review
REVIEW PERIOD: 2 months
MANUSCRIPT WORD LENGTH: Not cited
MANUSCRIPT COPIES: 2
PUBLICATION LAG TIME: 3 months
EARLY PUBLICATION OPTION: No
ACCEPTANCE RATE: 70%
AUTHORSHIP RESTRICTIONS: No

PAGE CHARGES: No
STYLE REQUIREMENTS: AMA
STYLE SHEET: Yes
REVISED THESES: Yes
STUDENT PAPERS: No
REPRINT POLICY: None free

SUBSCRIPTION ADDRESS: Parenteral Drug Association, Inc.
Western Savings Bank Building
Broad & Chestnut Streets, Philadelphia PA 19107
ANNUAL SUBSCRIPTION RATE: $20
FREQUENCY: Bimonthly   **CIRCULATION:** 4500
AFFILIATION: Parenteral Drug Association, Inc.
INDEXED/ABSTRACTED IN: IPA

◆

JOURNAL TITLE: Journal of Pediatric Psychology

MANUSCRIPT ADDRESS: Department of Psychology
The University of Iowa
Iowa City IA 52242
TYPES OF ARTICLES: Research, theoretical, review, case studies

MAJOR CONTENT AREAS: abuse (child/spouse), accidents, adolescence, children, death & dying, eating disorders, growth/ development, handicapping conditions, mental retardation, pain, parenting, patient teaching, pediatric nursing, psychology, rehabilitation
TOPICS PREFERRED: Topics of interest to psychologists working in pediatric or medical group practice settings
INAPPROPRIATE TOPICS: Program descriptions

REVIEW PROCEDURE: Editorial board and external review
REVIEW PERIOD: 3 months
MANUSCRIPT WORD LENGTH: 4000
MANUSCRIPT COPIES: 3
PUBLICATION LAG TIME: 12 months
EARLY PUBLICATION OPTION: No
ACCEPTANCE RATE: 50%
AUTHORSHIP RESTRICTIONS: No

PAGE CHARGES: No
STYLE REQUIREMENTS: APA
STYLE SHEET: Yes
REVISED THESES: Yes
STUDENT PAPERS: No
REPRINT POLICY: None free

SUBSCRIPTION ADDRESS: Plenum Publishing Corporation
227 West 17th Street
New York NY 10011
ANNUAL SUBSCRIPTION RATE: Individuals: $19.50 Institutions: $39.00
FREQUENCY: Quarterly   **CIRCULATION:** 1000
AFFILIATION: Society of Pediatric Psychology; APA
INDEXED/ABSTRACTED IN: PA

JOURNAL TITLE: Journal of Pediatrics

MANUSCRIPT ADDRESS: Joseph M. Garfunkel, M.D.
P.O. Box 3307
Springfield IL 62708

TYPES OF ARTICLES: Research, case studies, review, commentaries

MAJOR CONTENT AREAS: abuse, accidents, adaptation, cancer, genetics, growth/development, handicapping conditions, health sciences, human behavior, immunization, mental health/illness, mental retardation, nutrition, parenting, primary care, rehabilitation

TOPICS PREFERRED: None cited

INAPPROPRIATE TOPICS: None cited

REVIEW PROCEDURE: Editorial board and external review
REVIEW PERIOD: 4-6 weeks

MANUSCRIPT WORD LENGTH: 1000-3000	**PAGE CHARGES:** No
MANUSCRIPT COPIES: 2	**STYLE REQUIREMENTS:** IM
PUBLICATION LAG TIME: 6 months	**STYLE SHEET:** No (in journal)
EARLY PUBLICATION OPTION: Yes	**REVISED THESES:** No
ACCEPTANCE RATE: 29%	**STUDENT PAPERS:** No
AUTHORSHIP RESTRICTIONS: No	**REPRINT POLICY:** None free

SUBSCRIPTION ADDRESS: C.V. Mosby Company
11830 Westline Industrial Drive
St. Louis MO 63141

ANNUAL SUBSCRIPTION RATE: Individuals - $33.50   Institutions - $54.50
FREQUENCY: Monthly   **CIRCULATION:** 30,000
AFFILIATION: None
INDEXED/ABSTRACTED IN: BA, CA, CINAHL, HLI, IPA, IM, INI, NAR

◆

JOURNAL TITLE: Journal of Personality Assessment

MANUSCRIPT ADDRESS: 7840 S.W. 51st Street
Portland OR 97219

TYPES OF ARTICLES: Research, theoretical, review, case studies, commentaries

MAJOR CONTENT AREAS: counseling, crisis intervention/theory, human sexuality, leadership, marriage & divorce, mental health/illness, parenting, psych/mental health nursing, testing/measurement

TOPICS PREFERRED: Personality assessment

INAPPROPRIATE TOPICS: None

REVIEW PROCEDURE: 2 consultants, editor
REVIEW PERIOD: 3 months

MANUSCRIPT WORD LENGTH: Varies	**PAGE CHARGES:** No
MANUSCRIPT COPIES: 2	**STYLE REQUIREMENTS:** APA
PUBLICATION LAG TIME: 10 months	**STYLE SHEET:** No
EARLY PUBLICATION OPTION: No	**REVISED THESES:** Yes
ACCEPTANCE RATE: 35%	**STUDENT PAPERS:** No
AUTHORSHIP RESTRICTIONS: No	**REPRINT POLICY:** None Free

SUBSCRIPTION ADDRESS: Ms. Marilyn Graves
1070 E. Angelino Avenue
Burbank CA 91501

ANNUAL SUBSCRIPTION RATE: $22.50
FREQUENCY: Bimonthly   **CIRCULATION:** 2700
AFFILIATION: Society for Personality Assessment
INDEXED/ABSTRACTED IN: CC, PA, IM, INI

JOURNAL TITLE: Journal of Physiology

MANUSCRIPT ADDRESS: The Distributing Editors
Shaftesbury Road
Cambridge   CB2 2BS   England

TYPES OF ARTICLES: Research

MAJOR CONTENT AREAS: physiology (not anatomy)

TOPICS PREFERRED: Experimental physiology

INAPPROPRIATE TOPICS: None cited

REVIEW PROCEDURE: Editorial board
REVIEW PERIOD: 6 weeks
MANUSCRIPT WORD LENGTH: Not cited   **PAGE CHARGES:** No
MANUSCRIPT COPIES: 2   **STYLE REQUIREMENTS:** Own
PUBLICATION LAG TIME: 4 months   **STYLE SHEET:** Yes
EARLY PUBLICATION OPTION: No   **REVISED THESES:** No
ACCEPTANCE RATE: 65%   **STUDENT PAPERS:** No
AUTHORSHIP RESTRICTIONS: No   **REPRINT POLICY:** 50 free

SUBSCRIPTION ADDRESS: Cambridge University Press
32 East 57th Street
New York   NY   10022

ANNUAL SUBSCRIPTION RATE: $800
FREQUENCY: Monthly   **CIRCULATION:** 4000
AFFILIATION: Physiological Society
INDEXED/ABSTRACTED IN: BA, CA, IM, NAR, SA, INI

◆

JOURNAL TITLE: Journal of Practical Nursing

MANUSCRIPT ADDRESS: National Association for Practical Nurse Education
and Service, 254 West 31st Street
New York   NY   10001

TYPES OF ARTICLES: Research, clinic nursing care studies, case
studies, clinical review

MAJOR CONTENT AREAS: Most areas listed in Appendix A including:
all nursing areas, communication, continuity of
care, crisis intervention/theory, death & dying,
mental health/illness, pain, physical therapy,
primary care, public health, sensory deprivation

TOPICS PREFERRED: Long term care, diseases of geriatrics, nursing
care, nontraditional fields of nursing

INAPPROPRIATE TOPICS: Poetry, humor

REVIEW PROCEDURE: Editorial board; external review if appropriate
REVIEW PERIOD: 6-8 weeks
MANUSCRIPT WORD LENGTH: 500-2000   **PAGE CHARGES:** No
MANUSCRIPT COPIES: 1   **STYLE REQUIREMENTS:** Own
PUBLICATION LAG TIME: 6 months   **STYLE SHEET:** Yes
EARLY PUBLICATION OPTION: No   **REVISED THESES:** No
ACCEPTANCE RATE: 40%   **STUDENT PAPERS:** No
AUTHORSHIP RESTRICTIONS: No   **REPRINT POLICY:** 5 free journals

SUBSCRIPTION ADDRESS: NAPNES
Box 580
Martinsville NJ 08836

ANNUAL SUBSCRIPTION RATE: Individuals: $12.00 special rates for students
FREQUENCY: 10 times yearly   **CIRCULATION:** 40,000
AFFILIATION: National Assoc. Practical Nurse Education & Service
INDEXED/ABSTRACTED IN: CINAHL, HLI, INI

JOURNAL TITLE: Journal of Prevention

MANUSCRIPT ADDRESS: P.O. Box 297
Glastonbury CT 06033

TYPES OF ARTICLES: Research, theoretical, review

MAJOR CONTENT AREAS: abuse (child/spouse), all age groups, alcoholism & drug abuse, crisis intervention/theory, growth/ development, health promotion, marriage & divorce, mental health, parenting, psychology, psychopath- ology, suicide, systems theory, women's issues
TOPICS PREFERRED: Research

INAPPROPRIATE TOPICS: Student manuscripts

REVIEW PROCEDURE: Editorial board		
REVIEW PERIOD: 2 weeks		
MANUSCRIPT WORD LENGTH: 3000-4000	**PAGE CHARGES:** No	
MANUSCRIPT COPIES: 4	**STYLE REQUIREMENTS:** APA	
PUBLICATION LAG TIME: 8-12 months	**STYLE SHEET:** Yes	
EARLY PUBLICATION OPTION: No	**REVISED THESES:** No	
ACCEPTANCE RATE: 15%	**STUDENT PAPERS:** No	
AUTHORSHIP RESTRICTIONS: No	**REPRINT POLICY:** 1 free journal	

SUBSCRIPTION ADDRESS: Human Sciences Press
72 Fifth Avenue
New York NY 10011
ANNUAL SUBSCRIPTION RATE: Individuals: $18 Institutions: $35
FREQUENCY: Quarterly   **CIRCULATION:** New journal
AFFILIATION: National Association of Prevention Professionals
INDEXED/ABSTRACTED IN: New journal

◆

JOURNAL TITLE: Journal of Psychiatric Education

MANUSCRIPT ADDRESS: Robert Cranco, M.D.
New York University Medical Center
550 First Avenue, New York NY 10016
TYPES OF ARTICLES: Research, review, theoretical, case studies, commentaries, unsolicited book reviews
MAJOR CONTENT AREAS: teaching/learning, testing/measurement; any topic in Appendix A if related to psychiatric education

TOPICS PREFERRED: Topics related to psychiatric education

INAPPROPRIATE TOPICS: None cited

REVIEW PROCEDURE: Editorial board, external review		
REVIEW PERIOD: 3 months		
MANUSCRIPT WORD LENGTH: 3000	**PAGE CHARGES:** No	
MANUSCRIPT COPIES: 3	**STYLE REQUIREMENTS:** AMA	
PUBLICATION LAG TIME: 1 year	**STYLE SHEET:** Yes	
EARLY PUBLICATION OPTION: Yes	**REVISED THESES:** No	
ACCEPTANCE RATE: 15%	**STUDENT PAPERS:** No	
AUTHORSHIP RESTRICTIONS: No	**REPRINT POLICY:** None free	

SUBSCRIPTION ADDRESS: Human Sciences Press
72 Fifth Avenue
New York NY 10011
ANNUAL SUBSCRIPTION RATE: Individuals: $25 Institutions: $52
FREQUENCY: Quarterly   **CIRCULATION:** 600
AFFILIATION: Amer.Assoc.of Directors of Psych.Residency Training
INDEXED/ABSTRACTED IN: PA, EM, CPI, SSCI, CC/SBS

131

JOURNAL TITLE: Journal of Psychiatric Nursing and Mental Health †
              Services
MANUSCRIPT ADDRESS: Charles B. Slack, Inc.
                    6900 Grove Rd.
                    Thorofare NJ 08086
TYPES OF ARTICLES: Research, theoretical, case studies

MAJOR CONTENT AREAS: Any subject related to psychiatric nursing and
                     mental health services

TOPICS PREFERRED: None cited

INAPPROPRIATE TOPICS: None cited

REVIEW PROCEDURE: Editorial board
REVIEW PERIOD: 4-6 weeks

MANUSCRIPT WORD LENGTH: 3000	PAGE CHARGES: No
MANUSCRIPT COPIES: 2	STYLE REQUIREMENTS: AMA
PUBLICATION LAG TIME: 6 months	STYLE SHEET: Yes
EARLY PUBLICATION OPTION: Yes	REVISED THESES: No
ACCEPTANCE RATE: Not Cited	STUDENT PAPERS: Yes
AUTHORSHIP RESTRICTIONS: No	REPRINT POLICY: None free

SUBSCRIPTION ADDRESS: Charles B. Slack, Inc.
                      6900 Grove Rd.
                      Thorofare NJ 08086
ANNUAL SUBSCRIPTION RATE: $18
FREQUENCY: Monthly   CIRCULATION: 6500
AFFILIATION: None
INDEXED/ABSTRACTED IN: CINAHL, INI, IM

◄►

JOURNAL TITLE: Journal of Psychological Anthropology

MANUSCRIPT ADDRESS: Star Route A
                    Box 89-P
                    Anchorage Alaska 99507
TYPES OF ARTICLES: Research, theoretical, review, case studies

MAJOR CONTENT AREAS: adaptation, anthropology, change theory,
                     children, growth/development, human behavior,
                     human sexuality, life span, mental health/illness,
                     perception, psychology, psychopathology

TOPICS PREFERRED: Child socialization, culture and personality,
                  culture change
INAPPROPRIATE TOPICS: None cited

REVIEW PROCEDURE: Editorial board and external review
REVIEW PERIOD: 6 months

MANUSCRIPT WORD LENGTH: 5000-7000	PAGE CHARGES: No
MANUSCRIPT COPIES: 3	STYLE REQUIREMENTS: C
PUBLICATION LAG TIME: 1 year	STYLE SHEET: Yes
EARLY PUBLICATION OPTION: Yes	REVISED THESES: Yes
ACCEPTANCE RATE: 35%	STUDENT PAPERS: No
AUTHORSHIP RESTRICTIONS: No	REPRINT POLICY: 40 free

SUBSCRIPTION ADDRESS: Journal of Psychological Anthropology
                      2315 Broadway
                      New York NY 10024
ANNUAL SUBSCRIPTION RATE: Individuals: $18   Institutions: $26
FREQUENCY: Quarterly   CIRCULATION: 1800
AFFILIATION: Association and Institute of Psychohistory
INDEXED/ABSTRACTED IN: None cited

JOURNAL TITLE: Journal of Psychology

MANUSCRIPT ADDRESS: The Managing Editor
Box 543
Provincetown MA 02657
TYPES OF ARTICLES: Research, theoretical

MAJOR CONTENT AREAS: any content areas listed in Appendix A, but only
if related to psychological theory; particular
interest is general field of psychology

TOPICS PREFERRED: None cited

INAPPROPRIATE TOPICS: Essays that are not related to psychological
theory
REVIEW PROCEDURE: Editorial board and external review
REVIEW PERIOD: 4 weeks
MANUSCRIPT WORD LENGTH: Not cited   PAGE CHARGES: Yes
MANUSCRIPT COPIES: 2   STYLE REQUIREMENTS: Own
PUBLICATION LAG TIME: Immediate pub.   STYLE SHEET: Yes
EARLY PUBLICATION OPTION: Immediate pub.   REVISED THESES: No
ACCEPTANCE RATE: 50%   STUDENT PAPERS: No
AUTHORSHIP RESTRICTIONS: No   REPRINT POLICY: 200 free

SUBSCRIPTION ADDRESS: The Journal Press
Box 543
Provincetown MA 02657
ANNUAL SUBSCRIPTION RATE: $54
FREQUENCY: Bimonthly   CIRCULATION: 1660
AFFILIATION: None
INDEXED/ABSTRACTED IN: PA, PRG, ECER, EM, IM, IndPA, LLBA, SSI, SSCI, INI

◆

JOURNAL TITLE: Journal of Rehabilitation

MANUSCRIPT ADDRESS: Dr. Jack Sink
413 Aderhold
University of Georgia, Athens GA 30602
TYPES OF ARTICLES: Research, case studies, theoretical

MAJOR CONTENT AREAS: cancer, compliance, continuing education, counseling, handicapping conditions, human sexuality,
mental retardation, nursing: medical/surgical,
occupational; physical therapy, quality of life,
rehabilitation, teaching/learning, testing
TOPICS PREFERRED: Any type of article dealing with rehabilitation
of handicapped persons
INAPPROPRIATE TOPICS: None cited

REVIEW PROCEDURE: Editorial board and external review
REVIEW PERIOD: 2-3 months
MANUSCRIPT WORD LENGTH: 3000   PAGE CHARGES: No
MANUSCRIPT COPIES: 3   STYLE REQUIREMENTS: APA
PUBLICATION LAG TIME: 4 months   STYLE SHEET: Yes
EARLY PUBLICATION OPTION: No   REVISED THESES: Yes
ACCEPTANCE RATE: 60%   STUDENT PAPERS: Yes
AUTHORSHIP RESTRICTIONS: No   REPRINT POLICY: 4 free journals

SUBSCRIPTION ADDRESS: National Rehabilitation Association
633 South Washington St.
Alexandria VA 22314
ANNUAL SUBSCRIPTION RATE: $20
FREQUENCY: Quarterly   CIRCULATION: 30,000
AFFILIATION: National Rehabilitation Association
INDEXED/ABSTRACTED IN: PA, CC(SBS), CIJE, DSHA, LLBA, HLI, IM, SSCI,
CINAHL, SWRA, ECER

JOURNAL TITLE: Journal of Religion and Health

MANUSCRIPT ADDRESS: Box 1066
Southwest Harbor ME 04679

TYPES OF ARTICLES: Theoretical, research, commentaries, review, case studies

MAJOR CONTENT AREAS: aging and aged, alcoholism & drug abuse, biomedical research, counseling, ethics, health sciences, human behavior, mental health, nursing: philosophy, theory, psychiatric; psychology, psychopathology, quality of life, stress, suicide

TOPICS PREFERRED: None cited

INAPPROPRIATE TOPICS: None cited

REVIEW PROCEDURE: Editorial board
REVIEW PERIOD: 6 months

MANUSCRIPT WORD LENGTH: 2500	**PAGE CHARGES:** No
MANUSCRIPT COPIES: 3	**STYLE REQUIREMENTS:** C, Own
PUBLICATION LAG TIME: 1 year	**STYLE SHEET:** Yes
EARLY PUBLICATION OPTION: No	**REVISED THESES:** No
ACCEPTANCE RATE: 50%	**STUDENT PAPERS:** No
AUTHORSHIP RESTRICTIONS: No	**REPRINT POLICY:** None free

SUBSCRIPTION ADDRESS: Human Sciences Press
72 Fifth Avenue
New York NY 10011

ANNUAL SUBSCRIPTION RATE: Individuals: $16   Institutions: $35
FREQUENCY: Quarterly   **CIRCULATION:** 3500
AFFILIATION: None
INDEXED/ABSTRACTED IN: RTA, CC(SBS), SSCI, PCCA, GSSRPL, EM, PA

JOURNAL TITLE: The Journal of School Health

MANUSCRIPT ADDRESS: Gay E. Groomes, Editor
P.O. Box 708
Kent OH 44240

TYPES OF ARTICLES: Research, review, commentaries, case studies, unsolicited book reviews, practical

MAJOR CONTENT AREAS: immunization, nursing: clinical specialties, maternal/child, education, research, theory, pediatric, public health, school; nutrition, parenting, safety/first aid, stress, suicide, teaching/learning; most age groups and disorders

TOPICS PREFERRED: Topics related to the cited content areas

INAPPROPRIATE TOPICS: None cited

REVIEW PROCEDURE: External review
REVIEW PERIOD: 6-8 weeks

MANUSCRIPT WORD LENGTH: 2500-3000	**PAGE CHARGES:** No
MANUSCRIPT COPIES: 3	**STYLE REQUIREMENTS:** AMA
PUBLICATION LAG TIME: 3-6 months	**STYLE SHEET:** Yes
EARLY PUBLICATION OPTION: No	**REVISED THESES:** May submit
ACCEPTANCE RATE: 45%	**STUDENT PAPERS:** No
AUTHORSHIP RESTRICTIONS: Not cited	**REPRINT POLICY:** 2 free

SUBSCRIPTION ADDRESS: American School Health Association
P.O. Box 708
Kent OH 44240

ANNUAL SUBSCRIPTION RATE: Individuals: $40   Institutions: $35
FREQUENCY: 10 times yearly   **CIRCULATION:** 10,000
AFFILIATION: American School Health Association
INDEXED/ABSTRACTED IN: CINAHL, INI, BA, EI, IM, PA, SSCI

JOURNAL TITLE: Journal of Sex and Marital Therapy

MANUSCRIPT ADDRESS: Dr. Clifford Sager
65 East 67th Street, Suite 1A
New York NY 10021
TYPES OF ARTICLES: Research, theoretical, review

MAJOR CONTENT AREAS: counseling, human sexuality, marriage & divorce, medicine,
testing/measurement

TOPICS PREFERRED: Sexual functioning and marital relationships (Theoretical,
research, clinical and therapeutic aspects)
INAPPROPRIATE TOPICS: None cited

REVIEW PROCEDURE: Editorial board, external review
REVIEW PERIOD: 3 months
MANUSCRIPT WORD LENGTH: Not cited   PAGE CHARGES: No
MANUSCRIPT COPIES: 3   STYLE REQUIREMENTS: IM
PUBLICATION LAG TIME: 6 months   STYLE SHEET: Yes
EARLY PUBLICATION OPTION: No   REVISED THESES: Yes
ACCEPTANCE RATE: 35%   STUDENT PAPERS: No
AUTHORSHIP RESTRICTIONS: No   REPRINT POLICY: None free

SUBSCRIPTION ADDRESS: Helen Mack, Bruner/Mazel
19 Union Square West
New York NY 10003
ANNUAL SUBSCRIPTION RATE: Individuals: $24   Institutions: $52
FREQUENCY: Quarterly   CIRCULATION: 2000
AFFILIATION: None
INDEXED/ABSTRACTED IN: PA, EM, SSCI, CC, SocA, IM, CIJE

◆

JOURNAL TITLE: Journal of Studies on Alcohol

MANUSCRIPT ADDRESS: Rutgers Center of Alcohol Studies
P.O. Box 969
Piscataway NJ 08854
TYPES OF ARTICLES: Research, review, theoretical, case studies,
commentaries, unsolicited book reviews
MAJOR CONTENT AREAS: Most areas listed in Appendix A including:
alcoholism & drug abuse, nursing: clinical
specialties, community/public health, critical
care, diagnosis, education, psychiatric/mental
health; life span, patient teaching, stigma
TOPICS PREFERRED: Any topic relating to alcohol use and problems

INAPPROPRIATE TOPICS: Naive articles

REVIEW PROCEDURE: External review
REVIEW PERIOD: 4-6 months
MANUSCRIPT WORD LENGTH: Not cited   PAGE CHARGES: No
MANUSCRIPT COPIES: 2   STYLE REQUIREMENTS: CBE
PUBLICATION LAG TIME: 3-6 months   STYLE SHEET: Yes
EARLY PUBLICATION OPTION: No   REVISED THESES: Yes
ACCEPTANCE RATE: 35-40%   STUDENT PAPERS: No
AUTHORSHIP RESTRICTIONS: No   REPRINT POLICY: 25 free

SUBSCRIPTION ADDRESS: Publications Division
Rutgers Center of Alcohol Studies
P.O. Box 969 Piscataway NJ 08854
ANNUAL SUBSCRIPTION RATE: Individuals: $75 Foreign: $85
FREQUENCY: Monthly   CIRCULATION: 3700
AFFILIATION: None
INDEXED/ABSTRACTED IN: CC(LS), CC(SBS), IM, PAIS, ACP, SWRA, BA, BS, CA,
EM, HA, NR, PA, OSHA, SocA, HLI, INI, NAR, PPA

JOURNAL TITLE: Journal of Toxicology and Environmental Health

MANUSCRIPT ADDRESS: Rob S. McCutcheon
703 Morgan Creek Road
Chapel Hill NC 27514

TYPES OF ARTICLES: Research, theoretical, review, unsolicited book reviews

MAJOR CONTENT AREAS: biochemistry, biology, biomedical research, cancer, epidemiology, genetics, health sciences, health policies, medicine, microbiology, natural science, public health, research methodology, respiratory diseases, testing/measurement

TOPICS PREFERRED: Pollutants, carcinogenesis, mutagenesis, teratology, neurotoxicity, human health in workplace

INAPPROPRIATE TOPICS: None cited

REVIEW PROCEDURE: Editorial board and external review
REVIEW PERIOD: 60 days
MANUSCRIPT WORD LENGTH: 5500
MANUSCRIPT COPIES: 4
PUBLICATION LAG TIME: 7 months
EARLY PUBLICATION OPTION: No
ACCEPTANCE RATE: 50%
AUTHORSHIP RESTRICTIONS: No

PAGE CHARGES: Yes
STYLE REQUIREMENTS: C
STYLE SHEET: Yes
REVISED THESES: No
STUDENT PAPERS: No
REPRINT POLICY: None free

SUBSCRIPTION ADDRESS: Hemisphere Publishing Corporation
1025 Vermont Avenue, N.W.
Washington DC 20005
ANNUAL SUBSCRIPTION RATE: Individuals: $33.75 Institutions: $76.50
FREQUENCY: Nine times yearly **CIRCULATION:** 850
AFFILIATION: None
INDEXED/ABSTRACTED IN: CC(LS), CC(ABES), SCI, IM, BA, CA, EM

JOURNAL TITLE: Journal of Tropical Pediatrics and Environmental Child Health

MANUSCRIPT ADDRESS: Dr. G.J. Ebrahim
Institute of Child Health
30 Guilford Street, London WC1N 1EH England

TYPES OF ARTICLES: Research, theoretical, review, case studies,

MAJOR CONTENT AREAS: accidents, change theory, communication, counseling, eating disorders, family planning, genetics, immunization, nursing: clinical specialties, maternal/child, occupational, public health, school; parenting, stress, teaching/learning

TOPICS PREFERRED: Child nutrition, primary health care, infectious diseases, community health programmes

INAPPROPRIATE TOPICS: None cited

REVIEW PROCEDURE: Editorial board and external review
REVIEW PERIOD: 1 month
MANUSCRIPT WORD LENGTH: 2000
MANUSCRIPT COPIES: 1
PUBLICATION LAG TIME: 18 months
EARLY PUBLICATION OPTION: No
ACCEPTANCE RATE: 60-75%
AUTHORSHIP RESTRICTIONS: No

PAGE CHARGES: No
STYLE REQUIREMENTS: IM
STYLE SHEET: No
REVISED THESES: Yes
STUDENT PAPERS: Yes
REPRINT POLICY: 25 free

SUBSCRIPTION ADDRESS: JMP Services, Ltd.
2 Drayson Mews
Kensington London W8 England
ANNUAL SUBSCRIPTION RATE: $62.50
FREQUENCY: Bimonthly **CIRCULATION:** 1000
AFFILIATION: None
INDEXED/ABSTRACTED IN: IM, INI

JOURNAL TITLE: Journal of Verbal Learning & Verbal Behavior

MANUSCRIPT ADDRESS: Dr. Fergus I.M. Craik
Department of Psychology, Erindale College
Mississauga Ontario Canada L5L 1C6
TYPES OF ARTICLES: Research, review, theoretical, experimental

MAJOR CONTENT AREAS: problems of verbal learning, human memory, psycholinguistics and other verbal processes

TOPICS PREFERRED: Verbal learning and verbal behavior

INAPPROPRIATE TOPICS: None cited

REVIEW PROCEDURE: Editorial board		
REVIEW PERIOD: Not cited		
MANUSCRIPT WORD LENGTH: Not cited	**PAGE CHARGES:** No	
MANUSCRIPT COPIES: 3	**STYLE REQUIREMENTS:** APA, Own	
PUBLICATION LAG TIME: Not cited	**STYLE SHEET:** Not cited	
EARLY PUBLICATION OPTION: Not cited	**REVISED THESES:** Not cited	
ACCEPTANCE RATE: Not cited	**STUDENT PAPERS:** Not cited	
AUTHORSHIP RESTRICTIONS: No	**REPRINT POLICY:** 50 free	

SUBSCRIPTION ADDRESS: Academic Press
111 Fifth Avenue
New York   NY   10003
ANNUAL SUBSCRIPTION RATE: $72
FREQUENCY: Bimonthly   **CIRCULATION:** Not cited
AFFILIATION: None cited
INDEXED/ABSTRACTED IN: PA, SSI, SSCI

◆

JOURNAL TITLE: Journal of Youth and Adolescence

MANUSCRIPT ADDRESS: Daniel Offer, M.D., Dept. of Psychiatry
Michael Reese Hospital and Medical Center
2959 S. Cottage Grove, Chicago IL   60616
TYPES OF ARTICLES: Research, theoretical, review, commentaries

MAJOR CONTENT AREAS: adaptation, body image, crisis, dependency, eating disorders, human behavior & sexuality, loss/grief, marriage & divorce, parenting, psychiatric/mental health nursing, research methodology, sleep, stress, suicide
TOPICS PREFERRED: Normal and pathological issues in growth and development of adolescents and youth
INAPPROPRIATE TOPICS: Case studies

REVIEW PROCEDURE: Editorial board and external review		
REVIEW PERIOD: 2-3 months		
MANUSCRIPT WORD LENGTH: 5000	**PAGE CHARGES:** No	
MANUSCRIPT COPIES: 3	**STYLE REQUIREMENTS:** AIBS	
PUBLICATION LAG TIME: 9 months	**STYLE SHEET:** Yes	
EARLY PUBLICATION OPTION: No	**REVISED THESES:** No	
ACCEPTANCE RATE: 35%	**STUDENT PAPERS:** Yes	
AUTHORSHIP RESTRICTIONS: No	**REPRINT POLICY:** None free	

SUBSCRIPTION ADDRESS: Plenum Publishing Corporation
227 W. 17th Street
New York   NY   10011
ANNUAL SUBSCRIPTION RATE: Individuals: $28   Institutions: $56
FREQUENCY: Quarterly   **CIRCULATION:** 1000
AFFILIATION: None
INDEXED/ABSTRACTED IN: PA, SocA, IM, ACP, CC, EM, SUSA, SSCI

JOURNAL TITLE: Kenya Nursing Journal

MANUSCRIPT ADDRESS: The Editor
National Nurses' Association of Kenya
Nairobi Kenya

TYPES OF ARTICLES: Case studies, research, review

MAJOR CONTENT AREAS: Most areas in Appendix A including: nursing:
public health, critical care, maternal/child,
medical/surgical, neurological, assessment,
education, history, process, research,
occupational, OR, orthopedic, psychiatric, school

TOPICS PREFERRED: Those pertaining to major content areas listed

INAPPROPRIATE TOPICS: None cited

REVIEW PROCEDURE: Editorial board
REVIEW PERIOD: 6-8 weeks
MANUSCRIPT WORD LENGTH: 3000-5000   PAGE CHARGES: Yes
MANUSCRIPT COPIES: 3   STYLE REQUIREMENTS: Free style
PUBLICATION LAG TIME: 6 months   STYLE SHEET: Yes
EARLY PUBLICATION OPTION: No   REVISED THESES: No
ACCEPTANCE RATE: 60%   STUDENT PAPERS: Yes
AUTHORSHIP RESTRICTIONS: No   REPRINT POLICY: 1 free

SUBSCRIPTION ADDRESS: Subscription Officer
Kenya Nursing Journal
P.O. Box 49422, Nairobi Kenya
ANNUAL SUBSCRIPTION RATE: $12.00
FREQUENCY: Biannually   CIRCULATION: 3000
AFFILIATION: National Nurses' Association of Kenya
INDEXED/ABSTRACTED IN: INI

◆

JOURNAL TITLE: Lab World

MANUSCRIPT ADDRESS: A.E. Wooley, Ph.D., Editorial Director
401 North Broad Street
Philadelphia PA 19108
TYPES OF ARTICLES: Clinical laboratory orientation, commentaries

MAJOR CONTENT AREAS: aging & aged, cancer, circulatory diseases, continuing education, family planning, genetics, health: promotion, sciences, policies; hospitals, human behavior & sexuality, immunization, mental health, professionalism, quality of life, stress
TOPICS PREFERRED: People working in clinical labs

INAPPROPRIATE TOPICS: None cited

REVIEW PROCEDURE: Editorial board
REVIEW PERIOD: 2 weeks
MANUSCRIPT WORD LENGTH: 2000
MANUSCRIPT COPIES: 1
PUBLICATION LAG TIME: 3-6 months
EARLY PUBLICATION OPTION: Not cited
ACCEPTANCE RATE: Not cited
AUTHORSHIP RESTRICTIONS: No

PAGE CHARGES: No
STYLE REQUIREMENTS: AMA, NT
STYLE SHEET: Yes, SASE
REVISED THESES: No
STUDENT PAPERS: No
REPRINT POLICY: 5 free

SUBSCRIPTION ADDRESS: Lab World
401 North Broad Street
Philadelphia PA 19108
ANNUAL SUBSCRIPTION RATE: $18
FREQUENCY: Monthly
AFFILIATION: None
INDEXED/ABSTRACTED IN: CINAHL

CIRCULATION: 60,200

◆

JOURNAL TITLE: Lactation Review

MANUSCRIPT ADDRESS: 666 Sturges Highway
Westport CT 06880

TYPES OF ARTICLES: Research, review, case studies, commentaries

MAJOR CONTENT AREAS: anthropology, body image, children, community/public health nursing, cultural diversity, human behavior, human sexuality, maternal/child nursing, midwifery, nutrition, parenting, women's issues, lactation, infant & maternal nutrition
TOPICS PREFERRED: Lactation; infant maternal nutrition, development in Third World
INAPPROPRIATE TOPICS: None cited

REVIEW PROCEDURE: Editorial board
REVIEW PERIOD: 2 weeks
MANUSCRIPT WORD LENGTH: 600
MANUSCRIPT COPIES: 2
PUBLICATION LAG TIME: No set pattern
EARLY PUBLICATION OPTION: No
ACCEPTANCE RATE: 5%
AUTHORSHIP RESTRICTIONS: No

PAGE CHARGES: No
STYLE REQUIREMENTS: AA
STYLE SHEET: No
REVISED THESES: No
STUDENT PAPERS: No
REPRINT POLICY: 5 free

SUBSCRIPTION ADDRESS: 666 Sturges Highway
Westport CT 06880

ANNUAL SUBSCRIPTION RATE: Individuals: $15   Institutions: $25
FREQUENCY: 2-3 times yearly
AFFILIATION: None
INDEXED/ABSTRACTED IN: CINAHL

CIRCULATION: 2-3000

JOURNAL TITLE: Lancet

MANUSCRIPT ADDRESS: 7 Adam Street
London WC2N 6AD England

TYPES OF ARTICLES: Research, review, commentaries, theoretical, case
studies, unsolicited book reviews

MAJOR CONTENT AREAS: medicine

TOPICS PREFERRED: None cited

INAPPROPRIATE TOPICS: None cited

REVIEW PROCEDURE: Editorial board and external review		
REVIEW PERIOD: 4-8 weeks		
MANUSCRIPT WORD LENGTH: Not cited	PAGE CHARGES:	No
MANUSCRIPT COPIES: 1	STYLE REQUIREMENTS:	IM
PUBLICATION LAG TIME: 6 weeks	STYLE SHEET:	No
EARLY PUBLICATION OPTION: No	REVISED THESES:	No
ACCEPTANCE RATE: Not cited	STUDENT PAPERS:	No
AUTHORSHIP RESTRICTIONS: No	REPRINT POLICY:	100 free

SUBSCRIPTION ADDRESS: Little Brown and Company, Subscriptions Department
34 Beacon St.
Boston MA 02106

ANNUAL SUBSCRIPTION RATE: $55.00

FREQUENCY: Weekly   CIRCULATION: Not cited

AFFILIATION: Not cited

INDEXED/ABSTRACTED IN: Not cited

◆

JOURNAL TITLE: Legal Aspects of Medical Practice

MANUSCRIPT ADDRESS: Editor
747 Third Avenue
New York NY 10017

TYPES OF ARTICLES: Theoretical, review, case studies, commentaries,
unsolicited book reviews

MAJOR CONTENT AREAS: ethics, health policies, hospitals, mental
health/illness

TOPICS PREFERRED: Medical jurisprudence or forensic medicine

INAPPROPRIATE TOPICS: None cited

REVIEW PROCEDURE: Editorial board		
REVIEW PERIOD: Not cited		
MANUSCRIPT WORD LENGTH: Not cited	PAGE CHARGES:	Not cited
MANUSCRIPT COPIES: 1	STYLE REQUIREMENTS:	IM
PUBLICATION LAG TIME: Not cited	STYLE SHEET:	Not cited
EARLY PUBLICATION OPTION: Not cited	REVISED THESES:	Not cited
ACCEPTANCE RATE: Not cited	STUDENT PAPERS:	Not cited
AUTHORSHIP RESTRICTIONS: Not cited	REPRINT POLICY:	50 free

SUBSCRIPTION ADDRESS: 747 Third Avenue
New York NY 10017

ANNUAL SUBSCRIPTION RATE: $20

FREQUENCY: Monthly   CIRCULATION: Not cited

AFFILIATION: American College of Legal Medicine

INDEXED/ABSTRACTED IN: Not cited

JOURNAL TITLE: Life and Health

MANUSCRIPT ADDRESS: Review and Herald Publishing Association
6856 Eastern Avenue, NW
Washington DC 20012
TYPES OF ARTICLES: Health-related, emphasizing prevention (in
layman's terms), research
MAJOR CONTENT AREAS: accidents, adaptation, alcoholism & drug abuse,
biofeedback, counseling, crisis, fatigue, health
promotion, human behavior, mental health,
nutrition, parenting, public health, quality of
life, relaxation, sleep, stress, teaching/learning
TOPICS PREFERRED: Articles designed to motivate persons to adopt
and practice a better life style
INAPPROPRIATE TOPICS: Cultish or faddish material (rolfing, yoga, etc.)
or undocumented material
REVIEW PROCEDURE: Editorial consultants in specialty fields
REVIEW PERIOD: 2-6 weeks

MANUSCRIPT WORD LENGTH: 1250-1500	**PAGE CHARGES:** No
MANUSCRIPT COPIES: 1	**STYLE REQUIREMENTS:** Own
PUBLICATION LAG TIME: 5 months	**STYLE SHEET:** Yes
EARLY PUBLICATION OPTION: No	**REVISED THESES:** No
ACCEPTANCE RATE: 10%	**STUDENT PAPERS:** No
AUTHORSHIP RESTRICTIONS: No	**REPRINT POLICY:** 2 free

SUBSCRIPTION ADDRESS: Circulation Department
Review and Herald Publishing Association
6856 Eastern Avenue, NW, Washington DC 20012
ANNUAL SUBSCRIPTION RATE: $9.95
FREQUENCY: Monthly   **CIRCULATION:** 100,000
AFFILIATION: Seventh-day Adventist
INDEXED/ABSTRACTED IN: CINAHL

◆

JOURNAL TITLE: Long-term Care and Health Services Administration
Quarterly
MANUSCRIPT ADDRESS: 135 SE Spanish Trail
Boca Raton FL 33432

TYPES OF ARTICLES: Research, theoretical, review, case studies,
commentaries, unsolicited book reviews
MAJOR CONTENT AREAS: aging & aged, continuing education, continuity of
care, death and dying, health promotion, life
span, loss/grief, mental health/illness, nursing:
care, geriatric, psychiatric; nursing homes,
nutrition, physical therapy, psychology, suicide
TOPICS PREFERRED: Long-term care

INAPPROPRIATE TOPICS: None cited

REVIEW PROCEDURE: External review
REVIEW PERIOD: 1-2 weeks

MANUSCRIPT WORD LENGTH: 7500 max.	**PAGE CHARGES:** No
MANUSCRIPT COPIES: 2	**STYLE REQUIREMENTS:** APA
PUBLICATION LAG TIME: 6-9 months	**STYLE SHEET:** Yes
EARLY PUBLICATION OPTION: No	**REVISED THESES:** Yes
ACCEPTANCE RATE: 33%	**STUDENT PAPERS:** No
AUTHORSHIP RESTRICTIONS: No	**REPRINT POLICY:** 100 free

SUBSCRIPTION ADDRESS: Panel Publishers
14 Plaza Road
Greenvale NY 11548
ANNUAL SUBSCRIPTION RATE: $36
FREQUENCY: Quarterly   **CIRCULATION:** 3000
AFFILIATION: None
INDEXED/ABSTRACTED IN: CINAHL

JOURNAL TITLE: Lung

MANUSCRIPT ADDRESS: M.W. Williams, Jr., M.D.
Van Etten Hospital, Room 612, Pelham Parkway
and Eastchester Road, Bronx   NY   10461

TYPES OF ARTICLES: Research, review, theoretical, case studies,
short communications, technical notes

MAJOR CONTENT AREAS: anatomy and physiology, biochemistry, biomedical
research, cancer, children, epidemiology, health
sciences, medicine, pharmacology, research
methodology, respiratory diseases

TOPICS PREFERRED: Healthy and diseased lungs: epidemiological,
clinical, pathophysiological, biochemical studies

INAPPROPRIATE TOPICS: Manuscripts that have been published or submitted
for publication elsewhere

REVIEW PROCEDURE: Editorial board and external review
REVIEW PERIOD: 2 months

MANUSCRIPT WORD LENGTH: 4000	PAGE CHARGES: No	
MANUSCRIPT COPIES: 3	STYLE REQUIREMENTS: AMA, CBE, IM, Own	
PUBLICATION LAG TIME: 4-6 months	STYLE SHEET: Yes	
EARLY PUBLICATION OPTION: No	REVISED THESES: No	
ACCEPTANCE RATE: 50%	STUDENT PAPERS: No	
AUTHORSHIP RESTRICTIONS: No	REPRINT POLICY: 50 free	

SUBSCRIPTION ADDRESS: Springer-Verlag, Inc.
175 Fifth Ave.
New York   NY   10010

ANNUAL SUBSCRIPTION RATE: $131
FREQUENCY: Bimonthly   CIRCULATION: 800
AFFILIATION: None
INDEXED/ABSTRACTED IN: IM, CC, SCI, BA, CA

◆

142

JOURNAL TITLE: Man and Medicine: Journal of Values and Ethics †
in Health Care
MANUSCRIPT ADDRESS: Michael Meyer, Executive Editor
Columbia University College of Physicians &
Surgeons, 630 West 168th St., New York NY 10032
TYPES OF ARTICLES: Theoretical, review, case studies, commentaries,
unsolicited book reviews
MAJOR CONTENT AREAS: change theory, children, death & dying, ethics,
health policies, hospitals, human behavior,
medicine, professionalism, suicide, systems theory

TOPICS PREFERRED: None cited

INAPPROPRIATE TOPICS: None cited

REVIEW PROCEDURE: External review
REVIEW PERIOD: Not cited
MANUSCRIPT WORD LENGTH: 9000-10,000   PAGE CHARGES: No
MANUSCRIPT COPIES: 1   STYLE REQUIREMENTS: Not cited
PUBLICATION LAG TIME: Not cited   STYLE SHEET: Not cited
EARLY PUBLICATION OPTION: Not cited   REVISED THESES: Not cited
ACCEPTANCE RATE: Not cited   STUDENT PAPERS: Not cited
AUTHORSHIP RESTRICTIONS: No   REPRINT POLICY: Not cited

SUBSCRIPTION ADDRESS: Columbia University College of Physicians &
Surgeons
630 West 168th St., New York NY 10032
ANNUAL SUBSCRIPTION RATE: Individuals: $14   Institutions: $16.50
FREQUENCY: Quarterly   CIRCULATION: Not cited
AFFILIATION: None cited
INDEXED/ABSTRACTED IN: Not cited

◆

JOURNAL TITLE: Maternal-Child Nursing Journal

MANUSCRIPT ADDRESS: 437 Victoria Building
3500 Victoria Street
Pittsburgh PA 15261
TYPES OF ARTICLES: Research, theoretical, case studies, review of
literature
MAJOR CONTENT AREAS: accidents, body image, change theory, crisis,
death & dying, handicapping conditions, loss/
grief, midwifery, nursing: clinical specialties,
maternal/child, research, trauma; pain, parenting,
perception, sleep, stigma, stress, suicide
TOPICS PREFERRED: Research reports and case studies of mothers and
children
INAPPROPRIATE TOPICS: None cited

REVIEW PROCEDURE: Editorial board
REVIEW PERIOD: 6 weeks
MANUSCRIPT WORD LENGTH: Variable   PAGE CHARGES: No
MANUSCRIPT COPIES: 3   STYLE REQUIREMENTS: APA
PUBLICATION LAG TIME: Next issue   STYLE SHEET: Yes
EARLY PUBLICATION OPTION: No   REVISED THESES: Yes
ACCEPTANCE RATE: 50%   STUDENT PAPERS: Yes
AUTHORSHIP RESTRICTIONS: No   REPRINT POLICY: 50 free

SUBSCRIPTION ADDRESS: 437 Victoria Building
3500 Victoria Street
Pittsburgh PA 15261
ANNUAL SUBSCRIPTION RATE: $12
FREQUENCY: Quarterly   CIRCULATION: 1300
AFFILIATION: None
INDEXED/ABSTRACTED IN: CINAHL, INI, PA

JOURNAL TITLE: MCN: The American Journal of Maternal Child Nursing

MANUSCRIPT ADDRESS: Barbara E. Bishop, Editor
555 W. 57th Street
New York NY 10019

TYPES OF ARTICLES: Clinical, research, theoretical

MAJOR CONTENT AREAS: Most diseases and disorders listed in Appendix A; nursing: community health, critical care, assessment, maternal/child, audit, care, diagnosis, process, research, office, pediatric, school; midwifery, parenting, health promotion methodologies

TOPICS PREFERRED: None cited

INAPPROPRIATE TOPICS: Review of literature

REVIEW PROCEDURE: External review
REVIEW PERIOD: 6 weeks
MANUSCRIPT WORD LENGTH: Not cited
MANUSCRIPT COPIES: 3
PUBLICATION LAG TIME: 1 year
EARLY PUBLICATION OPTION: Not cited
ACCEPTANCE RATE: 25%
AUTHORSHIP RESTRICTIONS: No

PAGE CHARGES: No
STYLE REQUIREMENTS: Own
STYLE SHEET: Yes
REVISED THESES: Yes
STUDENT PAPERS: No
REPRINT POLICY: 100 free

SUBSCRIPTION ADDRESS: 555 W. 57th Street
New York NY 10019

ANNUAL SUBSCRIPTION RATE: $15
FREQUENCY: Bimonthly
AFFILIATION: None
INDEXED/ABSTRACTED IN: INI, CINAHL

CIRCULATION: 29,000

JOURNAL TITLE: Medical Anthropology

MANUSCRIPT ADDRESS: University of Connecticut
Box U-58
Storrs CT 06268

TYPES OF ARTICLES: Research, theoretical, case studies, review, commentaries, unsolicited book reviews

MAJOR CONTENT AREAS: health care and healing behavior, cultural diversity, family planning, midwifery, quality of life, health sciences & policies, genetics, community/public health nursing, patient teaching, women's issues

TOPICS PREFERRED: Empirical studies linking social/cultural factors to diseases, health care/utilization

INAPPROPRIATE TOPICS: None cited

REVIEW PROCEDURE: Editorial board and external review
REVIEW PERIOD: 2 months
MANUSCRIPT WORD LENGTH: Varies
MANUSCRIPT COPIES: 3
PUBLICATION LAG TIME: 6-12 months
EARLY PUBLICATION OPTION: Yes
ACCEPTANCE RATE: 30%
AUTHORSHIP RESTRICTIONS: No

PAGE CHARGES: No
STYLE REQUIREMENTS: AA
STYLE SHEET: Yes
REVISED THESES: Yes
STUDENT PAPERS: Yes
REPRINT POLICY: 10 free

SUBSCRIPTION ADDRESS: Docent Corporation, Redgrave Publishing Co.
P.O. Box 67
South Salem NY 10590

ANNUAL SUBSCRIPTION RATE: Individuals: $21   Institutions: $29
FREQUENCY: Quarterly   **CIRCULATION:** 800-1000
AFFILIATION: None
INDEXED/ABSTRACTED IN: International Bibliography of Periodical Literature

JOURNAL TITLE: Medical and Biological Engineering and Computing

MANUSCRIPT ADDRESS: Mr. D. Mackin
Peter Peregrinus, Ltd., P.O. Box 8
Southgate House, Stevenage, Herts SG1 1HQ England

TYPES OF ARTICLES: Research, theoretical, review, case studies

MAJOR CONTENT AREAS: anatomy & physiology, biofeedback, biomedical
research, body image, circulatory diseases, health
sciences, medicine, physical therapy, respiratory
diseases, sensory deprivation, systems theory,
testing/measurement

TOPICS PREFERRED: Research in biomedical engineering

INAPPROPRIATE TOPICS: None cited

REVIEW PROCEDURE: Editorial board and external review
REVIEW PERIOD: 2 months
MANUSCRIPT WORD LENGTH: 4000
MANUSCRIPT COPIES: 3
PUBLICATION LAG TIME: 7-8 months
EARLY PUBLICATION OPTION: No
ACCEPTANCE RATE: Not cited
AUTHORSHIP RESTRICTIONS: No

PAGE CHARGES: No
STYLE REQUIREMENTS: Own
STYLE SHEET: Yes
REVISED THESES: Yes
STUDENT PAPERS: No
REPRINT POLICY: 25 free

SUBSCRIPTION ADDRESS: Peter Peregrinus, Ltd.
c/o ISPEC/IEEE Service Center
445 Hoes Lane, Piscataway NJ 08854

ANNUAL SUBSCRIPTION RATE: $132
FREQUENCY: Bimonthly
AFFILIATION: Int. Fed. for Medical & Biological Engineering
INDEXED/ABSTRACTED IN: AMR, ASTI, BA, CA, Engl

CIRCULATION: 2000

JOURNAL TITLE: Medical Care

MANUSCRIPT ADDRESS: Donald C. Riedel, Ph.D., Editor, Dept. of Health
Services SC-37, School of Public Health
University of Washington, Seattle WA 98195

TYPES OF ARTICLES: Research, theoretical, review, case studies,
commentaries

MAJOR CONTENT AREAS: communication, compliance, cultural diversity,
allied health, mental health/illness, health promotion & policies, hospitals, human behavior,
nursing: audit, care, community/public health,
research; primary care, professionalism

TOPICS PREFERRED: Organization, utilization, financing and quality
of health services

INAPPROPRIATE TOPICS: Clinical care

REVIEW PROCEDURE: Editorial board and external review
REVIEW PERIOD: 4-6 weeks
MANUSCRIPT WORD LENGTH: 3000-5000
MANUSCRIPT COPIES: 4
PUBLICATION LAG TIME: 4-9 months
EARLY PUBLICATION OPTION: Yes
ACCEPTANCE RATE: 20%
AUTHORSHIP RESTRICTIONS: No

PAGE CHARGES: No
STYLE REQUIREMENTS: Own
STYLE SHEET: Yes
REVISED THESES: Yes
STUDENT PAPERS: No
REPRINT POLICY: None free

SUBSCRIPTION ADDRESS: Lippincott/Harper
2350 Virginia Avenue
Hagerstown MD 21740

ANNUAL SUBSCRIPTION RATE: $40 (Students: $23)
FREQUENCY: Monthly
AFFILIATION: Amer. Public Health Assoc. (Medical Care Section)
INDEXED/ABSTRACTED IN: AHM, MCR, IM, HLI, IPA, INI, SSCI, CINAHL

CIRCULATION: 4000

145

JOURNAL TITLE: Medical Self-Care

MANUSCRIPT ADDRESS: Managing Editor
P.O. Box 715
Inverness CA 94937
TYPES OF ARTICLES: Review, commentaries, unsolicited book reviews

MAJOR CONTENT AREAS: accidents, adaptation, death & dying, eating
disorders, family planning, health promotion,
health policies, human behavior, life span,
patient teaching, quality of life, relaxation,
safety/first aid, stress, women's issues
TOPICS PREFERRED: Self-care for the consumer; health care costs

INAPPROPRIATE TOPICS: None cited

REVIEW PROCEDURE: Editorial board
REVIEW PERIOD: Not cited
MANUSCRIPT WORD LENGTH: 500-700   PAGE CHARGES: No
MANUSCRIPT COPIES: 1   STYLE REQUIREMENTS: Own
PUBLICATION LAG TIME: Not cited   STYLE SHEET: Yes, SASE
EARLY PUBLICATION OPTION: Not cited   REVISED THESES: Not cited
ACCEPTANCE RATE: Not cited   STUDENT PAPERS: Not cited
AUTHORSHIP RESTRICTIONS: Not cited   REPRINT POLICY: Not cited

SUBSCRIPTION ADDRESS: Pam Boyd, Manager
P.O. Box 717
Inverness CA 94937
ANNUAL SUBSCRIPTION RATE: $15
FREQUENCY: Quarterly   CIRCULATION: 6000
AFFILIATION: None
INDEXED/ABSTRACTED IN: Not cited

◆

JOURNAL TITLE: Michigan Nurse

MANUSCRIPT ADDRESS: The Editor
120 Spartan Avenue
E. Lansing MI 48823
TYPES OF ARTICLES: Research, review

MAJOR CONTENT AREAS: Most areas listed in Appendix A including:
All nursing areas, all age groups, allied health,
alcoholism & drug abuse, change theory, cultural
diversity, dependency, discharge planning, ethics,
family planning, instructional technology
TOPICS PREFERRED: Michigan nursing

INAPPROPRIATE TOPICS: None cited

REVIEW PROCEDURE: Editorial board
REVIEW PERIOD: 3 months
MANUSCRIPT WORD LENGTH: 3000   PAGE CHARGES: No
MANUSCRIPT COPIES: 1   STYLE REQUIREMENTS: C
PUBLICATION LAG TIME: 3 months   STYLE SHEET: Yes
EARLY PUBLICATION OPTION: Yes   REVISED THESES: Yes
ACCEPTANCE RATE: 50%   STUDENT PAPERS: Yes
AUTHORSHIP RESTRICTIONS: No   REPRINT POLICY: 5 free

SUBSCRIPTION ADDRESS: Michigan Nurse
120 Spartan Avenue
E. Lansing MI 48823
ANNUAL SUBSCRIPTION RATE: $5
FREQUENCY: 11 issues yearly   CIRCULATION: 9000
AFFILIATION: Michigan Nurses' Association
INDEXED/ABSTRACTED IN: CINAHL, INI

JOURNAL TITLE: Midwife, Health Visitor & Community Nurse

MANUSCRIPT ADDRESS: Professor N. Morris, M.D., FRCOG
Recorder House, Church Street
London N16   England

TYPES OF ARTICLES: Research, review, commentaries, theoretical, case studies, unsolicited book reviews

MAJOR CONTENT AREAS: adolescence, children, community/public health nursing, growth/development, handicapping conditions, maternal/child nursing, midwifery, parenting

TOPICS PREFERRED: Special needs and common interests of midwives, health visitors, and community nurses

INAPPROPRIATE TOPICS: None cited

REVIEW PROCEDURE: Editorial board
REVIEW PERIOD: Not cited
MANUSCRIPT WORD LENGTH: 2000 4000   **PAGE CHARGES:** Not cited
MANUSCRIPT COPIES: Not cited   **STYLE REQUIREMENTS:** Not cited
PUBLICATION LAG TIME: Not cited   **STYLE SHEET:** Not cited
EARLY PUBLICATION OPTION: Not cited   **REVISED THESES:** Not cited
ACCEPTANCE RATE: Not cited   **STUDENT PAPERS:** Not cited
AUTHORSHIP RESTRICTIONS: Not cited   **REPRINT POLICY:** Not cited

SUBSCRIPTION ADDRESS: Recorder House
Church Street
London N16.01-254 7231   England
ANNUAL SUBSCRIPTION RATE: Free to clinics and health centers; $50.00
FREQUENCY: Monthly   **CIRCULATION:** 26,000
AFFILIATION: None
INDEXED/ABSTRACTED IN: CINAHL, INI

◆

JOURNAL TITLE: Midwives Chronicle

MANUSCRIPT ADDRESS: Miss A. Graveley, Editor
98 Belsize Lane
Hampstead, London NW3 5BB   England

TYPES OF ARTICLES: Case studies, research

MAJOR CONTENT AREAS: abuse (child), children, continuity of care, family planning, genetics, handicapping conditions, health promotion, immunization, inservice education, midwifery, nursing: public health, education, research; patient teaching, primary care

TOPICS PREFERRED: Midwifery and allied subjects

INAPPROPRIATE TOPICS: None cited

REVIEW PROCEDURE: Editorial board and external review
REVIEW PERIOD: 4 weeks
MANUSCRIPT WORD LENGTH: 2000-2500   **PAGE CHARGES:** Not cited
MANUSCRIPT COPIES: 1   **STYLE REQUIREMENTS:** Not cited
PUBLICATION LAG TIME: 6 months   **STYLE SHEET:** Yes
EARLY PUBLICATION OPTION: Yes   **REVISED THESES:** Yes
ACCEPTANCE RATE: 75%   **STUDENT PAPERS:** Yes
AUTHORSHIP RESTRICTIONS: No   **REPRINT POLICY:** Author purchase

SUBSCRIPTION ADDRESS: 98 Belsize Lane
Hampstead
London NW3 5BB   England
ANNUAL SUBSCRIPTION RATE: $6
FREQUENCY: Monthly   **CIRCULATION:** 20,000
AFFILIATION: Royal College of Midwives
INDEXED/ABSTRACTED IN: CINAHL, INI

147

JOURNAL TITLE: Milbank Memorial Fund Quarterly: Health and Society

MANUSCRIPT ADDRESS: The Editor
1 East 75th Street
New York NY 10021

TYPES OF ARTICLES: Theoretical, review, national interest for policy

MAJOR CONTENT AREAS: aging & aged, change theory, cultural diversity, death, dependency, epidemiology, ethics, health promotion & policies, hospitals, mental health, nursing homes, professionalism, public health, quality of life, systems theory, women's issues

TOPICS PREFERRED: Public policy regarding health, epidemiology of illness, health services' cost-benefit & efficacy

INAPPROPRIATE TOPICS: Case studies; inter-professional turf-building

REVIEW PROCEDURE: External review
REVIEW PERIOD: 8 weeks
MANUSCRIPT WORD LENGTH: 5000-7000
MANUSCRIPT COPIES: 3
PUBLICATION LAG TIME: 6 months
EARLY PUBLICATION OPTION: Yes
ACCEPTANCE RATE: 20%
AUTHORSHIP RESTRICTIONS: No

PAGE CHARGES: No
STYLE REQUIREMENTS: C
STYLE SHEET: Yes
REVISED THESES: No
STUDENT PAPERS: No
REPRINT POLICY: 25 free

SUBSCRIPTION ADDRESS: Journals Division
MIT Press
28 Carleton Street, Cambridge MA 02142
ANNUAL SUBSCRIPTION RATE: Individuals: $20 Institutions: $40
FREQUENCY: Quarterly CIRCULATION: 3000
AFFILIATION: None
INDEXED/ABSTRACTED IN: IM, MCR, BA, CA, CC, NAR, PAIS, SSCI

◆

JOURNAL TITLE: Mineral and Electrolyte Metabolism

MANUSCRIPT ADDRESS: Shaul G. Massry, M.D., University of Southern California, School of Medicine
2025 Zonal Avenue, Los Angeles CA 90033

TYPES OF ARTICLES: Research, review, case studies

MAJOR CONTENT AREAS: physiology, biochemistry, biomedical research, circulatory diseases, medicine, nutrition, pharmmacology

TOPICS PREFERRED: Fluid, electrolytes, minerals, hormones, bone, vitamins, kidney & endocrine glands, trace metals

INAPPROPRIATE TOPICS: None cited

REVIEW PROCEDURE: Editorial board and external review
REVIEW PERIOD: 2 months
MANUSCRIPT WORD LENGTH: 3000-4000
MANUSCRIPT COPIES: 3
PUBLICATION LAG TIME: 5-6 months
EARLY PUBLICATION OPTION: No
ACCEPTANCE RATE: 40%
AUTHORSHIP RESTRICTIONS: No

PAGE CHARGES: Yes
STYLE REQUIREMENTS: Own
STYLE SHEET: Yes
REVISED THESES: No
STUDENT PAPERS: No
REPRINT POLICY: None free

SUBSCRIPTION ADDRESS: S. Karger AG.
Arnold-Bocklin Strasse 25
CH-4011 Basel Switzerland
ANNUAL SUBSCRIPTION RATE: Individuals: $48.00 Institutions: $96
FREQUENCY: Monthly CIRCULATION: 1000
AFFILIATION: None
INDEXED/ABSTRACTED IN: CC

JOURNAL TITLE: Modern Healthcare

MANUSCRIPT ADDRESS: Donald E.L. Johnson, Editor
Crain Communications, Inc.
740 Rush Street, Chicago IL 60611

TYPES OF ARTICLES: Commentaries

MAJOR CONTENT AREAS: health policies, hospitals, nursing service
administration

TOPICS PREFERRED: Staffing, classification of patients

INAPPROPRIATE TOPICS: Case studies

REVIEW PROCEDURE: Editors
REVIEW PERIOD: 1-3 months
MANUSCRIPT WORD LENGTH: 700
MANUSCRIPT COPIES: 2
PUBLICATION LAG TIME: 1 month
EARLY PUBLICATION OPTION: Not cited
ACCEPTANCE RATE: 2-3%
AUTHORSHIP RESTRICTIONS: No

PAGE CHARGES: No
STYLE REQUIREMENTS: NT, AP
STYLE SHEET: Yes
REVISED THESES: Yes
STUDENT PAPERS: Yes
REPRINT POLICY: 2-3 free journals

SUBSCRIPTION ADDRESS: Circulation Department
740 Rush Street
Chicago IL 60611

ANNUAL SUBSCRIPTION RATE: $25
FREQUENCY: Monthly
AFFILIATION: None
INDEXED/ABSTRACTED IN: HLI, CINAHL, IPA, IM, INI

CIRCULATION: 65,000

JOURNAL TITLE: NATNEWS

MANUSCRIPT ADDRESS: Newton Mann Ltd.
Sherwood House
Matlock   Derbyshire   DE4 3LT   England
TYPES OF ARTICLES: Research, theoretical, case studies, commentaries

MAJOR CONTENT AREAS: anesthesiology, continuing education, inservice
education, nursing: assessment, audit, care,
education, history, process, research, operating
room, orthopedic, pediatric, surgical; pain,
professionalism, teaching/learning
TOPICS PREFERRED: Topics relating to the operating department

INAPPROPRIATE TOPICS: None cited

REVIEW PROCEDURE: Editorial board
REVIEW PERIOD: 2-3 weeks
MANUSCRIPT WORD LENGTH: 2000   **PAGE CHARGES:** No
MANUSCRIPT COPIES: 2   **STYLE REQUIREMENTS:** None cited
PUBLICATION LAG TIME: 6-12 weeks   **STYLE SHEET:** Yes
EARLY PUBLICATION OPTION: Yes   **REVISED THESES:** No
ACCEPTANCE RATE: 70-85%   **STUDENT PAPERS:** Yes
AUTHORSHIP RESTRICTIONS: No   **REPRINT POLICY:** Author purchase

SUBSCRIPTION ADDRESS: Newton Mann Ltd.
Sherwood House
Matlock   Derbyshire   DE4   3LT   England
ANNUAL SUBSCRIPTION RATE: $20
FREQUENCY: Monthly   **CIRCULATION:** 3000
AFFILIATION: National Association of Theatre Nurses
INDEXED/ABSTRACTED IN: CINAHL, INI

JOURNAL TITLE: Neuroscience

MANUSCRIPT ADDRESS: Dr. A.D. Smith
University Department of Pharmacology
South Parks Road, Oxford   OX1   3QT   England
TYPES OF ARTICLES: Research, review, commentaries

MAJOR CONTENT AREAS: anatomy and physiology, biology, biomedical
research, natural science, pharmacology, psychopathology

TOPICS PREFERRED: Nervous system and neurology

INAPPROPRIATE TOPICS: None cited

REVIEW PROCEDURE: Editorial board and external review
REVIEW PERIOD: 6 weeks
MANUSCRIPT WORD LENGTH: 3000-10,000   **PAGE CHARGES:** No
MANUSCRIPT COPIES: 3   **STYLE REQUIREMENTS:** CBE
PUBLICATION LAG TIME: 4 months   **STYLE SHEET:** Yes
EARLY PUBLICATION OPTION: No   **REVISED THESES:** No
ACCEPTANCE RATE: 35%   **STUDENT PAPERS:** No
AUTHORSHIP RESTRICTIONS: No   **REPRINT POLICY:** 25 free

SUBSCRIPTION ADDRESS: Pergamon Press, Inc.
Maxwell House, Fairview Park, Elmsford
New York   NY   10523
ANNUAL SUBSCRIPTION RATE: Members: $50   Institutions: $400
FREQUENCY: Monthly   **CIRCULATION:** 1200
AFFILIATION: International Brain Research Organization
INDEXED/ABSTRACTED IN: CC, IM, BA

JOURNAL TITLE: The New England Journal of Medicine

MANUSCRIPT ADDRESS: 10 Shattuck Street
Boston MA 02115

TYPES OF ARTICLES: Research, theoretical, review, case studies, commentaries
MAJOR CONTENT AREAS: clinical-scientific appealing to internal medicine thinking physician

TOPICS PREFERRED: None cited

INAPPROPRIATE TOPICS: None cited

REVIEW PROCEDURE: Editorial board and external review
REVIEW PERIOD: 2-6 weeks
MANUSCRIPT WORD LENGTH: Varies
MANUSCRIPT COPIES: 2
PUBLICATION LAG TIME: Not cited
EARLY PUBLICATION OPTION: No
ACCEPTANCE RATE: 8-10%
AUTHORSHIP RESTRICTIONS: No
PAGE CHARGES: No
STYLE REQUIREMENTS: CBE
STYLE SHEET: Yes
REVISED THESES: No
STUDENT PAPERS: No
REPRINT POLICY: None free

SUBSCRIPTION ADDRESS: The New England Journal of Medicine
10 Shattuck Street
Boston MA 02115
ANNUAL SUBSCRIPTION RATE: $48
FREQUENCY: Weekly
CIRCULATION: 196,000
AFFILIATION: Massachusetts Medical Society
INDEXED/ABSTRACTED IN: BA, CA, CINAHL, HLI, IPA, IM, INI, NAR, PA

◆

JOURNAL TITLE: New York State Journal of Medicine

MANUSCRIPT ADDRESS: The Editor
420 Lakeville Rd.
Lake Success NY 11042
TYPES OF ARTICLES: Research, review, commentaries, case studies

MAJOR CONTENT AREAS: Most areas listed in Appendix A including: abuse, continuity of care, continuing education, emergency services, epidemiology, ethics, health promotion, medicine, mental health, nursing education, patient teaching, public health, quality of life
TOPICS PREFERRED: Topics pertaining to practice of medicine

INAPPROPRIATE TOPICS: None cited

REVIEW PROCEDURE: Editorial board
REVIEW PERIOD: 2 months
MANUSCRIPT WORD LENGTH: 4000
MANUSCRIPT COPIES: 2
PUBLICATION LAG TIME: 3 months
EARLY PUBLICATION OPTION: No
ACCEPTANCE RATE: 60%
AUTHORSHIP RESTRICTIONS: No
PAGE CHARGES: No
STYLE REQUIREMENTS: AMA, C, IM
STYLE SHEET: Yes
REVISED THESES: Not cited
STUDENT PAPERS: No
REPRINT POLICY: None free

SUBSCRIPTION ADDRESS: New York State Journal of Medicine
420 Lakeville Rd.
Lake Success NY 11042
ANNUAL SUBSCRIPTION RATE: $3.50
FREQUENCY: Monthly
CIRCULATION: 29,000
AFFILIATION: Medical Society of the State of New York
INDEXED/ABSTRACTED IN: BA, CA, HLI, IM, INI, PA

JOURNAL TITLE: New Zealand Nursing Journal

MANUSCRIPT ADDRESS: P.O. Box 2128
Wellington
New Zealand
TYPES OF ARTICLES: Case studies

MAJOR CONTENT AREAS: communication, midwifery, nursing: care, critical care, diagnosis, geriatric, maternal/child, medical/ surgical, neurological, occupational health, operating room, orthopedic, pediatric, psychiatric, public health; pain, primary care
TOPICS PREFERRED: None cited

INAPPROPRIATE TOPICS: None cited

REVIEW PROCEDURE: Editorial board
REVIEW PERIOD: 2 months
MANUSCRIPT WORD LENGTH: 2000-3000   **PAGE CHARGES:** No
MANUSCRIPT COPIES: 2   **STYLE REQUIREMENTS:** Not cited
PUBLICATION LAG TIME: 6-9 months   **STYLE SHEET:** No
EARLY PUBLICATION OPTION: No   **REVISED THESES:** No
ACCEPTANCE RATE: 75%   **STUDENT PAPERS:** Yes
AUTHORSHIP RESTRICTIONS: No   **REPRINT POLICY:** 1 free

SUBSCRIPTION ADDRESS: P.O. Box 2128
Wellington
New Zealand
ANNUAL SUBSCRIPTION RATE: $27.00
FREQUENCY: Monthly   **CIRCULATION:** 12,750
AFFILIATION: New Zealand Nurses' Association
INDEXED/ABSTRACTED IN: CINAHL, INI

JOURNAL TITLE: The Nigerian Nurse

MANUSCRIPT ADDRESS: P.O. Box 60, Suoulere
Lagos
Nigeria, Africa
TYPES OF ARTICLES: Case studies, research, theoretical, review, commentaries, unsolicited book reviews
MAJOR CONTENT AREAS: Most areas listed in Appendix A including all nursing areas, age groups, diseases & disorders, health professions, treatment modalities, education topics; professionalism, quality of life, ethics, research methodology, women's issues
TOPICS PREFERRED: Medical, nursing and allied professions

INAPPROPRIATE TOPICS: None cited

REVIEW PROCEDURE: Editorial Board and external review
REVIEW PERIOD: 6-12 weeks
MANUSCRIPT WORD LENGTH: 2000-3000   **PAGE CHARGES:** Yes
MANUSCRIPT COPIES: 2   **STYLE REQUIREMENTS:** Not cited
PUBLICATION LAG TIME: 6-24 months   **STYLE SHEET:** Yes
EARLY PUBLICATION OPTION: Yes   **REVISED THESES:** Yes
ACCEPTANCE RATE: 75%   **STUDENT PAPERS:** Yes
AUTHORSHIP RESTRICTIONS: No   **REPRINT POLICY:** 2 free

SUBSCRIPTION ADDRESS: Nigerian Nurse
P.O. Box 60, Suoulere
Lagos, Nigeria, Africa
ANNUAL SUBSCRIPTION RATE: $13.50
FREQUENCY: Quarterly   **CIRCULATION:** 10,000
AFFILIATION: National Association of Nigeria Nurses & Midwives
INDEXED/ABSTRACTED IN: INI, CINAHL

JOURNAL TITLE: NITA

MANUSCRIPT ADDRESS: Mary Larkin, Editor
93 Concord Avenue, Suite 4
Belmont MA 02178
TYPES OF ARTICLES: Research, theoretical, review, case studies,
commentaries, unsolicited book reviews
MAJOR CONTENT AREAS: Many areas listed in Appendix A including:
nursing: assessment, audit, care, clinical
specialties, critical care, geriatric,
medical/surgical, neurological, pediatric,
philosophy, research, science, theory, trauma
TOPICS PREFERRED: Intravenous therapy

INAPPROPRIATE TOPICS: None cited

REVIEW PROCEDURE: Editorial board
REVIEW PERIOD: 3 months
MANUSCRIPT WORD LENGTH: Not cited   PAGE CHARGES: No
MANUSCRIPT COPIES: 3   STYLE REQUIREMENTS: CBE, Own
PUBLICATION LAG TIME: 6-12 months   STYLE SHEET: Yes
EARLY PUBLICATION OPTION: No   REVISED THESES: No
ACCEPTANCE RATE: 65-80%   STUDENT PAPERS: No
AUTHORSHIP RESTRICTIONS: No   REPRINT POLICY: None free

SUBSCRIPTION ADDRESS: Lippincott/Harper
2350 Virginia Avenue
Hagerstown MD 21740
ANNUAL SUBSCRIPTION RATE: $35
FREQUENCY: Bimonthly   CIRCULATION: 5000
AFFILIATION: National Intravenous Therapy Association
INDEXED/ABSTRACTED IN: CINAHL

◆

JOURNAL TITLE: Nurse Educator

MANUSCRIPT ADDRESS: 12 Lakeside Park
607 North Avenue
Wakefield MA 01880
TYPES OF ARTICLES: Thoorotical, commentaries, research, review

MAJOR CONTENT AREAS: continuing education, health promotion, inservice
education, instructional technology, nursing
assessment, nursing diagnosis, nursing education,
nursing research, research methodology

TOPICS PREFERRED: Innovations in nursing education: evaluation,
current issues, discussion of teaching strategies
INAPPROPRIATE TOPICS: Descriptions of "new" course which is not very
significant; "my personal experience"
REVIEW PROCEDURE: Editorial board and external review
REVIEW PERIOD: 6 weeks
MANUSCRIPT WORD LENGTH: 2500-5000   PAGE CHARGES: No
MANUSCRIPT COPIES: 3   STYLE REQUIREMENTS: C
PUBLICATION LAG TIME: 6-12 months   STYLE SHEET: Yes
EARLY PUBLICATION OPTION: Yes   REVISED THESES: Yes
ACCEPTANCE RATE: 10%   STUDENT PAPERS: No
AUTHORSHIP RESTRICTIONS: No   REPRINT POLICY: 2 free journals

SUBSCRIPTION ADDRESS: Subscription Services
12 Lakeside Park, 607 North Avenue
Wakefield MA 01880
ANNUAL SUBSCRIPTION RATE: $15
FREQUENCY: 7 times yearly   CIRCULATION: 32,000
AFFILIATION: None
INDEXED/ABSTRACTED IN: INI, CINAHL, CIJE, HLI

JOURNAL TITLE: Nurse Practitioner: The American Journal of
Primary Health Care

MANUSCRIPT ADDRESS: Editorial Director, Cynthia Jo Leitch
109 W. Mercer, C-19081
Seattle WA 98119

TYPES OF ARTICLES: Clinical, theoretical, review, research

MAJOR CONTENT AREAS: Most areas in Appendix A: nursing: assessment,
audit, care, diagnosis, geriatric, maternal/child,
medical/surgical, occupational, office, orthopedic, pediatric, psychiatric, public health, philosophy, process, research, science, theory, trauma

TOPICS PREFERRED: Major focus is on clinical information & practice
issues for the nurse in primary/ambulatory care

INAPPROPRIATE TOPICS: First person articles, humor, non scientific
papers

REVIEW PROCEDURE: Editorial board and external review

REVIEW PERIOD: 6-8 weeks

MANUSCRIPT WORD LENGTH: 2500-3000	**PAGE CHARGES:** No	
MANUSCRIPT COPIES: 3	**STYLE REQUIREMENTS:** Own	
PUBLICATION LAG TIME: 3-18 months	**STYLE SHEET:** Yes	
EARLY PUBLICATION OPTION: Not cited	**REVISED THESES:** Yes	
ACCEPTANCE RATE: 30-40%	**STUDENT PAPERS:** Yes	
AUTHORSHIP RESTRICTIONS: No	**REPRINT POLICY:** None free	

SUBSCRIPTION ADDRESS: Vernon Publications, Inc.
109 W. Mercer, C-19081
Seattle WA 98119

ANNUAL SUBSCRIPTION RATE: $23

FREQUENCY: Bimonthly   **CIRCULATION:** 5000

AFFILIATION: None

INDEXED/ABSTRACTED IN: CINAHL, INI, IM, HLI, IPA

JOURNAL TITLE: Nursing '81 [Title changes yearly]

MANUSCRIPT ADDRESS: Intermed Communications, Inc.
1111 Bethlehem Pike
Springhouse PA 19477

TYPES OF ARTICLES: Clinical "how-to" articles of interest to nurses

MAJOR CONTENT AREAS: Most areas listed in Appendix A: nursing: all
specialty areas, assessment, audit, care,
diagnosis, education, process, theory; patient
teaching, professionalism, health promotion,
hospitals, inservice education, leadership

TOPICS PREFERRED: Specific health problems or diseases with emphasis on nursing problems and their solution

INAPPROPRIATE TOPICS: None cited

REVIEW PROCEDURE: Editorial board and external review

REVIEW PERIOD: 6-8 weeks

MANUSCRIPT WORD LENGTH: 1400-4000	**PAGE CHARGES:** No	
MANUSCRIPT COPIES: 1	**STYLE REQUIREMENTS:** AMA	
PUBLICATION LAG TIME: Within 1 year	**STYLE SHEET:** Yes	
EARLY PUBLICATION OPTION: No	**REVISED THESES:** No	
ACCEPTANCE RATE: Not cited	**STUDENT PAPERS:** No	
AUTHORSHIP RESTRICTIONS: Primarily nurses	**REPRINT POLICY:** Author purchase	

SUBSCRIPTION ADDRESS: Fulfillment Department
1111 Bethlehem Pike
Springhouse PA 19477

ANNUAL SUBSCRIPTION RATE: $20

FREQUENCY: Monthly   **CIRCULATION:** 500,000

AFFILIATION: None

INDEXED/ABSTRACTED IN: CINAHL, HLI, INI

JOURNAL TITLE: Nursing Administation Quarterly

MANUSCRIPT ADDRESS: Aspen Systems Corporation
1600 Research Blvd.
Rockville MD 20850
TYPES OF ARTICLES: Case studies, applied research, commentaries

MAJOR CONTENT AREAS: nursing service administration

TOPICS PREFERRED: Nursing administration, management oriented

INAPPROPRIATE TOPICS: None cited

REVIEW PROCEDURE: Editorial board	
REVIEW PERIOD: 30-60 days	
MANUSCRIPT WORD LENGTH: 4500-6000	**PAGE CHARGES:** No
MANUSCRIPT COPIES: 3	**STYLE REQUIREMENTS:** C
PUBLICATION LAG TIME: 2-4 months	**STYLE SHEET:** Yes
EARLY PUBLICATION OPTION: No	**REVISED THESES:** No
ACCEPTANCE RATE: 1%	**STUDENT PAPERS:** No
AUTHORSHIP RESTRICTIONS: No	**REPRINT POLICY:** Author purchase

SUBSCRIPTION ADDRESS: Aspen Systems Corporation
16792 Oakmont Avenue
Gaithersburg MD 20877
ANNUAL SUBSCRIPTION RATE: $34.00
FREQUENCY: Quarterly   **CIRCULATION:** 5000
AFFILIATION: None
INDEXED/ABSTRACTED IN: CINAHL, INI

◆

JOURNAL TITLE: Nursing Careers

MANUSCRIPT ADDRESS: P.O. Box 617
Encino CA 91426

TYPES OF ARTICLES: Case studies, review, commentaries, theoretical,
research, unsolicited book reviews
MAJOR CONTENT AREAS: nursing: clinical specialties, community/public
health, critical care, education, geriatric,
history, occupational, operating room, orthopedic,
pediatric, philosophy, process, psychiatric/mental
health, school, service administration, theory
TOPICS PREFERRED: Career development/advancement

INAPPROPRIATE TOPICS: None cited

REVIEW PROCEDURE: Editorial board	
REVIEW PERIOD: 3 weeks	
MANUSCRIPT WORD LENGTH: 1000-1500	**PAGE CHARGES:** No
MANUSCRIPT COPIES: 2	**STYLE REQUIREMENTS:** Not cited
PUBLICATION LAG TIME: 2-3 months	**STYLE SHEET:** Yes
EARLY PUBLICATION OPTION: Not cited	**REVISED THESES:** No
ACCEPTANCE RATE: Not cited	**STUDENT PAPERS:** Yes
AUTHORSHIP RESTRICTIONS: No	**REPRINT POLICY:** Some free

SUBSCRIPTION ADDRESS: Nursing Careers
P.O. Box 617
Encino CA 91426
ANNUAL SUBSCRIPTION RATE: $18
FREQUENCY: Monthly   **CIRCULATION:** 100,000
AFFILIATION: None
INDEXED/ABSTRACTED IN: New publication

JOURNAL TITLE: Nursing Clinics of North America

MANUSCRIPT ADDRESS: Adele L. Morse,Editor
W.B. Saunders Company
W. Washington Square, Philadelphia PA 19105
TYPES OF ARTICLES: Clinical, practical reference; case studies

MAJOR CONTENT AREAS: nursing: assessment, audit, care, clinical
specialties, diagnosis, education, geriatric,
maternal/child, medical/surgical, neurological,
process, service administration, occupational,
OR, orthopedic, pediatric, psychiatric, trauma
TOPICS PREFERRED: Individual articles are not accepted, a symposium
format is used
INAPPROPRIATE TOPICS: Research; theory; reviews of literature; theses

REVIEW PROCEDURE: Editorial board
REVIEW PERIOD: 1 week
MANUSCRIPT WORD LENGTH: 3000-4000   PAGE CHARGES: No
MANUSCRIPT COPIES: 1   STYLE REQUIREMENTS: C
PUBLICATION LAG TIME: 1 year   STYLE SHEET: Yes
EARLY PUBLICATION OPTION: No   REVISED THESES: No
ACCEPTANCE RATE: 1%   STUDENT PAPERS: No
AUTHORSHIP RESTRICTIONS: No   REPRINT POLICY: 100 free

SUBSCRIPTION ADDRESS: W.B. Saunders Company
W. Washington Square
Philadelphia PA 19105
ANNUAL SUBSCRIPTION RATE: $20
FREQUENCY: Quarterly   CIRCULATION: 25,000
AFFILIATION: None
INDEXED/ABSTRACTED IN: CA, CINAHL, HLI, IM, INI

◆

JOURNAL TITLE: Nursing Dimensions Series †

MANUSCRIPT ADDRESS: 12 Lakeside Park
Wakefield MA 01880

TYPES OF ARTICLES: Guest editor compiles several articles focusing on
single topic
MAJOR CONTENT AREAS: nursing: assesssment, audit, care, clinical
specialties, diagnosis, education, history, philosophy, process, research, science, service administration, theory; health promotion & policies,
patient teaching, primary care, quality of life
TOPICS PREFERRED: None cited

INAPPROPRIATE TOPICS: None cited

REVIEW PROCEDURE: Editorial board and external review
REVIEW PERIOD: 2 weeks
MANUSCRIPT WORD LENGTH: Not applicable   PAGE CHARGES: No
MANUSCRIPT COPIES: 1   STYLE REQUIREMENTS: C
PUBLICATION LAG TIME: 6 months   STYLE SHEET: No
EARLY PUBLICATION OPTION: No   REVISED THESES: Yes
ACCEPTANCE RATE: Not applicable   STUDENT PAPERS: No
AUTHORSHIP RESTRICTIONS: No   REPRINT POLICY: 2 free

SUBSCRIPTION ADDRESS: The Nursing Dimensions Series
12 Lakeside Park
Wakefield MA 01880
ANNUAL SUBSCRIPTION RATE: $12
FREQUENCY: Quarterly   CIRCULATION: 9000
AFFILIATION: None
INDEXED/ABSTRACTED IN: CINAHL

JOURNAL TITLE: Nursing Focus

MANUSCRIPT ADDRESS: The Newbourne Group
91 Stoke Newington Church St.
London N16 OAU England
TYPES OF ARTICLES: Research, theoretical, book reviews

MAJOR CONTENT AREAS: Most areas listed in Appendix A

TOPICS PREFERRED: None cited

INAPPROPRIATE TOPICS: None cited

REVIEW PROCEDURE: Editorial board		
REVIEW PERIOD: New journal		
MANUSCRIPT WORD LENGTH: 2500	**PAGE CHARGES:** None cited	
MANUSCRIPT COPIES: 3	**STYLE REQUIREMENTS:** Own	
PUBLICATION LAG TIME: New journal	**STYLE SHEET:** Not cited	
EARLY PUBLICATION OPTION: Not cited	**REVISED THESES:** Not cited	
ACCEPTANCE RATE: New journal	**STUDENT PAPERS:** Not cited	
AUTHORSHIP RESTRICTIONS: No	**REPRINT POLICY:** Not cited	

SUBSCRIPTION ADDRESS: The Newbourne Group
91 Stoke Newington Church St.
London N16 OAU England
ANNUAL SUBSCRIPTION RATE: $30
FREQUENCY: monthly   **CIRCULATION:** New journal
AFFILIATION: None
INDEXED/ABSTRACTED IN: INI, CINAHL

◆

JOURNAL TITLE: Nursing Forum

MANUSCRIPT ADDRESS: Nursing Publications, Inc.
Box 218
Hillsdale NJ 07642
TYPES OF ARTICLES: Theoretical, research, clinical papers including
theory, review articles, unsolicited book reviews
MAJOR CONTENT AREAS: Nearly all areas listed in Appendix A

TOPICS PREFERRED: None cited

INAPPROPRIATE TOPICS: None

REVIEW PROCEDURE: Editorial board and external review		
REVIEW PERIOD: 4 months		
MANUSCRIPT WORD LENGTH: 4000	**PAGE CHARGES:** No	
MANUSCRIPT COPIES: 3	**STYLE REQUIREMENTS:** C, NT	
PUBLICATION LAG TIME: 6-12 months	**STYLE SHEET:** Yes	
EARLY PUBLICATION OPTION: No	**REVISED THESES:** Yes	
ACCEPTANCE RATE: 5%	**STUDENT PAPERS:** Yes	
AUTHORSHIP RESTRICTIONS: No	**REPRINT POLICY:** 6 free journals	

SUBSCRIPTION ADDRESS: Nursing Publications, Inc.
Box 218
Hillsdale NJ 07642
ANNUAL SUBSCRIPTION RATE: Individuals: $15   Institutions: $18
FREQUENCY: Quarterly   **CIRCULATION:** 6000
AFFILIATION: None
INDEXED/ABSTRACTED IN: CINAHL, INI, IM, HLI

JOURNAL TITLE: Nursing and Health Care

MANUSCRIPT ADDRESS: 265 Post Road West
Westport CT 06880

TYPES OF ARTICLES: Research, theoretical, review, case studies

MAJOR CONTENT AREAS: nursing: audit, community/public health,
diagnosis, education, history, philosophy, process,
research, science, service administration, theory;
public policy, legislation, business management
as they pertain to nursing and to health care

TOPICS PREFERRED: Nursing and health care

INAPPROPRIATE TOPICS: None cited (new journal)

REVIEW PROCEDURE:	Editorial board		
REVIEW PERIOD:	2 months		
MANUSCRIPT WORD LENGTH:	3600-4200	**PAGE CHARGES:**	No
MANUSCRIPT COPIES:	2	**STYLE REQUIREMENTS:**	IM
PUBLICATION LAG TIME:	Not cited (new)	**STYLE SHEET:**	Yes
EARLY PUBLICATION OPTION:	No	**REVISED THESES:**	Yes
ACCEPTANCE RATE:	New Journal	**STUDENT PAPERS:**	New journal
AUTHORSHIP RESTRICTIONS:	No	**REPRINT POLICY:**	100 free

SUBSCRIPTION ADDRESS: 265 Post Road West
Westport CT 06880

ANNUAL SUBSCRIPTION RATE:	$15		
FREQUENCY:	10 times yearly	**CIRCULATION:**	22,000
AFFILIATION:	National League for Nursing		
INDEXED/ABSTRACTED IN:	CINAHL		

JOURNAL TITLE: Nursing Homes

MANUSCRIPT ADDRESS: 4000 Albemarle St., N.W.
Washington DC 20016

TYPES OF ARTICLES: Not cited

MAJOR CONTENT AREAS: government relations, housekeeping, dietetics,
nursing, architecture, medicine, dentistry,
pharmacy, administration, rehabilitation and
social services

TOPICS PREFERRED: Topics of interest to administrators of nursing/
convalescent homes, retirement centers

INAPPROPRIATE TOPICS: None cited

REVIEW PROCEDURE:	Editorial board		
REVIEW PERIOD:	Not cited		
MANUSCRIPT WORD LENGTH:	Not cited	**PAGE CHARGES:**	Not cited
MANUSCRIPT COPIES:	Not cited	**STYLE REQUIREMENTS:**	Own
PUBLICATION LAG TIME:	Not cited	**STYLE SHEET:**	Not cited
EARLY PUBLICATION OPTION:	Not cited	**REVISED THESES:**	Not cited
ACCEPTANCE RATE:	Not cited	**STUDENT PAPERS:**	Not cited
AUTHORSHIP RESTRICTIONS:	Not cited	**REPRINT POLICY:**	Not cited

SUBSCRIPTION ADDRESS: Heldref Publications
4000 Albemarle St., N.W.
Washington DC 20016

ANNUAL SUBSCRIPTION RATE:	$20		
FREQUENCY:	Bimonthly	**CIRCULATION:**	5000
AFFILIATION:	American College of Nursing Home Administrators		
INDEXED/ABSTRACTED IN:	CINAHL, HLI, IPA, RL		

JOURNAL TITLE: Nursing Insights

MANUSCRIPT ADDRESS: Colleen V. Trody, R.N., M.S., Editor
Creative Nursing Publications
1 Adler Drive, East Syracuse NY 13057
TYPES OF ARTICLES: Self-instructional materials for continuing education units
MAJOR CONTENT AREAS: Many areas listed in Appendix A including:
nursing: assessment, audit, care, community/public
health, critical care, diagnosis, geriatric,
maternal/child, medical/surgical, psychiatric/
mental health, research, school, theory, trauma
TOPICS PREFERRED: Continuing education for nurses; each issue
offers nurses opportunity to earn .5 CEU
INAPPROPRIATE TOPICS: Manuscripts solicited

REVIEW PROCEDURE: Editorial board
REVIEW PERIOD: 3 months
MANUSCRIPT WORD LENGTH: Not applicable   PAGE CHARGES: No
MANUSCRIPT COPIES: 3   STYLE REQUIREMENTS: AMA
PUBLICATION LAG TIME: 1 year   STYLE SHEET: Yes
EARLY PUBLICATION OPTION: No   REVISED THESES: No
ACCEPTANCE RATE: Solicited   STUDENT PAPERS: No
AUTHORSHIP RESTRICTIONS: Yes   REPRINT POLICY: 10 free

SUBSCRIPTION ADDRESS: Creative Nursing Publications, Inc.
1 Adler Drive
East Syracuse NY 13057
ANNUAL SUBSCRIPTION RATE: $15
FREQUENCY: Monthly   CIRCULATION: New publication
AFFILIATION: None
INDEXED/ABSTRACTED IN: New publication

◆

JOURNAL TITLE: The Nursing Journal of Singapore

MANUSCRIPT ADDRESS: 129-B, Block 23
Outram Park Complex
Singapore 3
TYPES OF ARTICLES: Theoretical, research

MAJOR CONTENT AREAS: Many areas listed in Appendix A including:
nursing: assessment, audit, care, education,
occupational health, operating room, orthopedic,
pediatric, process, psychiatric/mental health,
research, school, service administration, trauma
TOPICS PREFERRED: Advances and trends in medicine and nursing

INAPPROPRIATE TOPICS: None

REVIEW PROCEDURE: Editorial board
REVIEW PERIOD: Manuscripts solicited
MANUSCRIPT WORD LENGTH: 1500-2000   PAGE CHARGES: No
MANUSCRIPT COPIES: 1   STYLE REQUIREMENTS: None
PUBLICATION LAG TIME: 6 months   STYLE SHEET: Yes
EARLY PUBLICATION OPTION: No   REVISED THESES: No
ACCEPTANCE RATE: 90%   STUDENT PAPERS: Yes
AUTHORSHIP RESTRICTIONS: No   REPRINT POLICY: 25 free

SUBSCRIPTION ADDRESS: No subscription orders; complimentary to
nursing school libraries and professional
associations
ANNUAL SUBSCRIPTION RATE:
FREQUENCY: Biyearly   CIRCULATION: 2000
AFFILIATION: None
INDEXED/ABSTRACTED IN: INI, CINAHL

JOURNAL TITLE: Nursing Law & Ethics †

MANUSCRIPT ADDRESS: 765 Commonwealth Avenue
16th Floor
Boston MA 02215

TYPES OF ARTICLES: Commentaries, unsolicited book reviews

MAJOR CONTENT AREAS: nursing law and ethics

TOPICS PREFERRED: Articles involving law, ethics & nursing practice

INAPPROPRIATE TOPICS: None cited

REVIEW PROCEDURE: Editorial board
REVIEW PERIOD: 3-4 months
MANUSCRIPT WORD LENGTH: Not cited
MANUSCRIPT COPIES: 2
PUBLICATION LAG TIME: 2-3 months
EARLY PUBLICATION OPTION: No
ACCEPTANCE RATE: 30%
AUTHORSHIP RESTRICTIONS: No

PAGE CHARGES: No
STYLE REQUIREMENTS: IM
STYLE SHEET: Yes
REVISED THESES: Yes
STUDENT PAPERS: May submit
REPRINT POLICY: 3 free

SUBSCRIPTION ADDRESS: 765 Commonwealth Avenue
16th Floor
Boston MA 02215

ANNUAL SUBSCRIPTION RATE: $30
FREQUENCY: Bimonthly
AFFILIATION: American Society of Law and Medicine
INDEXED/ABSTRACTED IN: New journal

CIRCULATION: 2000

◆

JOURNAL TITLE: Nursing Leadership

MANUSCRIPT ADDRESS: Charles B. Slack, Inc.
6900 Grove Rd.
Thorofare NJ 08086

TYPES OF ARTICLES: Research, theoretical

MAJOR CONTENT AREAS: Any nursing subject that denotes leadership

TOPICS PREFERRED: None cited

INAPPROPRIATE TOPICS: None cited

REVIEW PROCEDURE: Editorial board
REVIEW PERIOD: 6 weeks or less
MANUSCRIPT WORD LENGTH: 3000
MANUSCRIPT COPIES: 2
PUBLICATION LAG TIME: 2 months
EARLY PUBLICATION OPTION: Yes
ACCEPTANCE RATE: Not cited
AUTHORSHIP RESTRICTIONS: No

PAGE CHARGES: No
STYLE REQUIREMENTS: AMA
STYLE SHEET: Yes
REVISED THESES: No
STUDENT PAPERS: Yes
REPRINT POLICY: None free

SUBSCRIPTION ADDRESS: Charles B. Slack, Inc.
6900 Grove Rd.
Thorofare NJ 08086

ANNUAL SUBSCRIPTION RATE: $12
FREQUENCY: Quarterly
AFFILIATION: None
INDEXED/ABSTRACTED IN: INI, CINAHL

CIRCULATION: 3000

JOURNAL TITLE: Nursing Mirror

MANUSCRIPT ADDRESS: Surrey House
1 Throwley Way
Sutton, Surrey, SM1 4QQ England
TYPES OF ARTICLES: Case studies, commentaries, review, research
theoretical, unsolicited book reviews
MAJOR CONTENT AREAS: Most areas listed in Appendix A including:
nursing: assessment, care, clinical specialties,
diagnosis, education, history, philosophy,
process, research, science, service
administration, theory; midwifery
TOPICS PREFERRED: Nursing/midwifery

INAPPROPRIATE TOPICS: Non-nursing articles

REVIEW PROCEDURE: Editors decision
REVIEW PERIOD: Short time
MANUSCRIPT WORD LENGTH: 1500-2000   **PAGE CHARGES:** No
MANUSCRIPT COPIES: 1   **STYLE REQUIREMENTS:** Own
PUBLICATION LAG TIME: 1-6 months   **STYLE SHEET:** No
EARLY PUBLICATION OPTION: No   **REVISED THESES:** No
ACCEPTANCE RATE: 10%   **STUDENT PAPERS:** Yes
AUTHORSHIP RESTRICTIONS: No   **REPRINT POLICY:** None free

SUBSCRIPTION ADDRESS: Oakfield House
Perryimount Road
Haywards Heath, Sussex RH16 3DH   England
ANNUAL SUBSCRIPTION RATE: $78.00
FREQUENCY: Weekly   **CIRCULATION:** 60,000
AFFILIATION: None
INDEXED/ABSTRACTED IN: CINAHL, HLI, INI

◆

JOURNAL TITLE: Nursing Outlook

MANUSCRIPT ADDRESS: American Journal of Nursing Company
555 West 57th Street
New York NY 10019
TYPES OF ARTICLES: Theoretical, trends and issues in professional
nursing, commentaries, research
MAJOR CONTENT AREAS: Many areas listed in Appendix A including: nursing:
assessment, audit, public health, education, his-
tory, philosophy, process, research, science, service administration, theory; primary care, profes-
ionalism, teaching/learning, women's issues
TOPICS PREFERRED: Trends and issues in the nursing profession

INAPPROPRIATE TOPICS: Clinical, direct patient care articles

REVIEW PROCEDURE: Editorial staff (nurses), external review
REVIEW PERIOD: 6-8 weeks
MANUSCRIPT WORD LENGTH: 3000-5000   **PAGE CHARGES:** No
MANUSCRIPT COPIES: 2   **STYLE REQUIREMENTS:** C
PUBLICATION LAG TIME: 4-6 months   **STYLE SHEET:** Yes
EARLY PUBLICATION OPTION: No   **REVISED THESES:** No
ACCEPTANCE RATE: 10-12%   **STUDENT PAPERS:** No
AUTHORSHIP RESTRICTIONS: No   **REPRINT POLICY:** 100 free

SUBSCRIPTION ADDRESS: American Journal of Nursing Company
555 West 57th Street
New York NY 10019
ANNUAL SUBSCRIPTION RATE: $17
FREQUENCY: Monthly   **CIRCULATION:** 28,000
AFFILIATION: None
INDEXED/ABSTRACTED IN: AHM, CINAHL, ECER, HLI, IM, INI, IPA, PA, SSI, SWRA

JOURNAL TITLE: Nursing Papers: Perspectives in Nursing

MANUSCRIPT ADDRESS: School of Nursing, McGill University
3506 University Avenue
Montreal   Quebec   Canada

TYPES OF ARTICLES: Research, theoretical, commentaries, review, case
studies, unsolicited book reviews

MAJOR CONTENT AREAS: Most areas listed in Appendix A including all
nursing areas

TOPICS PREFERRED: Clinical nursing practice, health, learning

INAPPROPRIATE TOPICS: Bandwagon topics i.e. death and dying - too much
education

REVIEW PROCEDURE: External review

REVIEW PERIOD: 3 months

MANUSCRIPT WORD LENGTH: Not cited	PAGE CHARGES: Not cited
MANUSCRIPT COPIES: 3	STYLE REQUIREMENTS: Not cited
PUBLICATION LAG TIME: 6 months	STYLE SHEET: Yes
EARLY PUBLICATION OPTION: No	REVISED THESES: Yes
ACCEPTANCE RATE: Not cited	STUDENT PAPERS: No
AUTHORSHIP RESTRICTIONS: No	REPRINT POLICY: Not cited

SUBSCRIPTION ADDRESS: School of Nursing, Mc Gill University
3506 University Avenue
Montreal   P.Q.   H3A 2A7 Canada

ANNUAL SUBSCRIPTION RATE: Individuals: $10   Institutions: $15

FREQUENCY: Quarterly   CIRCULATION: 800

AFFILIATION: Canadian Assoc. of University Schools of Nursing

INDEXED/ABSTRACTED IN: CINAHL, INI

◆

JOURNAL TITLE: Nursing Research

MANUSCRIPT ADDRESS: Dr. Florence S. Downs, Associate Dean, Editor
School of Nursing, University of Pennsylvania
420 Service Drive S2, Philadelphia PA 19104

TYPES OF ARTICLES: Research, theoretical, review

MAJOR CONTENT AREAS: nursing: assessment, audit, care, diagnosis,
education, history, philosophy, process, research,
science, service administration, theory; research
methodology

TOPICS PREFERRED: Theoretical or practical approaches to solution of
nursing problems, replications, literature reviews

INAPPROPRIATE TOPICS: None cited

REVIEW PROCEDURE: External review

REVIEW PERIOD: 2 months

MANUSCRIPT WORD LENGTH: 3500-5000	PAGE CHARGES: No
MANUSCRIPT COPIES: 4	STYLE REQUIREMENTS: APA
PUBLICATION LAG TIME: 10-12 months	STYLE SHEET: Yes
EARLY PUBLICATION OPTION: Yes	REVISED THESES: May submit
ACCEPTANCE RATE: 15-20%	STUDENT PAPERS: No
AUTHORSHIP RESTRICTIONS: No	REPRINT POLICY: free tear sheets

SUBSCRIPTION ADDRESS: Nursing Research
555 West 57th Street
New York NY 10019

ANNUAL SUBSCRIPTION RATE: Individuals: $20.00   Institutions: $30.00

FREQUENCY: Bimonthly   CIRCULATION: 7500

AFFILIATION: None

INDEXED/ABSTRACTED IN: CINAHL, CC, EM, HLI, IPA, IM, INI, MSRS, MCR,
MRA, NSA, SSCI

JOURNAL TITLE: Nursing Times

MANUSCRIPT ADDRESS: The Editor
4 Little Essex St.
London WC2R 3LF England

TYPES OF ARTICLES: Research, theoretical, case studies, commentaries

MAJOR CONTENT AREAS: Not specified

TOPICS PREFERRED: None cited

INAPPROPRIATE TOPICS: None cited

REVIEW PROCEDURE: Internal review
REVIEW PERIOD: 1 month

MANUSCRIPT WORD LENGTH: 1000-2000	PAGE CHARGES:	No
MANUSCRIPT COPIES: 2	STYLE REQUIREMENTS:	Not cited
PUBLICATION LAG TIME: 1 year	STYLE SHEET:	Yes
EARLY PUBLICATION OPTION: Yes	REVISED THESES:	No
ACCEPTANCE RATE: 30%	STUDENT PAPERS:	No
AUTHORSHIP RESTRICTIONS: No	REPRINT POLICY:	None free

SUBSCRIPTION ADDRESS: MacMillan Journals Ltd.
4 Little Essex St.
London WC2R 3LF England
ANNUAL SUBSCRIPTION RATE: $85
FREQUENCY: Weekly   CIRCULATION: 57,000
AFFILIATION: None
INDEXED/ABSTRACTED IN: CINAHL, HosA, HLI, IM, INI

◆

JOURNAL TITLE: Nutrition Reports International

MANUSCRIPT ADDRESS: Dr. Anthony A. Albanese, Editor
Burke Rehabilitation Center
White Plains NY 10605

TYPES OF ARTICLES: Research

MAJOR CONTENT AREAS: biochemistry, biomedical research, nutrition,
research methodology

TOPICS PREFERRED: Basic and pragmatic research in human nutrition

INAPPROPRIATE TOPICS: Food processing

REVIEW PROCEDURE: Editorial board and external review
REVIEW PERIOD: 30-60 days

MANUSCRIPT WORD LENGTH: 2000-4000	PAGE CHARGES:	Yes
MANUSCRIPT COPIES: 3	STYLE REQUIREMENTS:	Own
PUBLICATION LAG TIME: 30-60 days	STYLE SHEET:	Yes
EARLY PUBLICATION OPTION: No	REVISED THESES:	Yes
ACCEPTANCE RATE: 70%	STUDENT PAPERS:	No
AUTHORSHIP RESTRICTIONS: No	REPRINT POLICY:	None free

SUBSCRIPTION ADDRESS: Geron-X, Inc.
Publishers, P.O. Box 1108
Los Altos CA 94022
ANNUAL SUBSCRIPTION RATE: Individuals: $70   Institutions: $110
FREQUENCY: Monthly   CIRCULATION: 1000
AFFILIATION: None
INDEXED/ABSTRACTED IN: CC, BA, CA, CC, NAR

JOURNAL TITLE: Obstetrics and Gynecology

MANUSCRIPT ADDRESS: Richard F. Mattinly, M.D., Editor
Medical College of Wisconsin
8700 W. Wisconsin Ave., Milwaukee WI 53226

TYPES OF ARTICLES: Clinical, research, review, case studies, letters
to the editor, unsolicited book reviews

MAJOR CONTENT AREAS: anesthesiology (ob/gyn), biochemistry (ob/gyn),
cancer, family planning, genetics, pathology
(ob/gyn)

TOPICS PREFERRED: Field of obstetrics and gynecology

INAPPROPRIATE TOPICS: None cited

REVIEW PROCEDURE: Editorial board and special consultants
REVIEW PERIOD: 4-6 weeks
MANUSCRIPT WORD LENGTH: Not cited   PAGE CHARGES: Not cited
MANUSCRIPT COPIES: 2   STYLE REQUIREMENTS: IM
PUBLICATION LAG TIME: 8 months   STYLE SHEET: Yes
EARLY PUBLICATION OPTION: No   REVISED THESES: No
ACCEPTANCE RATE: 47%   STUDENT PAPERS: No
AUTHORSHIP RESTRICTIONS: No   REPRINT POLICY: None free

SUBSCRIPTION ADDRESS: Elsevier North Holland
52 Vanderbilt Avenue
New York NY 10017
ANNUAL SUBSCRIPTION RATE: Individuals: $47.50 Institutions: $70.00
FREQUENCY: Monthly   CIRCULATION: 27,000
AFFILIATION: American College of Obstetricians & Gynecologists
INDEXED/ABSTRACTED IN: BA, CA, CINAHL, IPA, IM, INI, NAR

◆

JOURNAL TITLE: Occupational Health

MANUSCRIPT ADDRESS: 35 Red Lion Square
London WC1R 4SG
England

TYPES OF ARTICLES: Commentaries, case studies, research, review,
theoretical

MAJOR CONTENT AREAS: Many areas listed in Appendix A including:
accidents, alcoholism & drug abuse, nursing: care,
community/public health, diagnosis, education,
history, research, science, occupational health,
office; primary care, rehabilitation, stress

TOPICS PREFERRED: Any concerned with health, safety and welfare at
work

INAPPROPRIATE TOPICS: None cited

REVIEW PROCEDURE: External review
REVIEW PERIOD: 1 month
MANUSCRIPT WORD LENGTH: 2000   PAGE CHARGES: No
MANUSCRIPT COPIES: 7   STYLE REQUIREMENTS: Own
PUBLICATION LAG TIME: 2 months   STYLE SHEET: Yes
EARLY PUBLICATION OPTION: No   REVISED THESES: No
ACCEPTANCE RATE: 60-70%   STUDENT PAPERS: Yes
AUTHORSHIP RESTRICTIONS: No   REPRINT POLICY: 12 free journals

SUBSCRIPTION ADDRESS: 35 Red Lion Square
London WC1R 4SG
England
ANNUAL SUBSCRIPTION RATE: $40
FREQUENCY: Monthly   CIRCULATION: 3500
AFFILIATION: Royal Coll. of Nursing Soc. of Occ. Health Nursing
INDEXED/ABSTRACTED IN: CINAHL, INI

164

JOURNAL TITLE: Occupational Health Nursing

MANUSCRIPT ADDRESS: Charles B. Slack, Inc.
6900 Grove Rd.
Thorofare NJ 08086

TYPES OF ARTICLES: Research, theoretical, case studies

MAJOR CONTENT AREAS: All subjects related to field of occupational health

TOPICS PREFERRED: None cited

INAPPROPRIATE TOPICS: None cited

REVIEW PROCEDURE: Editorial board and external review
REVIEW PERIOD: 4 weeks
MANUSCRIPT WORD LENGTH: 3000
MANUSCRIPT COPIES: 2
PUBLICATION LAG TIME: 2-3 months
EARLY PUBLICATION OPTION: Yes
ACCEPTANCE RATE: Not cited
AUTHORSHIP RESTRICTIONS: No

PAGE CHARGES: No
STYLE REQUIREMENTS: AMA
STYLE SHEET: Yes
REVISED THESES: No
STUDENT PAPERS: Yes
REPRINT POLICY: None free

SUBSCRIPTION ADDRESS: Charles B. Slack, Inc.
6900 Grove Rd.
Thorofare NJ 08086

ANNUAL SUBSCRIPTION RATE: $20
FREQUENCY: Monthly   **CIRCULATION:** 12,000
AFFILIATION: American Assoc. of Occupational Health Nurses, Inc.
INDEXED/ABSTRACTED IN: CINAHL, INI

JOURNAL TITLE: Occupational Health and Safety

MANUSCRIPT ADDRESS: Editorial Review Board, OSH
Stevens Publishing Corp.
P.O. Box 7573, Waco TX 76710

TYPES OF ARTICLES: Commentaries, research, case studies, theoretical, review, unsolicited book reviews

MAJOR CONTENT AREAS: Most areas listed in Appendix A including: nursing: assessment, audit, care, all clinical specialties, diagnosis, education, research, service administration; accidents, compliance, counseling, rehabilitation

TOPICS PREFERRED: Occupational health and safety, industrial hygiene, environmental health

INAPPROPRIATE TOPICS: None cited

REVIEW PROCEDURE: Editorial board
REVIEW PERIOD: 2 weeks
MANUSCRIPT WORD LENGTH: 500 words
MANUSCRIPT COPIES: 1
PUBLICATION LAG TIME: Negligible
EARLY PUBLICATION OPTION: No
ACCEPTANCE RATE: 90%
AUTHORSHIP RESTRICTIONS: No

PAGE CHARGES: No
STYLE REQUIREMENTS: IM
STYLE SHEET: Yes
REVISED THESES: Yes
STUDENT PAPERS: Yes
REPRINT POLICY: Negotiable

SUBSCRIPTION ADDRESS: Managing Editor
P.O. Box 7573
Waco TX 76710

ANNUAL SUBSCRIPTION RATE: $18
FREQUENCY: Monthly   **CIRCULATION:** 35,000
AFFILIATION: None
INDEXED/ABSTRACTED IN: CA, CINAHL, HLI, IM, INI

JOURNAL TITLE: Omega

MANUSCRIPT ADDRESS: Robert Kastenbaum, Ph.D.
Department of Communications, Stauffer Hall
Arizona State Univ., Tempe   AZ   85281
TYPES OF ARTICLES: Research

MAJOR CONTENT AREAS: death & dying, suicide & other lethal behaviors, bereavement

TOPICS PREFERRED: Death & dying

INAPPROPRIATE TOPICS: None cited

REVIEW PROCEDURE:	Editorial board		
REVIEW PERIOD:	Not cited		
MANUSCRIPT WORD LENGTH:	Not cited	PAGE CHARGES:	Not cited
MANUSCRIPT COPIES:	3	STYLE REQUIREMENTS:	APA, Own
PUBLICATION LAG TIME:	Not cited	STYLE SHEET:	Not cited
EARLY PUBLICATION OPTION:	Not cited	REVISED THESES:	Not cited
ACCEPTANCE RATE:	Not cited	STUDENT PAPERS:	Not cited
AUTHORSHIP RESTRICTIONS:	Not cited	REPRINT POLICY:	20 free

SUBSCRIPTION ADDRESS: Baywood Publishing Co.
43 Central Drive
Farmingdale NY 11735
ANNUAL SUBSCRIPTION RATE: Individuals: $27   Institutions: $51
FREQUENCY: Quarterly   CIRCULATION: Not cited
AFFILIATION: None cited
INDEXED/ABSTRACTED IN: BA, EM, PA, SA, ASW

◆

JOURNAL TITLE: Oncology Nursing Forum

MANUSCRIPT ADDRESS: Susan B. Baird, R.N., M.P.H., Editor
Room B2, Building 50, Dartmouth-Hitchcock
Medical Center, Hanover NH 03755
TYPES OF ARTICLES: Research, clinical practice, theoretical, review

MAJOR CONTENT AREAS: cancer in all age groups in all settings; adaptation, biofeedback, chronicity, communication, compliance, counseling, death & dying, nursing: assessment, audit, care, diagnosis, education, process, research, science, theory; quality of life
TOPICS PREFERRED: Nursing research in oncology

INAPPROPRIATE TOPICS: Manuscripts often too general for a very specialized audience

REVIEW PROCEDURE:	Editorial board, blind referee system		
REVIEW PERIOD:	5 weeks		
MANUSCRIPT WORD LENGTH:	Not cited (new)	PAGE CHARGES:	No
MANUSCRIPT COPIES:	3	STYLE REQUIREMENTS:	IM
PUBLICATION LAG TIME:	1-3 months	STYLE SHEET:	Yes
EARLY PUBLICATION OPTION:	No	REVISED THESES:	Yes
ACCEPTANCE RATE:	50%	STUDENT PAPERS:	Yes
AUTHORSHIP RESTRICTIONS:	No	REPRINT POLICY:	None free

SUBSCRIPTION ADDRESS: Oncology Nursing Society
701 Washington Road
Pittsburgh PA 15228
ANNUAL SUBSCRIPTION RATE: Individuals: $15   Institutions: $35
FREQUENCY: Quarterly   CIRCULATION: 2600
AFFILIATION: Oncology Nursing Society
INDEXED/ABSTRACTED IN: CINAHL, INI

JOURNAL TITLE: The PA Journal

MANUSCRIPT ADDRESS: Martha L. Wilson, Managing Editor
AAPA National Office, 2341 Jefferson Highway
Suite 700, Arlington VA 22202
TYPES OF ARTICLES: Clinical articles, case studies

MAJOR CONTENT AREAS: abuse (child/spouse), accidents, all age groups, allied health, cancer, compliance, counseling, emergency services, family planning, human sexuality, medicine, mental health, pain, patient teaching, pharmacology, primary care, stress
TOPICS PREFERRED: Primary care

INAPPROPRIATE TOPICS: Too many research articles on various demographic aspects of the PA profession
REVIEW PROCEDURE: Editorial board
REVIEW PERIOD: 4-6 weeks
MANUSCRIPT WORD LENGTH: Not cited   **PAGE CHARGES:** No
MANUSCRIPT COPIES: 3   **STYLE REQUIREMENTS:** IM
PUBLICATION LAG TIME: 6-8 weeks   **STYLE SHEET:** Yes
EARLY PUBLICATION OPTION: No   **REVISED THESES:** No
ACCEPTANCE RATE: Not cited   **STUDENT PAPERS:** Yes
AUTHORSHIP RESTRICTIONS: No   **REPRINT POLICY:** 1 free journal

SUBSCRIPTION ADDRESS: AAPA National Office
2341 Jefferson Highway, Suite 700
Arlington VA 22202
ANNUAL SUBSCRIPTION RATE: Individuals: $14   Institutions: $20
FREQUENCY: Quarterly   **CIRCULATION:** 7000
AFFILIATION: American Academy of Physician Assistants
INDEXED/ABSTRACTED IN: CINAHL, CC

◆

JOURNAL TITLE: Pain

MANUSCRIPT ADDRESS: Professor P.D. Wall, Dept. of Anatomy
University College London
Gower St. London WC1E 6BT England
TYPES OF ARTICLES: Research, review, case studies

MAJOR CONTENT AREAS: pain

TOPICS PREFERRED: All aspects of pain problems

INAPPROPRIATE TOPICS: None cited

REVIEW PROCEDURE: External review
REVIEW PERIOD: 2-3 months
MANUSCRIPT WORD LENGTH: 5000   **PAGE CHARGES:** No
MANUSCRIPT COPIES: 3   **STYLE REQUIREMENTS:** Own
PUBLICATION LAG TIME: 2-3 months   **STYLE SHEET:** Not cited
EARLY PUBLICATION OPTION: No   **REVISED THESES:** Yes
ACCEPTANCE RATE: 50%   **STUDENT PAPERS:** No
AUTHORSHIP RESTRICTIONS: No   **REPRINT POLICY:** 50 free

SUBSCRIPTION ADDRESS: Journal Division
Elesevier/North Holland, P.O. Box 211, 1000 AE
Amsterdam Netherlands
ANNUAL SUBSCRIPTION RATE: $156.30
FREQUENCY: Bimonthly   **CIRCULATION:** 2200
AFFILIATION: International Association for the Study of Pain
INDEXED/ABSTRACTED IN: CC, BA, EM, PA

JOURNAL TITLE: Paraplegia

MANUSCRIPT ADDRESS: Longman Group Ltd.
6th Floor, Westgate House
The High, Harlow, Essex CM20 1NE England

TYPES OF ARTICLES: Research, theoretical, review, case studies, commentaries

MAJOR CONTENT AREAS: clinical, physiological and pathological aspects of spinal cord injuries and diseases; nursing: assessment, care, education, process, science, service administration, most clinical specialties; rehabilitation

TOPICS PREFERRED: All aspects of spinal cord physiology and pathology

INAPPROPRIATE TOPICS: None cited

REVIEW PROCEDURE: Editorial board
REVIEW PERIOD: 4-6 months
MANUSCRIPT WORD LENGTH: 2500-4000
MANUSCRIPT COPIES: 2
PUBLICATION LAG TIME: 4-6 months
EARLY PUBLICATION OPTION: Yes
ACCEPTANCE RATE: 80%
AUTHORSHIP RESTRICTIONS: No

PAGE CHARGES: Yes
STYLE REQUIREMENTS: AMA
STYLE SHEET: Yes
REVISED THESES: Yes
STUDENT PAPERS: Yes
REPRINT POLICY: 25 free

SUBSCRIPTION ADDRESS: Subscription Manager, Journals Dept.
Longman Group Ltd.
Fourth Avenue, Harlow, Essex, CM195AA England
ANNUAL SUBSCRIPTION RATE: $69
FREQUENCY: Bimonthly
AFFILIATION: International Medical Society of Paraplegia
INDEXED/ABSTRACTED IN: IM, INI

CIRCULATION: 1600

◆

JOURNAL TITLE: Patient Care

MANUSCRIPT ADDRESS: Patient Care Publications, Inc.
16 Thorndal Circle, P.O. Box 1245
Darien CT 06820

TYPES OF ARTICLES: Clinical articles based on interviews with medical authorities

MAJOR CONTENT AREAS: all clinical topics

TOPICS PREFERRED: None cited

INAPPROPRIATE TOPICS: Unsolicited manuscripts not welcome. Query first

REVIEW PROCEDURE: Editorial board
REVIEW PERIOD: Not cited
MANUSCRIPT WORD LENGTH: 3000
MANUSCRIPT COPIES: Not cited
PUBLICATION LAG TIME: Not cited
EARLY PUBLICATION OPTION: No
ACCEPTANCE RATE: Not cited
AUTHORSHIP RESTRICTIONS: Yes

PAGE CHARGES: No
STYLE REQUIREMENTS: AMA, Own
STYLE SHEET: Yes
REVISED THESES: No
STUDENT PAPERS: No
REPRINT POLICY: Not cited

SUBSCRIPTION ADDRESS: Patient Care Publications, Inc.
16 Thorndal Circle, P.O. Box 1245
Darien CT 06820
ANNUAL SUBSCRIPTION RATE: $42
FREQUENCY: 21 times yearly
AFFILIATION: None
INDEXED/ABSTRACTED IN: CINAHL

CIRCULATION: 108,000

JOURNAL TITLE: Patient Counseling and Health Education

MANUSCRIPT ADDRESS: Executive Editor, Jose L. Garcia
P.O. Box 3085
Princeton NJ 08540
TYPES OF ARTICLES: Research, theoretical, review, case studies, commentaries
MAJOR CONTENT AREAS: adaptation, aging and aged, counseling, health promotion, patient teaching, patient counseling and health education

TOPICS PREFERRED: None cited

INAPPROPRIATE TOPICS: None cited

REVIEW PROCEDURE: Editorial board and external review
REVIEW PERIOD: 4-6 weeks
MANUSCRIPT WORD LENGTH: Not cited   **PAGE CHARGES:** No
MANUSCRIPT COPIES: 3   **STYLE REQUIREMENTS:** Own
PUBLICATION LAG TIME: 3-4 months   **STYLE SHEET:** Yes
EARLY PUBLICATION OPTION: Not cited   **REVISED THESES:** No
ACCEPTANCE RATE: 80%   **STUDENT PAPERS:** No
AUTHORSHIP RESTRICTIONS: No   **REPRINT POLICY:** Author purchase

SUBSCRIPTION ADDRESS: P.O. Box 3085
Princeton
NJ 08540
ANNUAL SUBSCRIPTION RATE: Individuals: $19.50   Institutions: $38.00
FREQUENCY: Quarterly   **CIRCULATION:** 2000
AFFILIATION: None
INDEXED/ABSTRACTED IN: Not cited

JOURNAL TITLE: Pediatric Nursing

MANUSCRIPT ADDRESS: North Woodbury Road
P.O. Box 56
Pitman NJ 08071
TYPES OF ARTICLES: Research, theoretical, commentaries

MAJOR CONTENT AREAS: all topics must pertain to general subject of pediatric medicine or maternal child nursing; nursing: assessment, diagnosis, philosophy, research; accidents, body image, family planning, mental retardation, parenting, women's issues
TOPICS PREFERRED: Pediatric primary care

INAPPROPRIATE TOPICS: Job descriptions based on "N=1" and no hard data to validiate importance
REVIEW PROCEDURE: Editorial board and review panel
REVIEW PERIOD: 6 weeks
MANUSCRIPT WORD LENGTH: 3000   **PAGE CHARGES:** Yes
MANUSCRIPT COPIES: 2   **STYLE REQUIREMENTS:** AMA
PUBLICATION LAG TIME: 3-9 months   **STYLE SHEET:** Yes
EARLY PUBLICATION OPTION: No   **REVISED THESES:** Yes
ACCEPTANCE RATE: 80%   **STUDENT PAPERS:** Yes
AUTHORSHIP RESTRICTIONS: No   **REPRINT POLICY:** 5 free journals

SUBSCRIPTION ADDRESS: Box 56
North Woodbury Road
Pitman NJ 08071
ANNUAL SUBSCRIPTION RATE: Individuals: $15   Institutions: $18
FREQUENCY: Bimonthly   **CIRCULATION:** 13,000
AFFILIATION: Nat. Assoc. of Ped. Nurse Associates & Practitioners
INDEXED/ABSTRACTED IN: INI, CINAHL

JOURNAL TITLE: Pediatrics

MANUSCRIPT ADDRESS: Mary Fletcher Hospital
Colchester Avenue
Burlington VT 05401

TYPES OF ARTICLES: Research, review

MAJOR CONTENT AREAS: abuse(child/spouse), children, genetics, human
sexuality, immunization

TOPICS PREFERRED: None cited

INAPPROPRIATE TOPICS: None cited

REVIEW PROCEDURE: Editorial board
REVIEW PERIOD: Not cited

MANUSCRIPT WORD LENGTH: 4000	PAGE CHARGES:	No
MANUSCRIPT COPIES: 3	STYLE REQUIREMENTS:	CBE, IM
PUBLICATION LAG TIME: 6 months	STYLE SHEET:	Yes
EARLY PUBLICATION OPTION: Yes	REVISED THESES:	No
ACCEPTANCE RATE: 10%	STUDENT PAPERS:	No
AUTHORSHIP RESTRICTIONS: No	REPRINT POLICY:	None free

SUBSCRIPTION ADDRESS: American Academy of Pediatrics
Suite 2080, 1603 Orrington Avenue
Evanston IL 60201

ANNUAL SUBSCRIPTION RATE: $30
FREQUENCY: Monthly   CIRCULATION: 30,000
AFFILIATION: American Academy of Pediatrics
INDEXED/ABSTRACTED IN: BA, CA, CINAHL, HLI, IPA, IM, INI, NAR

◆

JOURNAL TITLE: Perceptual and Motor Skills

MANUSCRIPT ADDRESS: Box 9229
Missoula MT 59807

TYPES OF ARTICLES: Research, theoretical, review

MAJOR CONTENT AREAS: accidents, chronicity, communication, fatigue,
human behavior, pain, perception, physical
therapy, psychology, research methodology, sleep,
teaching/learning

TOPICS PREFERRED: None cited

INAPPROPRIATE TOPICS: None cited

REVIEW PROCEDURE: Editorial board and external review
REVIEW PERIOD: 3 weeks

MANUSCRIPT WORD LENGTH: No restriction	PAGE CHARGES:	Yes
MANUSCRIPT COPIES: 2	STYLE REQUIREMENTS:	APA
PUBLICATION LAG TIME: 5-6 weeks	STYLE SHEET:	Yes
EARLY PUBLICATION OPTION: Yes	REVISED THESES:	Yes
ACCEPTANCE RATE: Not cited	STUDENT PAPERS:	Yes
AUTHORSHIP RESTRICTIONS: No	REPRINT POLICY:	Author purchase

SUBSCRIPTION ADDRESS: Box 9229
Missoula MT 59807

ANNUAL SUBSCRIPTION RATE: $112.00
FREQUENCY: 2 volumes yearly   CIRCULATION: 1800
AFFILIATION: None
INDEXED/ABSTRACTED IN: BA, DSHA, EM, INI, PA, SSI

JOURNAL TITLE: Perinatology/Neonatology

MANUSCRIPT ADDRESS: 825 South Barrington Avenue
Los Angeles CA 90049

TYPES OF ARTICLES: Research, theoretical, review, case studies,
commentaries, equipment surveys
MAJOR CONTENT AREAS: anesthesiology, bioethics, maternal/child
nursing, pediatric nursing, respiratory diseases,
Ob/Gyn, radiology, pediatrics, cardiology, surgery

TOPICS PREFERRED: Diagnostic techniques, therapeutic procedures,
perinatal/neonatal pathology, managerial policies
INAPPROPRIATE TOPICS: None cited

REVIEW PROCEDURE: Editorial board, external review, in-house review
REVIEW PERIOD: 2-3 weeks
MANUSCRIPT WORD LENGTH: 3500   **PAGE CHARGES:** No
MANUSCRIPT COPIES: 2   **STYLE REQUIREMENTS:** C
PUBLICATION LAG TIME: Varies   **STYLE SHEET:** Yes
EARLY PUBLICATION OPTION: Yes   **REVISED THESES:** Yes
ACCEPTANCE RATE: 75%   **STUDENT PAPERS:** Yes
AUTHORSHIP RESTRICTIONS: No   **REPRINT POLICY:** 1 free journal

SUBSCRIPTION ADDRESS: Perinatology/Neonatology
825 South Barrington Avenue
Los Angeles CA 90049
ANNUAL SUBSCRIPTION RATE: $40
FREQUENCY: Bimonthly   **CIRCULATION:** 20,000-30,000
AFFILIATION: None cited
INDEXED/ABSTRACTED IN: CINAHL

JOURNAL TITLE: Perspectives in Psychiatric Care

MANUSCRIPT ADDRESS: Nursing Publications
Box 218
Hillsdale NJ 07642
TYPES OF ARTICLES: Theoretical, research, clinical papers including
observation and theory, unsolicited book reviews
MAJOR CONTENT AREAS: Nearly all areas listed in Appendix A, including
nursing: assessment, care, diagnosis, education,
history, process, research, science, theory,
clinical specialties, community health, geriatric

TOPICS PREFERRED: Psychiatric/mental health nursing issues

INAPPROPRIATE TOPICS: None

REVIEW PROCEDURE: Editorial board and external review
REVIEW PERIOD: 4 months
MANUSCRIPT WORD LENGTH: 4000   **PAGE CHARGES:** No
MANUSCRIPT COPIES: 3   **STYLE REQUIREMENTS:** C, NT
PUBLICATION LAG TIME: 6-12 months   **STYLE SHEET:** Yes
EARLY PUBLICATION OPTION: No   **REVISED THESES:** Yes
ACCEPTANCE RATE: 5%   **STUDENT PAPERS:** Yes
AUTHORSHIP RESTRICTIONS: No   **REPRINT POLICY:** 6 free journals

SUBSCRIPTION ADDRESS: Nursing Publications
Box 218
Hillsdale NJ 07642
ANNUAL SUBSCRIPTION RATE: Individuals: $16   Institutions: $19
FREQUENCY: Bimonthly   **CIRCULATION:** 6000
AFFILIATION: None
INDEXED/ABSTRACTED IN: CINAHL, INI, IM, HLI, PA

JOURNAL TITLE: Pharmacology and Therapeutics

MANUSCRIPT ADDRESS: Department of Pharmacology
Yale University School of Medicine
333 Cedar St., New Haven CT 06510

TYPES OF ARTICLES: Review

MAJOR CONTENT AREAS: pharmacology

TOPICS PREFERRED: Chemotherapy, toxicology, metabolic inhibitors,
clinical pharmacology, pharmacodynamics

INAPPROPRIATE TOPICS: None cited

REVIEW PROCEDURE: Editorial board and external review
REVIEW PERIOD: 6-10 weeks

MANUSCRIPT WORD LENGTH: Not cited	PAGE CHARGES: No
MANUSCRIPT COPIES: 2	STYLE REQUIREMENTS: Own
PUBLICATION LAG TIME: 6-7 months	STYLE SHEET: Yes
EARLY PUBLICATION OPTION: No	REVISED THESES: No
ACCEPTANCE RATE: New journal	STUDENT PAPERS: No
AUTHORSHIP RESTRICTIONS: No	REPRINT POLICY: None free

SUBSCRIPTION ADDRESS: Pergamon Press, Inc.
Maxwell House, Fairview Park
Elmsford NY 10523

ANNUAL SUBSCRIPTION RATE: Institutions: $700	
FREQUENCY: Monthly	CIRCULATION: New journal
AFFILIATION: None	
INDEXED/ABSTRACTED IN: IM	

◆

JOURNAL TITLE: Pharmacy Management

MANUSCRIPT ADDRESS: 43rd Street and Kingsessing Mall
Philadelphia PA 19104

TYPES OF ARTICLES: Research, case studies, review

MAJOR CONTENT AREAS: pharmacology

TOPICS PREFERRED: Management topics related to practice of pharmacy

INAPPROPRIATE TOPICS: None cited

REVIEW PROCEDURE: External review
REVIEW PERIOD: 4-6 weeks

MANUSCRIPT WORD LENGTH: 2000	PAGE CHARGES: No
MANUSCRIPT COPIES: 3	STYLE REQUIREMENTS: IM
PUBLICATION LAG TIME: 2-6 months	STYLE SHEET: Yes
EARLY PUBLICATION OPTION: No	REVISED THESES: No
ACCEPTANCE RATE: Not cited	STUDENT PAPERS: No
AUTHORSHIP RESTRICTIONS: Not cited	REPRINT POLICY: None free

SUBSCRIPTION ADDRESS: Pharmacy Management
43rd Street and Kingsessing Mall
Philadelphia PA 19104

ANNUAL SUBSCRIPTION RATE: $15	
FREQUENCY: Bimonthly	CIRCULATION: 2800
AFFILIATION: American Society for Pharmacy Law	
INDEXED/ABSTRACTED IN: Not cited	

JOURNAL TITLE: The Philippine Journal of Nursing

MANUSCRIPT ADDRESS: 1663 Kansas Avenue
Manila
Philippines D-2801

TYPES OF ARTICLES: Commentaries, theoretical, research, case studies, review, unsolicited book reviews, literary, news

MAJOR CONTENT AREAS: Most areas listed in appendix A including: projects, developmental plans, accomplishments of professional organizations

TOPICS PREFERRED: Economic and general welfare topics, experiences demonstrating new concepts, practices

INAPPROPRIATE TOPICS: Research articles (not very scientific and poorly written)

REVIEW PROCEDURE: External review

REVIEW PERIOD: 4 weeks

MANUSCRIPT WORD LENGTH: 2000-3500	**PAGE CHARGES:** No
MANUSCRIPT COPIES: 3	**STYLE REQUIREMENTS:** C
PUBLICATION LAG TIME: 2 months	**STYLE SHEET:** Yes
EARLY PUBLICATION OPTION: Not cited	**REVISED THESES:** No
ACCEPTANCE RATE: 80%	**STUDENT PAPERS:** No
AUTHORSHIP RESTRICTIONS: No	**REPRINT POLICY:** 3 free journals

SUBSCRIPTION ADDRESS: 1663 Kansas Avenue
Manila
Philippines D-2801

ANNUAL SUBSCRIPTION RATE: $10

FREQUENCY: Quarterly   **CIRCULATION:** 17,000

AFFILIATION: Philippine Nurses Association

INDEXED/ABSTRACTED IN: CINAHL, INI

◆

JOURNAL TITLE: Physical Therapy

MANUSCRIPT ADDRESS: 1156 15th Street, N.W.
Washington DC 20005

TYPES OF ARTICLES: Research, review, theoretical, case studies, clinical reports, clinical suggestions, commentaries

MAJOR CONTENT AREAS: physical therapy, rehabilitation

TOPICS PREFERRED: Demonstration of the implications of materials & findings to the improvement of patient services

INAPPROPRIATE TOPICS: None cited

REVIEW PROCEDURE: Editorial board

REVIEW PERIOD: 8-9 months

MANUSCRIPT WORD LENGTH: 3000-4000	**PAGE CHARGES:** No
MANUSCRIPT COPIES: 2	**STYLE REQUIREMENTS:** Own
PUBLICATION LAG TIME: Up to 1 year	**STYLE SHEET:** Yes
EARLY PUBLICATION OPTION: No	**REVISED THESES:** Yes
ACCEPTANCE RATE: 75-80%	**STUDENT PAPERS:** Not cited
AUTHORSHIP RESTRICTIONS: No	**REPRINT POLICY:** None free

SUBSCRIPTION ADDRESS: 1156 15th Street   NW
Washington   DC   20005

ANNUAL SUBSCRIPTION RATE: $24

FREQUENCY: Monthly   **CIRCULATION:** 34,000

AFFILIATION: American Physical Therapy Association

INDEXED/ABSTRACTED IN: IM, CC(CP), CINAHL, ECER, HLI, INI

JOURNAL TITLE: Physiotherapy Canada

MANUSCRIPT ADDRESS: Joan Cleather, Editor
3600 Barclay Avenue, Suite 300
Montreal, Quebec H3S 1K5, Canada

TYPES OF ARTICLES: Research, theoretical, review, case studies

MAJOR CONTENT AREAS: allied health personnel, biofeedback, biomedical
research, circulatory diseases, continuing
education, handicapping conditions, physical
therapy, rehabilitation

TOPICS PREFERRED: Research, clinical practice, education & public
issues related to the rehabilitation sciences

INAPPROPRIATE TOPICS: Personal opinion pieces and inadequately prepared
case reports

REVIEW PROCEDURE: Editorial board and external review

REVIEW PERIOD: 3 months

MANUSCRIPT WORD LENGTH: 4000	PAGE CHARGES: No	
MANUSCRIPT COPIES: 3	STYLE REQUIREMENTS: CBE, IM	
PUBLICATION LAG TIME: 4 months	STYLE SHEET: Yes	
EARLY PUBLICATION OPTION: No	REVISED THESES: Yes	
ACCEPTANCE RATE: 70%	STUDENT PAPERS: No	
AUTHORSHIP RESTRICTIONS: No	REPRINT POLICY: 10 free	

SUBSCRIPTION ADDRESS: Canadian Physiotherapy Association
25 Imperial St
Toronto, Ontario M5P 1B9, Canada

ANNUAL SUBSCRIPTION RATE: $18.00

FREQUENCY: Bimonthly   CIRCULATION: 6000

AFFILIATION: Canadian Physiotherapy Association

INDEXED/ABSTRACTED IN: CINAHL, RL

◆

JOURNAL TITLE: Point of View® Magazine

MANUSCRIPT ADDRESS: Ethicon, Inc.
Somerville NJ 08876

TYPES OF ARTICLES: Current trends, theoretical, research, case
studies, commentaries

MAJOR CONTENT AREAS: Many areas listed in Appendix A including:
nursing: assessment, audit, care, clinical
specialties, diagnosis, medical/surgical, process,
research, trauma

TOPICS PREFERRED: Topics pertinent to operating room, delivery room
and emergency department nursing personnel

INAPPROPRIATE TOPICS: None cited

REVIEW PROCEDURE: Editor and internal review

REVIEW PERIOD: 1-4 weeks

MANUSCRIPT WORD LENGTH: 2000	PAGE CHARGES: No	
MANUSCRIPT COPIES: 2	STYLE REQUIREMENTS: IM	
PUBLICATION LAG TIME: 8-12 months	STYLE SHEET: Yes	
EARLY PUBLICATION OPTION: Yes	REVISED THESES: No	
ACCEPTANCE RATE: 90%	STUDENT PAPERS: Yes	
AUTHORSHIP RESTRICTIONS: No	REPRINT POLICY: 6-10 free	

SUBSCRIPTION ADDRESS: Restricted subscriptions available from Ethicon,
Inc. to OR, DR and ED nursing personnel

ANNUAL SUBSCRIPTION RATE: No charge

FREQUENCY: Quarterly   CIRCULATION: 42,500

AFFILIATION: None

INDEXED/ABSTRACTED IN: CINAHL

JOURNAL TITLE: Practical Gastroenterology

MANUSCRIPT ADDRESS: Pharmaceutical Communications, Inc.
42-15 Crescent Street
Long Island City NY 11101

TYPES OF ARTICLES: Review, case studies

MAJOR CONTENT AREAS: aging and aged, alcoholism and drug abuse, cancer, medicine, nutrition, all diseases of the G.I. tract, emphasis on diagnosis, therapy, and management

TOPICS PREFERRED: Topics on digestive disorders and related disciplines

INAPPROPRIATE TOPICS: None cited

REVIEW PROCEDURE: Editorial board and occasionally external review
REVIEW PERIOD: 2 months
MANUSCRIPT WORD LENGTH: 3000-3500
MANUSCRIPT COPIES: 1
PUBLICATION LAG TIME: 4-6 months
EARLY PUBLICATION OPTION: Not cited
ACCEPTANCE RATE: 60-70%
AUTHORSHIP RESTRICTIONS: No

PAGE CHARGES: Not cited
STYLE REQUIREMENTS: IM
STYLE SHEET: Yes
REVISED THESES: Will review
STUDENT PAPERS: Possibly
REPRINT POLICY: 100 free

SUBSCRIPTION ADDRESS: Pharmaceutical Communications, Inc.
42-15 Crescent Street
Long Island City NY 11101

ANNUAL SUBSCRIPTION RATE: $30
FREQUENCY: Bimonthly
AFFILIATION: None
INDEXED/ABSTRACTED IN: CC, IM (pending)

CIRCULATION: 75,000

JOURNAL TITLE: Preventive Medicine

MANUSCRIPT ADDRESS: American Health Foundation
320 East 43rd St.
New York NY 10017

TYPES OF ARTICLES: Research, applied research

MAJOR CONTENT AREAS: accidents, cancer, circulatory diseases, death, respiratory diseases, suicide, infectious diseases, heart disease, stroke

TOPICS PREFERRED: Reduction of disease & death

INAPPROPRIATE TOPICS: None cited

REVIEW PROCEDURE: Editorial board
REVIEW PERIOD: Not cited
MANUSCRIPT WORD LENGTH: 5000
MANUSCRIPT COPIES: 3
PUBLICATION LAG TIME: Not cited
EARLY PUBLICATION OPTION: Not cited
ACCEPTANCE RATE: Not cited
AUTHORSHIP RESTRICTIONS: Not cited

PAGE CHARGES: No
STYLE REQUIREMENTS: Own
STYLE SHEET: Not cited
REVISED THESES: Not cited
STUDENT PAPERS: Not cited
REPRINT POLICY: 50 free

SUBSCRIPTION ADDRESS: Academic Press
111 Fifth Avenue
New York NY 10003

ANNUAL SUBSCRIPTION RATE: $98
FREQUENCY: Quarterly
AFFILIATION: American Health Foundation
INDEXED/ABSTRACTED IN: BA, CA, CC, IM, CINAHL

CIRCULATION: Not cited

JOURNAL TITLE: Professional Medical Assistant

MANUSCRIPT ADDRESS: One East Wacker Drive
Suite 2110
Chicago IL 60601
TYPES OF ARTICLES: Educational, research, review, theoretical, case
studies, commentaries, unsolicited book reviews
MAJOR CONTENT AREAS: all disease problems & conditions, allied health
personnel, emergency services, ethics, growth/
development, health: promotion, sciences, policies; human behavior & sexuality, immunization,
leadership, office nursing, pain, professionalism
TOPICS PREFERRED: Articles relating to medical office management
and clinical procedures, not hospital
INAPPROPRIATE TOPICS: "A day in the life of..."--too personal accounts

REVIEW PROCEDURE: External review
REVIEW PERIOD: 1 month
MANUSCRIPT WORD LENGTH: 2500-5000   PAGE CHARGES: No
MANUSCRIPT COPIES: 2   STYLE REQUIREMENTS: AMA, C, Own
PUBLICATION LAG TIME: 4-12 months   STYLE SHEET: Yes
EARLY PUBLICATION OPTION: No   REVISED THESES: Yes
ACCEPTANCE RATE: 90%   STUDENT PAPERS: No
AUTHORSHIP RESTRICTIONS: No   REPRINT POLICY: 5 free journals

SUBSCRIPTION ADDRESS: Membership Department, AAMA
One East Wacker Drive, Suite 2110
Chicago IL 60601
ANNUAL SUBSCRIPTION RATE: $8
FREQUENCY: Bimonthly   CIRCULATION: 22,000
AFFILIATION: American Association of Medical Assistants
INDEXED/ABSTRACTED IN: INI, CINAHL

◆

JOURNAL TITLE: Professional Nurse

MANUSCRIPT ADDRESS: Charles Blackwell, Managing Editor
130 John Street
New York NY 10038
TYPES OF ARTICLES: Theoretical, review, case studies, commentaries

MAJOR CONTENT AREAS: continuing & inservice education, hospitals,
medicine, nursing: care, critical care,
geriatric, maternal/child, neurological, operating
room, orthopedic, pediatric, service administration, trauma; primary care, professionalism
TOPICS PREFERRED: Current developments/issues of interest to nurses
in the major hospital services
INAPPROPRIATE TOPICS: None cited

REVIEW PROCEDURE: Editorial board and editor
REVIEW PERIOD: Not cited
MANUSCRIPT WORD LENGTH: 1500-2000   PAGE CHARGES: No
MANUSCRIPT COPIES: 1   STYLE REQUIREMENTS: Own
PUBLICATION LAG TIME: Not cited   STYLE SHEET: Yes
EARLY PUBLICATION OPTION: No   REVISED THESES: No
ACCEPTANCE RATE: New journal   STUDENT PAPERS: No
AUTHORSHIP RESTRICTIONS: No   REPRINT POLICY: Not cited

SUBSCRIPTION ADDRESS: Le Jacq Publishing Inc.
130 John St.
New York NY 10038
ANNUAL SUBSCRIPTION RATE: $14
FREQUENCY: Monthly   CIRCULATION: New journal
AFFILIATION: None
INDEXED/ABSTRACTED IN: New journal

JOURNAL TITLE: Psychiatric Opinion

MANUSCRIPT ADDRESS: RR 1
Box 396
Shelburne Falls   MA   01370
TYPES OF ARTICLES: Commentaries, case studies, research

MAJOR CONTENT AREAS: abuse (child/spouse), biofeedback, death and
dying, human behavior, human sexuality,
loss/grief, medicine, mental health/illness, mental retardation, psychiatric/mental health
nursing, stress, suicide, women's issues
TOPICS PREFERRED: None cited

INAPPROPRIATE TOPICS: None cited

REVIEW PROCEDURE: Editorial board and/or editorial staff
REVIEW PERIOD: 1-2 months
MANUSCRIPT WORD LENGTH: 1500-2500   PAGE CHARGES: Yes
MANUSCRIPT COPIES: 2   STYLE REQUIREMENTS: Own
PUBLICATION LAG TIME: Not cited   STYLE SHEET: Yes
EARLY PUBLICATION OPTION: Not cited   REVISED THESES: No
ACCEPTANCE RATE: Not cited   STUDENT PAPERS: No
AUTHORSHIP RESTRICTIONS: No   REPRINT POLICY: 10 free journals

SUBSCRIPTION ADDRESS: RR 1
Box 396
Shelburne Falls   MA   01370
ANNUAL SUBSCRIPTION RATE: $30
FREQUENCY: 10 times yearly   CIRCULATION: 32,000
AFFILIATION: None
INDEXED/ABSTRACTED IN: PA, CMHR

JOURNAL TITLE: Psychiatric Quarterly

MANUSCRIPT ADDRESS: Donald P. Kenefick, New York School of Psychiatry,
Hudson River Psychiatric Center, Branch B
Poughkeepsie NY   12601
TYPES OF ARTICLES: Research, theoretical, review

MAJOR CONTENT AREAS: abuse (child/spouse), all age groups, allied
health, counseling, crisis, death, health polic-
ies, human behavior & sexuality, mental health/
illness, mental retardation, perception, psychology, psychopathology, psychiatric nursing
TOPICS PREFERRED: Mental health and illness, therapy, law

INAPPROPRIATE TOPICS: Not cited

REVIEW PROCEDURE: Editorial board
REVIEW PERIOD: 1-3 months
MANUSCRIPT WORD LENGTH: 3750-5000   PAGE CHARGES: No
MANUSCRIPT COPIES: 3   STYLE REQUIREMENTS: IM
PUBLICATION LAG TIME: 6-12 months   STYLE SHEET: Yes
EARLY PUBLICATION OPTION: Yes   REVISED THESES: Yes
ACCEPTANCE RATE: 15%   STUDENT PAPERS: Yes
AUTHORSHIP RESTRICTIONS: No   REPRINT POLICY: 1 free journal

SUBSCRIPTION ADDRESS: Human Sciences Press
72 Fifth Avenue
New York   NY   10011
ANNUAL SUBSCRIPTION RATE: Individuals: $25   Institutions: $54
FREQUENCY: Quarterly   CIRCULATION: 2000
AFFILIATION: None
INDEXED/ABSTRACTED IN: AHM, CC(SBS), CC(CP), ASCA, CMHR, EM, SA, NAR,
HLI, INI, SSCI, CINAHL

JOURNAL TITLE: Psychiatry - Journal for the Study of
Interpersonal Processes
MANUSCRIPT ADDRESS: 1610 New Hampshire Avenue, N.W.
Washington DC 20009

TYPES OF ARTICLES: Research

MAJOR CONTENT AREAS: counseling, cultural diversity, epidemiology,
human behavior, mental health/illness, psychology,
psychopathology, psychiatric/mental health
nursing, sociology, psychotherapy

TOPICS PREFERRED: Research in psychotherapy and psychopathology

INAPPROPRIATE TOPICS: Systems theory, single case histories

REVIEW PROCEDURE: Editorial board
REVIEW PERIOD: 3-4 months
MANUSCRIPT WORD LENGTH: 7500   **PAGE CHARGES:** No
MANUSCRIPT COPIES: 2   **STYLE REQUIREMENTS:** Own
PUBLICATION LAG TIME: 9 months   **STYLE SHEET:** Yes
EARLY PUBLICATION OPTION: No   **REVISED THESES:** No
ACCEPTANCE RATE: 25%   **STUDENT PAPERS:** No
AUTHORSHIP RESTRICTIONS: No   **REPRINT POLICY:** None free

SUBSCRIPTION ADDRESS: 1610 New Hampshire Avenue NW
Washington DC 20009

ANNUAL SUBSCRIPTION RATE: Individuals: $20 Institutions: $30
FREQUENCY: Quarterly   **CIRCULATION:** 3100
AFFILIATION: William Alanson White Psychiatric Foundation
INDEXED/ABSTRACTED IN: IM, PA, SA, EM, HA, HLI, INI, SSCI, SCI, SocA

◆

JOURNAL TITLE: Psychological Medicine

MANUSCRIPT ADDRESS: Professor Michael Shepherd, Institute of Psychiatry
De Crespigny Park, Denmark Hill
London SE 5 8AF England
TYPES OF ARTICLES: Research, review, theoretical, commentaries, case
studies, editorials, signed book reviews
MAJOR CONTENT AREAS: alcoholism & drug abuse, eating disorders,
genetics, growth/development, health sciences,
human sexuality, mental health, mental
retardation, pain, primary care, psychopathology,
research methodology, sleep, sociology, suicide
TOPICS PREFERRED: Psychiatry and related sciences

INAPPROPRIATE TOPICS: Advice on living

REVIEW PROCEDURE: Editorial board and external review
REVIEW PERIOD: 10 weeks
MANUSCRIPT WORD LENGTH: 4000   **PAGE CHARGES:** No
MANUSCRIPT COPIES: 3   **STYLE REQUIREMENTS:** H
PUBLICATION LAG TIME: 6 months   **STYLE SHEET:** Yes
EARLY PUBLICATION OPTION: No   **REVISED THESES:** No
ACCEPTANCE RATE: 20%   **STUDENT PAPERS:** No
AUTHORSHIP RESTRICTIONS: No   **REPRINT POLICY:** 50 free

SUBSCRIPTION ADDRESS: Psychological Medicine
Cambridge University Press
32 East 57th St., New York NY 10022
ANNUAL SUBSCRIPTION RATE: Individuals: $75 Institutions: $147.50
FREQUENCY: Quarterly   **CIRCULATION:** Not cited
AFFILIATION: None
INDEXED/ABSTRACTED IN: CA, IM, PA, SSCI, INI

JOURNAL TITLE: Psychological Reports

MANUSCRIPT ADDRESS: Box 9229
Missoula MT 59807

TYPES OF ARTICLES: Research, theoretical, review, case studies

MAJOR CONTENT AREAS: all age groups, diseases and disorders related to psychology, abuse, biofeedback, biorhythms, body image, compliance, counseling, crisis, cultural diversity, human behavior & sexuality, leadership, loss/grief, nursing education, pain, perception

TOPICS PREFERRED: General psychology

INAPPROPRIATE TOPICS: Opinions, no data

REVIEW PROCEDURE: Editorial board and external review
REVIEW PERIOD: 3 weeks

MANUSCRIPT WORD LENGTH: No restriction	**PAGE CHARGES:** Yes	
MANUSCRIPT COPIES: 3	**STYLE REQUIREMENTS:** APA	
PUBLICATION LAG TIME: 5-6 weeks	**STYLE SHEET:** Yes	
EARLY PUBLICATION OPTION: Yes	**REVISED THESES:** Yes	
ACCEPTANCE RATE: Not cited	**STUDENT PAPERS:** Yes	
AUTHORSHIP RESTRICTIONS: No	**REPRINT POLICY:** Author purchase	

SUBSCRIPTION ADDRESS: Box 9229
Missoula MT 59807

ANNUAL SUBSCRIPTION RATE: $112.00
FREQUENCY: Bimonthly   **CIRCULATION:** Not cited
AFFILIATION: None
INDEXED/ABSTRACTED IN: BA, EM, LLBA, PA, SSCI, SCI, SSI, IM, INI

◆

JOURNAL TITLE: Psychosocial Rehabilitation Journal

MANUSCRIPT ADDRESS: 157 Belmont Street
Brockton MA 02401

TYPES OF ARTICLES: Research, theoretical, review

MAJOR CONTENT AREAS: change theory, crisis intervention/theory, dependency, discharge planning, handicapping conditions, human behavior, mental health/illness, psychopathology, psychiatric nursing, rehabilitation, stigma, systems theory

TOPICS PREFERRED: Psychosocial rehabilitation

INAPPROPRIATE TOPICS: Counseling theory

REVIEW PROCEDURE: Editorial board
REVIEW PERIOD: 6 months

MANUSCRIPT WORD LENGTH: Not cited	**PAGE CHARGES:** No	
MANUSCRIPT COPIES: 3	**STYLE REQUIREMENTS:** APA	
PUBLICATION LAG TIME: 6 months	**STYLE SHEET:** Yes	
EARLY PUBLICATION OPTION: Yes	**REVISED THESES:** No	
ACCEPTANCE RATE: 75%	**STUDENT PAPERS:** No	
AUTHORSHIP RESTRICTIONS: No	**REPRINT POLICY:** 2 free journals	

SUBSCRIPTION ADDRESS: 157 Belmont Street
Brockton MA 02401

ANNUAL SUBSCRIPTION RATE: Individuals: $18   Institutions: $26
FREQUENCY: 3 times yearly   **CIRCULATION:** 250
AFFILIATION: None
INDEXED/ABSTRACTED IN: PA, CMHR, CINAHL

JOURNAL TITLE: Psychosomatic Medicine

MANUSCRIPT ADDRESS: American Psychosomatic Society
265 Nassau Road
Roosevelt NY 11575

TYPES OF ARTICLES: Research, theoretical, review, case studies, unsolicited book reviews

MAJOR CONTENT AREAS: adaptation, biofeedback, biorhythms, body image, cancer, circulatory & respiratory diseases, dependency, eating disorders, health sciences, human behavior & sexuality, loss/grief, nursing research, pain, relaxation, sleep, stress

TOPICS PREFERRED: Socio-psycho-biological medicine, behavioral and psychobiological medicine and research

INAPPROPRIATE TOPICS: None

REVIEW PROCEDURE: Editorial board and external review
REVIEW PERIOD: 3-6 weeks

MANUSCRIPT WORD LENGTH: Not cited	PAGE CHARGES:	Yes
MANUSCRIPT COPIES: 3	STYLE REQUIREMENTS:	CBE, IM
PUBLICATION LAG TIME: 4 months	STYLE SHEET:	Yes
EARLY PUBLICATION OPTION: Yes	REVISED THESES:	Yes
ACCEPTANCE RATE: 20%	STUDENT PAPERS:	Yes
AUTHORSHIP RESTRICTIONS: No	REPRINT POLICY:	25 free

SUBSCRIPTION ADDRESS: Subscription Department
Elsevier North Holland, Inc.
52 Vanderbilt Avenue New York NY 10017

ANNUAL SUBSCRIPTION RATE: Individuals: $38 Institutions: $79
FREQUENCY: 8 times yearly   CIRCULATION: 3300
AFFILIATION: American Psychosomatic Society
INDEXED/ABSTRACTED IN: IM, BA, CA, NAR, PA, SSCI

◆

JOURNAL TITLE: Psychosomatics

MANUSCRIPT ADDRESS: Wilfred Dorfman, M.D., Editor-in-Chief
1921 Newkirk Avenue
Brooklyn NY 11226

TYPES OF ARTICLES: Research (clinical), review, case studies

MAJOR CONTENT AREAS: psychosomatic aspects of diseases and disorders; adolescence, aging and aged, biofeedback, compliance, crisis intervention/theory, fatigue, human behavior & sexuality, life span, pain, primary care, sleep, stress, suicide

TOPICS PREFERRED: Clinical psychosomatic medicine

INAPPROPRIATE TOPICS: None cited

REVIEW PROCEDURE: Editorial board and external review
REVIEW PERIOD: 2-3 months

MANUSCRIPT WORD LENGTH: 2000-2500	PAGE CHARGES:	No
MANUSCRIPT COPIES: 2	STYLE REQUIREMENTS:	AMA
PUBLICATION LAG TIME: 3-4 months	STYLE SHEET:	Yes
EARLY PUBLICATION OPTION: No	REVISED THESES:	No
ACCEPTANCE RATE: 20%	STUDENT PAPERS:	No
AUTHORSHIP RESTRICTIONS: No	REPRINT POLICY:	None free

SUBSCRIPTION ADDRESS: Psychosomatics
500 West Putnam Avenue
Greenwich CT 06830

ANNUAL SUBSCRIPTION RATE: $20
FREQUENCY: Monthly   CIRCULATION: 25,000
AFFILIATION: Academy of Psychosomatic Medicine
INDEXED/ABSTRACTED IN: IM, CA, CINAHL, PA, SSCI

JOURNAL TITLE: Public Health Reports

MANUSCRIPT ADDRESS: Center Building, Room 10-44
3700 East-West Highway
Hyattsville MD 20782

TYPES OF ARTICLES: Research articles; epidemiology, "how to" of a
successful program

MAJOR CONTENT AREAS: abuse, accidents, allied health personnel,
chronicity, emergency services, family planning,
genetics, health sciences & policies, immunization, mental health/illness, nursing homes,
nursing: community health, occupational, school

TOPICS PREFERRED: Topics that are pertinent to public health and
community medicine

INAPPROPRIATE TOPICS: Adolescent health care

REVIEW PROCEDURE: External review
REVIEW PERIOD: 3-4 months
MANUSCRIPT WORD LENGTH: 3500   PAGE CHARGES: No
MANUSCRIPT COPIES: 4   STYLE REQUIREMENTS: IM
PUBLICATION LAG TIME: 8-12 months   STYLE SHEET: Yes
EARLY PUBLICATION OPTION: No   REVISED THESES: No
ACCEPTANCE RATE: 40%   STUDENT PAPERS: No
AUTHORSHIP RESTRICTIONS: No   REPRINT POLICY: 120 free

SUBSCRIPTION ADDRESS: Superintendent of Documents
U.S. Government Printing Office
Washington DC 20402

ANNUAL SUBSCRIPTION RATE: $15
FREQUENCY: Bimonthly   CIRCULATION: 13,000
AFFILIATION: U.S. Public Health Service
INDEXED/ABSTRACTED IN: IM, HLI, CINAHL, SWRA, INI

JOURNAL TITLE: Public Health Reviews

MANUSCRIPT ADDRESS: Editorial Office
29 Reading Street
Tel Aviv Israel

TYPES OF ARTICLES: Review articles and unsolicited book reviews only

MAJOR CONTENT AREAS: aging & aged, cancer, epidemiology, ethics,
family planning, health promotion, health
policies, mental health/illness, nursing:
geriatric, maternal/child, psychiatric, public
health; quality of life, sociology

TOPICS PREFERRED: Role of nursing in prevention of diseases, health
and community health services

INAPPROPRIATE TOPICS: None cited

REVIEW PROCEDURE: Editorial board and external review
REVIEW PERIOD: 1 month
MANUSCRIPT WORD LENGTH: 10,000   PAGE CHARGES: No
MANUSCRIPT COPIES: 2   STYLE REQUIREMENTS: IM
PUBLICATION LAG TIME: Several months   STYLE SHEET: Yes
EARLY PUBLICATION OPTION: No   REVISED THESES: Reviews only
ACCEPTANCE RATE: 50%   STUDENT PAPERS: No
AUTHORSHIP RESTRICTIONS: No   REPRINT POLICY: 25 free

SUBSCRIPTION ADDRESS: Editorial Office
29 Reading Street
Tel Aviv Israel

ANNUAL SUBSCRIPTION RATE: $54
FREQUENCY: Quarterly   CIRCULATION: Undisclosed
AFFILIATION: None
INDEXED/ABSTRACTED IN: BA, CINAHL, CC(SBS), EM, HLI, SSCI

JOURNAL TITLE: QRB: Quality Review Bulletin

MANUSCRIPT ADDRESS: Joint Commission on Accreditation of Hospitals
875 North Michigan Avenue
Chicago IL 60611

TYPES OF ARTICLES: Evaluation of nursing care, research articles

MAJOR CONTENT AREAS: anesthesiology, cancer, continuing education, continuity of care, discharge planning, emergency services, epidemiology, nursing: assessment, audit, care, geriatric, maternal/child, medical/surgical, OR, research; patient teaching

TOPICS PREFERRED: Nursing care evaluation, utilization review, continuing education

INAPPROPRIATE TOPICS: None cited

REVIEW PROCEDURE: Editorial board and external review
REVIEW PERIOD: 6 weeks
MANUSCRIPT WORD LENGTH: 2000-3000
MANUSCRIPT COPIES: 2
PUBLICATION LAG TIME: 3-4 months
EARLY PUBLICATION OPTION: No
ACCEPTANCE RATE: 75%
AUTHORSHIP RESTRICTIONS: No

PAGE CHARGES: No
STYLE REQUIREMENTS: AMA
STYLE SHEET: Yes
REVISED THESES: No
STUDENT PAPERS: No
REPRINT POLICY: 25 free

SUBSCRIPTION ADDRESS: Joint Commission on Accreditation of Hospitals
875 North Michigan Avenue
Chicago IL 60611

ANNUAL SUBSCRIPTION RATE: Basic: $65
FREQUENCY: Monthly
CIRCULATION: 4000
AFFILIATION: Joint Commission on Accreditation of Hospitals
INDEXED/ABSTRACTED IN: IM, HLI, INI

JOURNAL TITLE: Radiography

MANUSCRIPT ADDRESS: The College of Radiographers
14 Upper Wimpole Street
London W1M 8BN England

TYPES OF ARTICLES: Research, technical, theoretical, review, case
studies

MAJOR CONTENT AREAS: cancer

TOPICS PREFERRED: Radiography and allied subjects

INAPPROPRIATE TOPICS: Many

REVIEW PROCEDURE: Editorial board
REVIEW PERIOD: Variable
MANUSCRIPT WORD LENGTH: 4000-6000
MANUSCRIPT COPIES: 1
PUBLICATION LAG TIME: Variable
EARLY PUBLICATION OPTION: Possibly
ACCEPTANCE RATE: 95%
AUTHORSHIP RESTRICTIONS: No

PAGE CHARGES: No
STYLE REQUIREMENTS: Own
STYLE SHEET: No
REVISED THESES: Yes
STUDENT PAPERS: Yes
REPRINT POLICY: 25 free

SUBSCRIPTION ADDRESS: The College of Radiographers
14 Upper Wimpole Street
London W1M 8NB England

ANNUAL SUBSCRIPTION RATE: $40
FREQUENCY: Monthly
AFFILIATION: College of Radiographers
INDEXED/ABSTRACTED IN: BA, IM, CINAHL

CIRCULATION: 9500

◆

JOURNAL TITLE: Radiology

MANUSCRIPT ADDRESS: William R. Eyler, M.D., Editor
Tower 14, Suite 835, 21700 Northwestern Highway
Southfield MI 48075

TYPES OF ARTICLES: Research, review

MAJOR CONTENT AREAS: radiology, nuclear medicine, ultrasound, computer
tomography, physics, radiation therapy,
radiobiology

TOPICS PREFERRED: As in content areas cited

INAPPROPRIATE TOPICS: None cited

REVIEW PROCEDURE: Editorial board and external review
REVIEW PERIOD: 4-12 weeks
MANUSCRIPT WORD LENGTH: 2500-4000
MANUSCRIPT COPIES: 2
PUBLICATION LAG TIME: 12 weeks
EARLY PUBLICATION OPTION: Yes
ACCEPTANCE RATE: 40%
AUTHORSHIP RESTRICTIONS: No

PAGE CHARGES: No
STYLE REQUIREMENTS: IM
STYLE SHEET: Yes
REVISED THESES: No
STUDENT PAPERS: No
REPRINT POLICY: 100 free

SUBSCRIPTION ADDRESS: Dues and Subscription Department
The Radiological Society of North America, Inc.
20th and Northampton Streets, Easton, PA 18042

ANNUAL SUBSCRIPTION RATE: $65
FREQUENCY: Monthly
AFFILIATION: Radiological Society of North America, Inc.
INDEXED/ABSTRACTED IN: BA, CA, IM, INI, SA

CIRCULATION: 26,000

JOURNAL TITLE: RC: Respiratory Care

MANUSCRIPT ADDRESS: American Association for Respiratory Therapy
1720 Regal Row
Dallas TX 75235

TYPES OF ARTICLES: Research, review, theoretical, case studies

MAJOR CONTENT AREAS: adaptation, allied health personnel, biomedical
research, continuity of care, death & dying,
emergency services, health sciences, hospitals,
loss/grief, medicine, rehabilitation, respiratory
diseases, teaching/learning

TOPICS PREFERRED: Cardiorespiratory disease and treatment

INAPPROPRIATE TOPICS: None cited

REVIEW PROCEDURE: External review
REVIEW PERIOD: 2-3 months

MANUSCRIPT WORD LENGTH: Not important	PAGE CHARGES: No	
MANUSCRIPT COPIES: 3	STYLE REQUIREMENTS: IM	
PUBLICATION LAG TIME: 3-4 months	STYLE SHEET: Yes	
EARLY PUBLICATION OPTION: No	REVISED THESES: No	
ACCEPTANCE RATE: 45%	STUDENT PAPERS: No	
AUTHORSHIP RESTRICTIONS: No	REPRINT POLICY: None free	

SUBSCRIPTION ADDRESS: American Association for Respiratory Therapy
1720 Regal Row
Dallas TX 75235

ANNUAL SUBSCRIPTION RATE: $25
FREQUENCY: Monthly   CIRCULATION: 25,000
AFFILIATION: American Association for Respiratory Therapy
INDEXED/ABSTRACTED IN: HLI, CINAHL

◆

JOURNAL TITLE: Research on Aging

MANUSCRIPT ADDRESS: CASE Center for Gerontological Studies
Graduate Center, CUNY, 33 West 42nd Street
New York NY 10036

TYPES OF ARTICLES: Not specified

MAJOR CONTENT AREAS: backgrounds of editorial board, sociology,
geriatrics, history, psychology, anthropology,
public health, economics, criminal justice, social
work

TOPICS PREFERRED: Interdisciplinary research on current issues, meth-
odological & research problems in studying the aged

INAPPROPRIATE TOPICS: None cited

REVIEW PROCEDURE: None cited
REVIEW PERIOD: New journal

MANUSCRIPT WORD LENGTH: Not cited	PAGE CHARGES: Not cited	
MANUSCRIPT COPIES: 3	STYLE REQUIREMENTS: APA, ASA	
PUBLICATION LAG TIME: New Journal	STYLE SHEET: Not cited	
EARLY PUBLICATION OPTION: Not cited	REVISED THESES: Not cited	
ACCEPTANCE RATE: Not cited	STUDENT PAPERS: Not cited	
AUTHORSHIP RESTRICTIONS: Not cited	REPRINT POLICY: Not cited	

SUBSCRIPTION ADDRESS: SAGE Publications, Inc.
P.O. Box 5024
Beverly Hills CA 90210

ANNUAL SUBSCRIPTION RATE: Individuals: $16.50 Institutions: $32.00
FREQUENCY: Quarterly   CIRCULATION: New journal
AFFILIATION: None
INDEXED/ABSTRACTED IN: New journal

JOURNAL TITLE: Research in Nursing and Health

MANUSCRIPT ADDRESS: Harriet H. Werley, Ph.D., Associate Dean
School of Nursing, University of Missouri -
Columbia, Columbia MO 65211

TYPES OF ARTICLES: Research, theoretical, review, research methods,
basic sciences research, implementation of research

MAJOR CONTENT AREAS: all nursing areas listed in Appendix A; aging and
aged, alcoholism and drug abuse, body image, con-
tinuity of care, death and dying, discharge plan-
ing, family planning, parenting, primary care,
quality of life, rehabilitation,

TOPICS PREFERRED: Research in nursing and health

INAPPROPRIATE TOPICS: None cited

REVIEW PROCEDURE: Editorial board and external review
REVIEW PERIOD: 4-8 weeks

MANUSCRIPT WORD LENGTH: 5000		**PAGE CHARGES:** No	
MANUSCRIPT COPIES: 4		**STYLE REQUIREMENTS:** APA	
PUBLICATION LAG TIME: 4-8 months		**STYLE SHEET:** Yes	
EARLY PUBLICATION OPTION: Not cited		**REVISED THESES:** Yes	
ACCEPTANCE RATE: 22%		**STUDENT PAPERS:** No	
AUTHORSHIP RESTRICTIONS: No		**REPRINT POLICY:** 100 free	

SUBSCRIPTION ADDRESS: Subscription Fulfillment Department
20th and Northampton Streets
Easton PA 18042

ANNUAL SUBSCRIPTION RATE: $25
FREQUENCY: Quarterly   **CIRCULATION:** 1000
AFFILIATION: None
INDEXED/ABSTRACTED IN: CINAHL, CC(LS), CC(SBS), CIJE, EI, SSI, HLI, IM,
INI, PA, PHR, SCI, SSCI, SocA

◆

JOURNAL TITLE: Research Quarterly for Exercise and Sports

MANUSCRIPT ADDRESS: 420 Lathrop Hall
University of Wisconsin
Madison WI 53706

TYPES OF ARTICLES: Research, review

MAJOR CONTENT AREAS: anatomy & physiology, body image, growth/
development, physical therapy, research
methodology, sociology of sports, testing/
measurement

TOPICS PREFERRED: Exercise physiology, sports, physical education

INAPPROPRIATE TOPICS: None cited

REVIEW PROCEDURE: Editorial board, external review
REVIEW PERIOD: 6-9 months

MANUSCRIPT WORD LENGTH: 2500-3000		**PAGE CHARGES:** Yes	
MANUSCRIPT COPIES: 3		**STYLE REQUIREMENTS:** APA	
PUBLICATION LAG TIME: 6 months		**STYLE SHEET:** Yes	
EARLY PUBLICATION OPTION: No		**REVISED THESES:** Yes	
ACCEPTANCE RATE: 40%		**STUDENT PAPERS:** No	
AUTHORSHIP RESTRICTIONS: No		**REPRINT POLICY:** 2 free journals	

SUBSCRIPTION ADDRESS: Research Quarterly for Exercise and Sports
1201 16th Street, N.W.
Washington DC 20036

ANNUAL SUBSCRIPTION RATE: Individuals: $35(with membership) Institutions:$30
FREQUENCY: Quarterly   **CIRCULATION:** 12,000
AFFILIATION: Amer. Alli. for Health, Phys. Ed., Recre. & Dance
INDEXED/ABSTRACTED IN: Not cited

JOURNAL TITLE: Respiratory Technology

MANUSCRIPT ADDRESS: Pennex Ltd.
107 Paramount Road
Winnipeg, Manitoba R2X 2W6 Canada
TYPES OF ARTICLES: Research, case studies, commentaries, review, unsolicited book reviews
MAJOR CONTENT AREAS: respiratory diseases

TOPICS PREFERRED: All aspects of respiratory disease as related to the role/function of a respiratory technologist
INAPPROPRIATE TOPICS: None cited

REVIEW PROCEDURE: Editorial board		
REVIEW PERIOD: 1 month		
MANUSCRIPT WORD LENGTH: 1500-2000	**PAGE CHARGES:** No	
MANUSCRIPT COPIES: 2	**STYLE REQUIREMENTS:** Own	
PUBLICATION LAG TIME: 2 months	**STYLE SHEET:** Yes	
EARLY PUBLICATION OPTION: No	**REVISED THESES:** Yes	
ACCEPTANCE RATE: 75%	**STUDENT PAPERS:** No	
AUTHORSHIP RESTRICTIONS: No	**REPRINT POLICY:** 2 free journals	

SUBSCRIPTION ADDRESS: Pennex Ltd.
107 Paramount Road
Winnipeg, Manitoba R2X 2W6 Canada
ANNUAL SUBSCRIPTION RATE: $9
FREQUENCY: Bimonthly   **CIRCULATION:** 2000-3000
AFFILIATION: Canadian Society of Respiratory Technologists
INDEXED/ABSTRACTED IN: CINAHL

◆

JOURNAL TITLE: Respiratory Therapy

MANUSCRIPT ADDRESS: 825 South Barrington Avenue
Los Angeles CA 90049

TYPES OF ARTICLES: Research, theoretical, review, case studies, equipment surveys, commentaries
MAJOR CONTENT AREAS: allied health personnel, anesthesiology, respiratory diseases, inhalation and cardiopulmonary therapy, medical equipment, accreditation, licensure, legal liability

TOPICS PREFERRED: Case histories, facility reports, professional advancements, therapy techniques
INAPPROPRIATE TOPICS: None cited

REVIEW PROCEDURE: Editorial board, external review, & inhouse review		
REVIEW PERIOD: 2-3 weeks		
MANUSCRIPT WORD LENGTH: 3500	**PAGE CHARGES:** No	
MANUSCRIPT COPIES: 2	**STYLE REQUIREMENTS:** C	
PUBLICATION LAG TIME: Varies	**STYLE SHEET:** Yes	
EARLY PUBLICATION OPTION: Yes	**REVISED THESES:** Yes	
ACCEPTANCE RATE: 75%	**STUDENT PAPERS:** Yes	
AUTHORSHIP RESTRICTIONS: No	**REPRINT POLICY:** 1 free journal	

SUBSCRIPTION ADDRESS: Respiratory Therapy
825 South Barrington Avenue
Los Angeles CA 90049
ANNUAL SUBSCRIPTION RATE: $30
FREQUENCY: Bimonthly   **CIRCULATION:** 20,000
AFFILIATION: None
INDEXED/ABSTRACTED IN: CINAHL

JOURNAL TITLE: RN Magazine

MANUSCRIPT ADDRESS: 680 Kinderkamack Road
Oradell NJ 07649

TYPES OF ARTICLES: Research, review, case studies, commentaries

MAJOR CONTENT AREAS: crisis, death & dying, discharge planning, human
sexuality, loss/grief, nursing: assessment, care,
clinical specialties, critical care, diagnosis,
geriatric, maternal/child, medical/surgical, neurological, research, OR, orthopedic, pediatric, trauma

TOPICS PREFERRED: None cited

INAPPROPRIATE TOPICS: Personal experiences of a nonclinical nature

REVIEW PROCEDURE: Editorial board and internal review
REVIEW PERIOD: 2-8 weeks
MANUSCRIPT WORD LENGTH: 2000   **PAGE CHARGES:** No
MANUSCRIPT COPIES: 2   **STYLE REQUIREMENTS:** AMA, IM, NT
PUBLICATION LAG TIME: 6 months   **STYLE SHEET:** Yes
EARLY PUBLICATION OPTION: Yes   **REVISED THESES:** No
ACCEPTANCE RATE: 5%   **STUDENT PAPERS:** No
AUTHORSHIP RESTRICTIONS: Yes   **REPRINT POLICY:** None free

SUBSCRIPTION ADDRESS: RN Magazine
Box 56
Oradell NJ 07649
ANNUAL SUBSCRIPTION RATE: $16
FREQUENCY: Monthly   **CIRCULATION:** 332,000
AFFILIATION: None
INDEXED/ABSTRACTED IN: CINAHL, HLI, INI

◆

JOURNAL TITLE: Santo Tomas Nursing Journal

MANUSCRIPT ADDRESS: University of Santo Tomas
Espana
Manila Philippines

TYPES OF ARTICLES: Research, theoretical, review, case studies

MAJOR CONTENT AREAS: nursing: assessment, audit, care, community/
public health, diagnosis, education, maternal/
child, medical/surgical, occupational, philosophy,
process, psychiatric, research, science, service
administration, theory; teaching/learning

TOPICS PREFERRED: Research and nursing education topics

INAPPROPRIATE TOPICS: None

REVIEW PROCEDURE: Editorial board
REVIEW PERIOD: 2 months
MANUSCRIPT WORD LENGTH: No maximum
MANUSCRIPT COPIES: 2
PUBLICATION LAG TIME: Varies
EARLY PUBLICATION OPTION: No
ACCEPTANCE RATE: 80%
AUTHORSHIP RESTRICTIONS: No

PAGE CHARGES: No
STYLE REQUIREMENTS: Own
STYLE SHEET: Yes
REVISED THESES: Yes
STUDENT PAPERS: Yes
REPRINT POLICY: 2 free

SUBSCRIPTION ADDRESS: University of Santo Tomas
Espana
Manila Philippines
ANNUAL SUBSCRIPTION RATE: $5
FREQUENCY: Biannual
AFFILIATION: None
INDEXED/ABSTRACTED IN: CINAHL, INI

CIRCULATION: 3000

◆

JOURNAL TITLE: Scandinavian Journal of Rehabilitation Medicine

MANUSCRIPT ADDRESS: Almquist & Wiksell International
P.O. Box 62
S-101 20 Stockholm 1 Sweden

TYPES OF ARTICLES: Research

MAJOR CONTENT AREAS: biofeedback, biomedical research, dependency,
handicapping conditions, neurological nursing,
pain, physical therapy, quality of life,
rehabilitation, teaching/learning

TOPICS PREFERRED: Rehabilitation including physical therapy

INAPPROPRIATE TOPICS: None cited

REVIEW PROCEDURE: Editorial board and external review
REVIEW PERIOD: 2-3 months
MANUSCRIPT WORD LENGTH: 5-6 pages
MANUSCRIPT COPIES: 3
PUBLICATION LAG TIME: 6-12 months
EARLY PUBLICATION OPTION: No
ACCEPTANCE RATE: 50%
AUTHORSHIP RESTRICTIONS: No

PAGE CHARGES: No
STYLE REQUIREMENTS: IM, Own
STYLE SHEET: Yes
REVISED THESES: Yes
STUDENT PAPERS: No
REPRINT POLICY: 100-200 free

SUBSCRIPTION ADDRESS: The Almquist & Wiksell Periodical Company
P.O. Box 62
S-101 20 Stockholm 1 Sweden
ANNUAL SUBSCRIPTION RATE: $35
FREQUENCY: Quarterly
AFFILIATION: None
INDEXED/ABSTRACTED IN: IM, EM, BA, CINAHL

CIRCULATION: 1000

JOURNAL TITLE: Scandinavian Journal of Social Medicine

MANUSCRIPT ADDRESS: Socialmedicinska Institutionen
Karolinska Institutet
S-104 01 Stockholm 60, Sweden

TYPES OF ARTICLES: Research, theoretical, case studies, review

MAJOR CONTENT AREAS: Most diseases and disorders listed in Appendix A,
health promotion, life span, nursing: care,
diagnosis, geriatric, research, science, service
administration; nutrition, patient teaching, primary care, quality of life

TOPICS PREFERRED: Epidemiology, health services research, preventive medicine and community health; addiction

INAPPROPRIATE TOPICS: None cited

REVIEW PROCEDURE: External review
REVIEW PERIOD: 2 months
MANUSCRIPT WORD LENGTH: 3000
MANUSCRIPT COPIES: 4
PUBLICATION LAG TIME: 1 year
EARLY PUBLICATION OPTION: Yes
ACCEPTANCE RATE: 50%
AUTHORSHIP RESTRICTIONS: No

PAGE CHARGES: Yes
STYLE REQUIREMENTS: Own, IM
STYLE SHEET: No
REVISED THESES: Yes
STUDENT PAPERS: No
REPRINT POLICY: None free

SUBSCRIPTION ADDRESS: The Almquist & Wiksell Periodical Company
P.O. Box 62
S-101 20 Stockholm 1, Sweden

ANNUAL SUBSCRIPTION RATE: $35
FREQUENCY: Quarterly
AFFILIATION: The Scandinavian Association for Social Medicine
INDEXED/ABSTRACTED IN: IM, SSCI, CINAHL, INI

CIRCULATION: 500

◆

JOURNAL TITLE: School Nurse

MANUSCRIPT ADDRESS: Barbara Jo Nerone, Managing Editor
New York Statler, 33rd St. & 7th Ave., Ste. 104,
New York NY 10001

TYPES OF ARTICLES: Research, case studies

MAJOR CONTENT AREAS: abuse, counseling, crisis, family planning,
growth/development, handicapping conditions
human behavior & sexuality, immunization,
nursing: assessment, clinical specialties, public
health, maternal/child, pediatric, school

TOPICS PREFERRED: Articles on issues directly related to the care
of children K-12

INAPPROPRIATE TOPICS: Not applicable

REVIEW PROCEDURE: Editorial board
REVIEW PERIOD: 3-4 months
MANUSCRIPT WORD LENGTH: 1200
MANUSCRIPT COPIES: 2
PUBLICATION LAG TIME: 1-2 years
EARLY PUBLICATION OPTION: No
ACCEPTANCE RATE: 50%
AUTHORSHIP RESTRICTIONS: No

PAGE CHARGES: No
STYLE REQUIREMENTS: C
STYLE SHEET: Yes
REVISED THESES: Yes
STUDENT PAPERS: No
REPRINT POLICY: 3 free

SUBSCRIPTION ADDRESS: National Association of School Nurses
New York Statler, 33rd St. & 7th Ave., Ste. 104
New York NY 10001

ANNUAL SUBSCRIPTION RATE: $20
FREQUENCY: Quarterly
AFFILIATION: National Association of School Nurses
INDEXED/ABSTRACTED IN: None

CIRCULATION: 2500

189

JOURNAL TITLE: Science

MANUSCRIPT ADDRESS: 1515 Massachusetts Avenue, N.W.
Washington DC 20005

TYPES OF ARTICLES: Research, review, theoretical

MAJOR CONTENT AREAS: anthropology, biochemistry, biology, biomedical.
research, genetics, medicine, microbiology,
natural science, pharmacology, physics, psychology

TOPICS PREFERRED: Research in all sciences

INAPPROPRIATE TOPICS: None cited

REVIEW PROCEDURE: External review
REVIEW PERIOD: 4-8 weeks

MANUSCRIPT WORD LENGTH: 1000-5000	PAGE CHARGES: No	
MANUSCRIPT COPIES: 3	STYLE REQUIREMENTS: C, AP, CBE	
PUBLICATION LAG TIME: 6-14 weeks	STYLE SHEET: Yes	
EARLY PUBLICATION OPTION: No	REVISED THESES: No	
ACCEPTANCE RATE: 20-25%	STUDENT PAPERS: No	
AUTHORSHIP RESTRICTIONS: No	REPRINT POLICY: None free	

SUBSCRIPTION ADDRESS: Science
1515 Massachusetts Avenue, N.W.
Washington DC 20005
ANNUAL SUBSCRIPTION RATE: Individuals: $34 Institutions: $70
FREQUENCY: Weekly   CIRCULATION: 155,000
AFFILIATION: American Assoc. for the Advancement of Science
INDEXED/ABSTRACTED IN: CA, BA, PA, IM, RGPL, MA, ASTI, BRD, MeA, MGA,
NAR, OA, SI, PoIA, CINAHL

◆

JOURNAL TITLE: Score

MANUSCRIPT ADDRESS: Bertha Yanis Litsky, Ph.D., Editor
9 Kettle Pond Road
Amherst MA 01002
TYPES OF ARTICLES: Case studies, research, theoretical,

MAJOR CONTENT AREAS: continuing education, epidemiology, health
sciences, inservice education, microbiology,
nursing education, nursing history, nursing homes,
nursing research, operating room nursing, central
service
TOPICS PREFERRED: Infection control

INAPPROPRIATE TOPICS: Manuscripts on subjects other than infection
control
REVIEW PROCEDURE: Editorial board and external review
REVIEW PERIOD: 2 months

MANUSCRIPT WORD LENGTH: 500 words	PAGE CHARGES: No	
MANUSCRIPT COPIES: 2	STYLE REQUIREMENTS: C	
PUBLICATION LAG TIME: Within 1 year	STYLE SHEET: Yes	
EARLY PUBLICATION OPTION: No	REVISED THESES: Yes	
ACCEPTANCE RATE: 70%	STUDENT PAPERS: Yes	
AUTHORSHIP RESTRICTIONS: No	REPRINT POLICY: Free journals	

SUBSCRIPTION ADDRESS: Surgicot, Inc., Medical Products Division
55 Kennedy Drive
Smithtown NY 11787
ANNUAL SUBSCRIPTION RATE: Individuals (allied health professionals): $12
FREQUENCY: 5 issues/year   CIRCULATION: 16,000
AFFILIATION: None
INDEXED/ABSTRACTED IN: CINAHL

JOURNAL TITLE: Sexuality and Disability

MANUSCRIPT ADDRESS: Susan M. Daniels, Ph.D.
Department of Rehabilitation Counseling
100 S. Derbigny St., New Orleans LA   70112
TYPES OF ARTICLES: Review, research, theoretical, case studies,
commentaries, unsolicited book reviews
MAJOR CONTENT AREAS: body image, communication, counseling, family
planning, genetics, instructional technology,
marriage & divorce, maternal/child nursing, mental
retardation, midwifery, pain, professionalism,
psych./mental health nursing, rehabilitation, stigma
TOPICS PREFERRED: Anything related to sexuality, health and illness

INAPPROPRIATE TOPICS: None cited

REVIEW PROCEDURE: Editorial board
REVIEW PERIOD: 3 months
MANUSCRIPT WORD LENGTH: Varies   PAGE CHARGES: No
MANUSCRIPT COPIES: 3   STYLE REQUIREMENTS: IM
PUBLICATION LAG TIME: 4-6 months   STYLE SHEET: Yes
EARLY PUBLICATION OPTION: No   REVISED THESES: Yes
ACCEPTANCE RATE: 30%   STUDENT PAPERS: Yes
AUTHORSHIP RESTRICTIONS: No   REPRINT POLICY: 3 free

SUBSCRIPTION ADDRESS: Human Sciences Press
72 Fifth Avenue
New York   NY   10011
ANNUAL SUBSCRIPTION RATE: Individuals: $23   Institutions: $50
FREQUENCY: Quarterly   CIRCULATION: Not cited
AFFILIATION: None
INDEXED/ABSTRACTED IN: SocA, EM, PCCA, CC(SBS), SSCI, SSA

JOURNAL TITLE: Sexually Transmitted Diseases

MANUSCRIPT ADDRESS: William M. McCormack, Editor
State Laboratory Institute - 305 South Street
Jamaica Plain MA 02130
TYPES OF ARTICLES: Research, case studies, review, commentaries

MAJOR CONTENT AREAS: abuse (child/spouse), adolescence, biomedical
research, epidemiology, health promotion, human
behavior, human sexuality, medicine, microbiology,
public health, research methodology, women's
issues
TOPICS PREFERRED: All aspects of sexually transmitted diseases

INAPPROPRIATE TOPICS: None

REVIEW PROCEDURE: Editorial board, external review
REVIEW PERIOD: 6 Weeks
MANUSCRIPT WORD LENGTH: 2000-2500   PAGE CHARGES: No
MANUSCRIPT COPIES: 3   STYLE REQUIREMENTS: C
PUBLICATION LAG TIME: 4 Months   STYLE SHEET: Yes
EARLY PUBLICATION OPTION: No   REVISED THESES: Yes
ACCEPTANCE RATE: 65%   STUDENT PAPERS: No
AUTHORSHIP RESTRICTIONS: No   REPRINT POLICY: None free

SUBSCRIPTION ADDRESS: J.B. Lippincott Co.
East Washington Square
Philadelphia PA 19105
ANNUAL SUBSCRIPTION RATE: $28
FREQUENCY: Quarterly   CIRCULATION: 1200
AFFILIATION: American Venereal Disease Association
INDEXED/ABSTRACTED IN: IM, CC(CP), CA

JOURNAL TITLE: SGA Journal

MANUSCRIPT ADDRESS: c/o Linda A. Lauretano, R.N.
9 Clifford Street, Box 322
Southboro MA 01772

TYPES OF ARTICLES: Research, theoretical, review, case studies

MAJOR CONTENT AREAS: anesthesiology, biomedical research, cancer, counseling, crisis, eating disorders, nursing: assessment, audit, care, clinical specialties, diagnosis, education, medical/surgical, process, research, service administration; patient teaching

TOPICS PREFERRED: Anything relating to the fields of GI endoscopy, medicine & surgery

INAPPROPRIATE TOPICS: None

REVIEW PROCEDURE: Editorial board
REVIEW PERIOD: 2 months
MANUSCRIPT WORD LENGTH: Not cited
MANUSCRIPT COPIES: 4
PUBLICATION LAG TIME: 4 to 6 months
EARLY PUBLICATION OPTION: No
ACCEPTANCE RATE: 90%
AUTHORSHIP RESTRICTIONS: No

PAGE CHARGES: No
STYLE REQUIREMENTS: Own
STYLE SHEET: Yes
REVISED THESES: Yes
STUDENT PAPERS: No
REPRINT POLICY: None

SUBSCRIPTION ADDRESS: SGA Inc.
211 East 43rd St.
New York NY 10017
ANNUAL SUBSCRIPTION RATE: $18
FREQUENCY: Quarterly
CIRCULATION: 1500
AFFILIATION: Society of Gastrointestinal Assistants, Inc.
INDEXED/ABSTRACTED IN: CINAHL

◆

JOURNAL TITLE: Sharing and Caring

MANUSCRIPT ADDRESS: American Health Care Association - CAC
1200 15th St., N.W.
Washington DC 20005

TYPES OF ARTICLES: Personal experiences of nursing home activity coordinators, unsolicited book reviews, research

MAJOR CONTENT AREAS: counseling, cultural diversity, dependency, discharge planning, ethics, handicapping conditions, human behavior & sexuality, life span, loss/grief, mental health/illness, pain, quality of life, rehabilitation, teaching/learning

TOPICS PREFERRED: None cited

INAPPROPRIATE TOPICS: None cited

REVIEW PROCEDURE: Editorial board
REVIEW PERIOD: 2 months
MANUSCRIPT WORD LENGTH: 500-1000
MANUSCRIPT COPIES: 1
PUBLICATION LAG TIME: 2-4 months
EARLY PUBLICATION OPTION: Not cited
ACCEPTANCE RATE: Not cited
AUTHORSHIP RESTRICTIONS: No

PAGE CHARGES: No
STYLE REQUIREMENTS: Own
STYLE SHEET: Yes
REVISED THESES: No
STUDENT PAPERS: No
REPRINT POLICY: None

SUBSCRIPTION ADDRESS: Membership in AHCA-CAC

ANNUAL SUBSCRIPTION RATE: Membership: $15
FREQUENCY: Bimonthly
CIRCULATION: 1500
AFFILIATION: American Health Care Association
INDEXED/ABSTRACTED IN: None cited

192

JOURNAL TITLE: Sleep

MANUSCRIPT ADDRESS: The Editors, TD-114
Stanford University School of Medicine
Stanford CA 94305
TYPES OF ARTICLES: Research, case studies, review, theoretical

MAJOR CONTENT AREAS: anatomy & physiology, biochemistry, biorhythms,
circulatory & respiratory diseases, genetics, handicapping conditions, life span, medicine, pharmacology, psychopathology, public health nursing,
research methodology, sleep, testing/measurement
TOPICS PREFERRED: Any aspect of sleep: clinical, experimental,
biochemical
INAPPROPRIATE TOPICS: None cited

REVIEW PROCEDURE: External review
REVIEW PERIOD: 5-20 weeks
MANUSCRIPT WORD LENGTH: 2000-6250   PAGE CHARGES: No
MANUSCRIPT COPIES: 3   STYLE REQUIREMENTS: CBE, IM
PUBLICATION LAG TIME: 2-5 months   STYLE SHEET: Yes
EARLY PUBLICATION OPTION: Not cited   REVISED THESES: Yes
ACCEPTANCE RATE: 40%   STUDENT PAPERS: No
AUTHORSHIP RESTRICTIONS: No   REPRINT POLICY: 25 free

SUBSCRIPTION ADDRESS: Raven Press
1140 Avenue of the Americas
New York NY 10036
ANNUAL SUBSCRIPTION RATE: Individuals: $45   Institutions: $50
FREQUENCY: Quarterly   CIRCULATION: 600 (New journal)
AFFILIATION: Assoc. for the Psychophysiological Study of Sleep
INDEXED/ABSTRACTED IN: CC

◆

JOURNAL TITLE: Social Biology

MANUSCRIPT ADDRESS: Arthur Falek, Editor
Georgia Mental Health Institute
1256 Briarcliff Road, Atlanta GA 30306
TYPES OF ARTICLES: Research, theoretical, review, commentaries

MAJOR CONTENT AREAS: anthropology, biology, biomedical research,
epidemiology, family planning, genetics, sociology

TOPICS PREFERRED: Social or biological factors influencing the evolution of human populations
INAPPROPRIATE TOPICS: None cited

REVIEW PROCEDURE: External review
REVIEW PERIOD: 4-6 months
MANUSCRIPT WORD LENGTH: 6500   PAGE CHARGES: No
MANUSCRIPT COPIES: 3   STYLE REQUIREMENTS: CBE
PUBLICATION LAG TIME: 6 months   STYLE SHEET: Yes
EARLY PUBLICATION OPTION: No   REVISED THESES: No
ACCEPTANCE RATE: 50%   STUDENT PAPERS: No
AUTHORSHIP RESTRICTIONS: No   REPRINT POLICY: None free

SUBSCRIPTION ADDRESS: 1180 Observatory Drive
Room 5440
Madison WI 53705
ANNUAL SUBSCRIPTION RATE: Members: $16   Institutions: $38.50
FREQUENCY: Quarterly   CIRCULATION: 1650
AFFILIATION: Society for the Study of Social Biology
INDEXED/ABSTRACTED IN: AA, BA, BAI, CA, IM, PAIS, PA, SSI, SSCI

JOURNAL TITLE: Social Psychiatry

MANUSCRIPT ADDRESS: Dr. R.S. Daniels, University of Cincinnati
Medical Center, College of Medicine
Cincinnati OH 45267
TYPES OF ARTICLES: Research, review, theoretical

MAJOR CONTENT AREAS: health sciences, mental health/illness, mental
retardation, psychopathology, psychiatric/mental
health nursing, research methodology

TOPICS PREFERRED: Social psychiatry

INAPPROPRIATE TOPICS: None cited

REVIEW PROCEDURE: Editorial board and external review
REVIEW PERIOD: 2-3 months
MANUSCRIPT WORD LENGTH: Not cited   **PAGE CHARGES:** No
MANUSCRIPT COPIES: 3   **STYLE REQUIREMENTS:** Own
PUBLICATION LAG TIME: 10-12 months   **STYLE SHEET:** Yes
EARLY PUBLICATION OPTION: No   **REVISED THESES:** No
ACCEPTANCE RATE: 50%   **STUDENT PAPERS:** No
AUTHORSHIP RESTRICTIONS: No   **REPRINT POLICY:** 50 free

SUBSCRIPTION ADDRESS: Department of Psychiatry
25 Park Street
New Haven CT 06519
ANNUAL SUBSCRIPTION RATE: $98
FREQUENCY: Quarterly   **CIRCULATION:** 1-2000
AFFILIATION: None
INDEXED/ABSTRACTED IN: BA, CC, PA, SSCI

◆

JOURNAL TITLE: Social Science and Medicine

MANUSCRIPT ADDRESS: Pergamon Press, Inc., Maxwell House
Fairview Park
Elmsford NY 10523
TYPES OF ARTICLES: Research, theoretical, review, commentaries, case
studies, unsolicited book reviews
MAJOR CONTENT AREAS: aging & aged, communication, compliance, cultural
diversity, death & dying, ethics, health:
promotion, sciences, policies, nursing philosophy,
pain, quality of life, stress, teaching/learning,
pharmacy, medical economics, medical services
TOPICS PREFERRED: None cited

INAPPROPRIATE TOPICS: None

REVIEW PROCEDURE: Editorial board and external review
REVIEW PERIOD: 2 months
MANUSCRIPT WORD LENGTH: 1000-6000   **PAGE CHARGES:** No
MANUSCRIPT COPIES: 3   **STYLE REQUIREMENTS:** Own
PUBLICATION LAG TIME: 2 months   **STYLE SHEET:** Yes
EARLY PUBLICATION OPTION: Yes   **REVISED THESES:** Yes
ACCEPTANCE RATE: 50%   **STUDENT PAPERS:** No
AUTHORSHIP RESTRICTIONS: No   **REPRINT POLICY:** 25 free

SUBSCRIPTION ADDRESS: Pergamon Press, Inc., Maxwell House
Fairview Park
Elmsford NY 10523
ANNUAL SUBSCRIPTION RATE: Individuals: $90 Institutions: $450
FREQUENCY: 26 issues yearly   **CIRCULATION:** 2000
AFFILIATION: None
INDEXED/ABSTRACTED IN: BA, CINAHL, IM, INI, PA, SSCI

JOURNAL TITLE: Social Work in Health Care

MANUSCRIPT ADDRESS: Sylvia S. Clarke, Editor, Consultant
Social Work Dept., The Mt. Sinai Medical Center
One Gustave L. Levy Pl., New York NY 10029

TYPES OF ARTICLES: Social aspects of health care, case studies, theoretical, research, review

MAJOR CONTENT AREAS: abuse, body image, chronicity, compliance, continuity of care, counseling, crisis, death, discharge planning, family planning, groups, handicapping conditions, health promotion, loss/grief, mental health, mental retardation, primary care

TOPICS PREFERRED: Collaborative, interdisciplinary aproaches to social work in health care

INAPPROPRIATE TOPICS: None cited

REVIEW PROCEDURE: Editorial board & external review
REVIEW PERIOD: 1-3 months
MANUSCRIPT WORD LENGTH: 3500-4000   **PAGE CHARGES:** No
MANUSCRIPT COPIES: 3   **STYLE REQUIREMENTS:** APA
PUBLICATION LAG TIME: 3-6 months   **STYLE SHEET:** Yes
EARLY PUBLICATION OPTION: Yes   **REVISED THESES:** Yes
ACCEPTANCE RATE: 25%   **STUDENT PAPERS:** Yes
AUTHORSHIP RESTRICTIONS: No   **REPRINT POLICY:** 10 free

SUBSCRIPTION ADDRESS: The Haworth Press
28 East 22nd Street
New York NY 10010
ANNUAL SUBSCRIPTION RATE: Individuals: $32   Institutions: $48-60
FREQUENCY: Quarterly   **CIRCULATION:** 4000
AFFILIATION: None
INDEXED/ABSTRACTED IN: AHM, CINAHL, HLI, IM, MCR, PA, SWRA, SocA

◆

JOURNAL TITLE: Southeast Asian Journal of Tropical Medicine and Public Health

MANUSCRIPT ADDRESS: Tropmed Central Office
420/6 Rajvithi Road
Bangkok 4 Thailand

TYPES OF ARTICLES: Research, case studies

MAJOR CONTENT AREAS: biomedical research, cancer, epidemiology, health promotion, health sciences, medicine, microbiology, pathology, pharmacology, public health

TOPICS PREFERRED: Tropical diseases

INAPPROPRIATE TOPICS: Basic sciences, veterinary medicine

REVIEW PROCEDURE: Editorial board and external review
REVIEW PERIOD: 1-2 months
MANUSCRIPT WORD LENGTH: 3000   **PAGE CHARGES:** No
MANUSCRIPT COPIES: 3   **STYLE REQUIREMENTS:** AMA, IM
PUBLICATION LAG TIME: 3 months   **STYLE SHEET:** Yes
EARLY PUBLICATION OPTION: No   **REVISED THESES:** Yes
ACCEPTANCE RATE: 70%   **STUDENT PAPERS:** Yes
AUTHORSHIP RESTRICTIONS: No   **REPRINT POLICY:** 30-50 free

SUBSCRIPTION ADDRESS: SEAMED-TROPMED Project
420/6 Rajvithi Road
Bangkok 4 Thailand
ANNUAL SUBSCRIPTION RATE: $12
FREQUENCY: Quarterly   **CIRCULATION:** 1000
AFFILIATION: Southeast Asian Ministers of Education Organization
INDEXED/ABSTRACTED IN: IM, BA, CA

JOURNAL TITLE: Studies in Family Planning

MANUSCRIPT ADDRESS: Population Council
One Dag Hammarskjold Plaza
New York NY 10017
TYPES OF ARTICLES: Research, case studies, theoretical

MAJOR CONTENT AREAS: family planning, health promotion, maternal/child
health

TOPICS PREFERRED: Safety issues in contraception; technology transfer
& diffusion; All aspects of family planning
INAPPROPRIATE TOPICS: None cited

REVIEW PROCEDURE: External review
REVIEW PERIOD: 2 months
MANUSCRIPT WORD LENGTH: 5000   PAGE CHARGES: No
MANUSCRIPT COPIES: 3   STYLE REQUIREMENTS: C
PUBLICATION LAG TIME: 6 months   STYLE SHEET: Yes
EARLY PUBLICATION OPTION: Not cited   REVISED THESES: Not cited
ACCEPTANCE RATE: 25%   STUDENT PAPERS: Not cited
AUTHORSHIP RESTRICTIONS: No   REPRINT POLICY: 20 free journals

SUBSCRIPTION ADDRESS: Circulation Department
One Dag Hammarskjold Plaza
New York NY 10017
ANNUAL SUBSCRIPTION RATE: No charge
FREQUENCY: Monthly   CIRCULATION: 12,500
AFFILIATION: None
INDEXED/ABSTRACTED IN: BA, IM, SSCI, INI

◆

JOURNAL TITLE: Suicide and Life Threatening Behavior

MANUSCRIPT ADDRESS: UCLA Neuropsychiatric Institute
760 Westwood Plaza
Los Angeles CA 90024
TYPES OF ARTICLES: Research, theoretical, review, case studies

MAJOR CONTENT AREAS: death and dying, suicide

TOPICS PREFERRED: Self destruction and life-threatening topics

INAPPROPRIATE TOPICS: Over-simplified cases, demographic studies of
small areas
REVIEW PROCEDURE: Editorial board
REVIEW PERIOD: 6 months
MANUSCRIPT WORD LENGTH: 3000-5000   PAGE CHARGES: No
MANUSCRIPT COPIES: 4   STYLE REQUIREMENTS: APA
PUBLICATION LAG TIME: 1 year   STYLE SHEET: Yes
EARLY PUBLICATION OPTION: No   REVISED THESES: Yes
ACCEPTANCE RATE: 40%   STUDENT PAPERS: Yes
AUTHORSHIP RESTRICTIONS: No   REPRINT POLICY: 1 free

SUBSCRIPTION ADDRESS: Human Sciences Press
72 Fifth Avenue
New York NY 10011
ANNUAL SUBSCRIPTION RATE: Individuals: $15   Institutions: $35
FREQUENCY: Quarterly   CIRCULATION: 1000
AFFILIATION: American Association of Suicidology
INDEXED/ABSTRACTED IN: IM, PA, ACP, CC, SSCI, INI

JOURNAL TITLE: Supervisor Nurse †

MANUSCRIPT ADDRESS: 3734 Glenway Avenue
Cincinnati OH 45205

TYPES OF ARTICLES: Commentaries, research, theoretical

MAJOR CONTENT AREAS: Most areas listed in Appendix A including:
nursing: assessment, audit, care, clinical
specialties, diagnosis, maternal/child, medical/
surgical, operating room, orthopedic, philosophy,
process, research, service administration, theory
TOPICS PREFERRED: Topics dealing with managerial and administrative
problems in health care facilities
INAPPROPRIATE TOPICS: Masters theses and dissertations

REVIEW PROCEDURE: Editorial board			
REVIEW PERIOD: 3-6 weeks			
MANUSCRIPT WORD LENGTH: 2500		**PAGE CHARGES:** No	
MANUSCRIPT COPIES: 2		**STYLE REQUIREMENTS:** C	
PUBLICATION LAG TIME: 12-18 months		**STYLE SHEET:** Yes	
EARLY PUBLICATION OPTION: Yes		**REVISED THESES:** No	
ACCEPTANCE RATE: 40-50%		**STUDENT PAPERS:** No	
AUTHORSHIP RESTRICTIONS: No		**REPRINT POLICY:** 6 free	

SUBSCRIPTION ADDRESS: 8 South Michigan Avenue
Chicago IL 60603

ANNUAL SUBSCRIPTION RATE: Individuals: $18 (Free to qualified supervisors)
FREQUENCY: Monthly   **CIRCULATION:** 100,000
AFFILIATION: None
INDEXED/ABSTRACTED IN: INI, CINAHL, HLI

◆

JOURNAL TITLE: The Surgical Technologist

MANUSCRIPT ADDRESS: Association of Surgical Technologists
Caller No. E.
Littleton CO 80120
TYPES OF ARTICLES: Research, theoretical

MAJOR CONTENT AREAS: allied health, anatomy & physiology, anesthesiology, cancer, continuing education, death &
dying, emergency services, epidemiology, health
promotion, health sciences, nursing: medical/
surgical, OR; pharmacology, professionalism, stress
TOPICS PREFERRED: Items that relate to the functioning of the
operating room
INAPPROPRIATE TOPICS: None cited

REVIEW PROCEDURE: Editorial board			
REVIEW PERIOD: 4-6 weeks			
MANUSCRIPT WORD LENGTH: 3000-5000		**PAGE CHARGES:** No	
MANUSCRIPT COPIES: 1		**STYLE REQUIREMENTS:** APA	
PUBLICATION LAG TIME: 3-5 months		**STYLE SHEET:** Yes	
EARLY PUBLICATION OPTION: No		**REVISED THESES:** No	
ACCEPTANCE RATE: 50%		**STUDENT PAPERS:** Yes	
AUTHORSHIP RESTRICTIONS: No		**REPRINT POLICY:** 10 free journals	

SUBSCRIPTION ADDRESS: Association of Surgical Technologists
Caller No. E
Littleton CO 80120
ANNUAL SUBSCRIPTION RATE: $12
FREQUENCY: Bimonthly   **CIRCULATION:** 14,000
AFFILIATION: Association of Surgical Technologists
INDEXED/ABSTRACTED IN: CINAHL

JOURNAL TITLE: Today's OR Nurse

MANUSCRIPT ADDRESS: Charles B. Slack, Inc.
6900 Grove Road
Thorofare NJ 08086
TYPES OF ARTICLES: Review, case studies, commentaries, abstracts of
articles from other journals
MAJOR CONTENT AREAS: clinical nurse specialties, operating room nursing

TOPICS PREFERRED: None cited

INAPPROPRIATE TOPICS: None cited

REVIEW PROCEDURE: Editorial board			
REVIEW PERIOD: Not cited			
MANUSCRIPT WORD LENGTH: 1500-2000		**PAGE CHARGES:** Not cited	
MANUSCRIPT COPIES: Not cited		**STYLE REQUIREMENTS:** Not cited	
PUBLICATION LAG TIME: Not cited		**STYLE SHEET:** Not cited	
EARLY PUBLICATION OPTION: Not cited		**REVISED THESES:** Not cited	
ACCEPTANCE RATE: Not cited		**STUDENT PAPERS:** Not cited	
AUTHORSHIP RESTRICTIONS: Not cited		**REPRINT POLICY:** Not cited	

SUBSCRIPTION ADDRESS: Charles B. Slack, Inc.
6900 Grove Road
Thorofare NJ 08086
ANNUAL SUBSCRIPTION RATE: Individuals: $12   Institutions: $18
FREQUENCY: Monthly   **CIRCULATION:** New journal
AFFILIATION: Not cited
INDEXED/ABSTRACTED IN: New journal

◆

JOURNAL TITLE: Topics in Clinical Nursing

MANUSCRIPT ADDRESS: Aspen Systems Corporation
1600 Research Boulevard
Rockville MD 20850
TYPES OF ARTICLES: Theoretical, commentaries, research

MAJOR CONTENT AREAS: nursing care, nursing philosophy

TOPICS PREFERRED: Journal is topical; submit articles concerning
specific topic, contact editor for upcoming topics
INAPPROPRIATE TOPICS: None cited

REVIEW PROCEDURE: Editorial board			
REVIEW PERIOD: 4-6 weeks			
MANUSCRIPT WORD LENGTH: Up to 5000		**PAGE CHARGES:** No	
MANUSCRIPT COPIES: 3		**STYLE REQUIREMENTS:** C	
PUBLICATION LAG TIME: 3 months		**STYLE SHEET:** Yes	
EARLY PUBLICATION OPTION: No		**REVISED THESES:** No	
ACCEPTANCE RATE: Not cited		**STUDENT PAPERS:** No	
AUTHORSHIP RESTRICTIONS: No		**REPRINT POLICY:** 2 free journals	

SUBSCRIPTION ADDRESS: Fulfillment Operations
Aspen Systems Corporation, 16792 Oakmont Avenue
Gaithersburg MD 20877
ANNUAL SUBSCRIPTION RATE: $36
FREQUENCY: Quarterly   **CIRCULATION:** 4000
AFFILIATION: None
INDEXED/ABSTRACTED IN: CINAHL

JOURNAL TITLE: Topics in Emergency Medicine

MANUSCRIPT ADDRESS: Aspen Systems Corporation
1600 Research Boulevard
Rockville MD 20850

TYPES OF ARTICLES: Technical articles geared toward emergency medicine clinicians' delivery of patient care

MAJOR CONTENT AREAS: Emergency services, intradisciplinary emergency
medical care

TOPICS PREFERRED: None cited

INAPPROPRIATE TOPICS: None cited

REVIEW PROCEDURE: Editorial board		
REVIEW PERIOD: 4-6 weeks		
MANUSCRIPT WORD LENGTH: Up to 5000	**PAGE CHARGES:** Not cited	
MANUSCRIPT COPIES: 3	**STYLE REQUIREMENTS:** AMA	
PUBLICATION LAG TIME: 3 months	**STYLE SHEET:** Yes	
EARLY PUBLICATION OPTION: No	**REVISED THESES:** No	
ACCEPTANCE RATE: Not cited	**STUDENT PAPERS:** No	
AUTHORSHIP RESTRICTIONS: No	**REPRINT POLICY:** 2 free journals	

SUBSCRIPTION ADDRESS: Fulfillment Operations
Aspen Systems Corporation
P.O. Box 486, Gaithersburg MD 20760

ANNUAL SUBSCRIPTION RATE: $36

FREQUENCY: Quarterly   **CIRCULATION:** 5000

AFFILIATION: None

INDEXED/ABSTRACTED IN: CINAHL

◆

JOURNAL TITLE: Training World

MANUSCRIPT ADDRESS: 60 East 42nd Street
Suite 1026
New York NY 10017

TYPES OF ARTICLES: Not cited

MAJOR CONTENT AREAS: communication, inservice education, instructional
technology, leadership, teaching/learning

TOPICS PREFERRED: Training and education methods for business and
industry for which proof of efficacy exists

INAPPROPRIATE TOPICS: None cited

REVIEW PROCEDURE: Editorial board and the editor's judgement		
REVIEW PERIOD: 1 week		
MANUSCRIPT WORD LENGTH: 750-1500	**PAGE CHARGES:** No	
MANUSCRIPT COPIES: 1	**STYLE REQUIREMENTS:** Own	
PUBLICATION LAG TIME: 2-4 months	**STYLE SHEET:** Yes	
EARLY PUBLICATION OPTION: No	**REVISED THESES:** No	
ACCEPTANCE RATE: 20%	**STUDENT PAPERS:** No	
AUTHORSHIP RESTRICTIONS: No	**REPRINT POLICY:** 20 free issues	

SUBSCRIPTION ADDRESS: Bill Robinson, Circulation Manager
60 East 42nd Street, Suite 1026
New York NY 10017

ANNUAL SUBSCRIPTION RATE: $18

FREQUENCY: Bimonthly   **CIRCULATION:** 20,000

AFFILIATION: None

INDEXED/ABSTRACTED IN: None cited

JOURNAL TITLE: Urban Health

MANUSCRIPT ADDRESS: P.O. Box 42409
Atlanta GA 30311

TYPES OF ARTICLES: Research, commentaries

MAJOR CONTENT AREAS: treatment of medical problems with high incidence in urban communities; innovations in urban health care delivery; clinical management of medical problems & issues in urban health care delivery, hospitals, private practice, community health

TOPICS PREFERRED: How economic problems affect specific segments of the urban health community

INAPPROPRIATE TOPICS: None cited

REVIEW PROCEDURE: Not cited		
REVIEW PERIOD: Not cited		
MANUSCRIPT WORD LENGTH: 2500-3000	**PAGE CHARGES:** Not cited	
MANUSCRIPT COPIES: 2	**STYLE REQUIREMENTS:** Own	
PUBLICATION LAG TIME: Not cited	**STYLE SHEET:** Not cited	
EARLY PUBLICATION OPTION: Not cited	**REVISED THESES:** Not cited	
ACCEPTANCE RATE: Not cited	**STUDENT PAPERS:** Not cited	
AUTHORSHIP RESTRICTIONS: Not cited	**REPRINT POLICY:** Not cited	

SUBSCRIPTION ADDRESS: Urban Publishing Co.
1868 Washington Rd., Suite B
East Point GA 30344

ANNUAL SUBSCRIPTION RATE: $12

FREQUENCY: 10 times yearly   **CIRCULATION:** 16,600

AFFILIATION: None cited

INDEXED/ABSTRACTED IN: Not cited

JOURNAL TITLE: Volunteer Leader

MANUSCRIPT ADDRESS: 211 E. Chicago Avenue
Chicago IL 60611

TYPES OF ARTICLES: Case studies, commentaries

MAJOR CONTENT AREAS: volunteer programs in hospitals

TOPICS PREFERRED: Volunteer programs in hospitals, feminism, career development, health legislation, health education

INAPPROPRIATE TOPICS: Stories about the work of single volunteers, rather than organized programs

REVIEW PROCEDURE: Editorial board		
REVIEW PERIOD: 4-6 weeks		
MANUSCRIPT WORD LENGTH: 1500	**PAGE CHARGES:** Not cited	
MANUSCRIPT COPIES: 2	**STYLE REQUIREMENTS:** Own	
PUBLICATION LAG TIME: $1^{1}/_{2}$-3 months	**STYLE SHEET:** Yes	
EARLY PUBLICATION OPTION: No	**REVISED THESES:** No	
ACCEPTANCE RATE: 50%	**STUDENT PAPERS:** No	
AUTHORSHIP RESTRICTIONS: Yes	**REPRINT POLICY:** 2 free	

SUBSCRIPTION ADDRESS: American Hospital Publishing, Inc.
211 East Chicago Avenue
Chicago IL 60611

ANNUAL SUBSCRIPTION RATE: $6

FREQUENCY: Quarterly   **CIRCULATION:** 8500

AFFILIATION: American Hospital Association

INDEXED/ABSTRACTED IN: HLI

200

JOURNAL TITLE: Wellness Newsletter

MANUSCRIPT ADDRESS: c/o Dr. Carolyn Chambers Clark
P.O.B. 132
Sloatsburg NY 10974

TYPES OF ARTICLES: Wellness assessments, unsolicited book reviews, research, theoretical

MAJOR CONTENT AREAS: biofeedback, body image, counseling, crisis intervention/theory, health promotion, loss/grief, nutrition, pain, patient teaching/ consumer education, relaxation, stress, self care; unity with the environment, fitness

TOPICS PREFERRED: Wellness, prevention of illness, nutrition, self-care, fitness, unity with the environment

INAPPROPRIATE TOPICS: None cited

REVIEW PROCEDURE: Editorial board
REVIEW PERIOD: 3-4 weeks
MANUSCRIPT WORD LENGTH: 120-500
MANUSCRIPT COPIES: 2
PUBLICATION LAG TIME: 1-12 months
EARLY PUBLICATION OPTION: No
ACCEPTANCE RATE: 50%
AUTHORSHIP RESTRICTIONS: No

PAGE CHARGES: No
STYLE REQUIREMENTS: Own
STYLE SHEET: Yes
REVISED THESES: No
STUDENT PAPERS: No
REPRINT POLICY: 5 free

SUBSCRIPTION ADDRESS: c/o The Wellness Institute
P.O.B. 132
Sloatsburg NY 10974
ANNUAL SUBSCRIPTION RATE: Individuals: $8 Institutions: $15
FREQUENCY: Bimonthly CIRCULATION: 2000
AFFILIATION: The Wellness Institute
INDEXED/ABSTRACTED IN: None cited

◆

JOURNAL TITLE: Western Journal of Nursing Research

MANUSCRIPT ADDRESS: Executive Editor, WJNR
UCLA School of Nursing
Los Angeles CA 90024

TYPES OF ARTICLES: Research, theoretical, review, case studies

MAJOR CONTENT AREAS: None specified

TOPICS PREFERRED: Anything relevant to nursing research

INAPPROPRIATE TOPICS: Unrelated to research

REVIEW PROCEDURE: External review
REVIEW PERIOD: 2-9 months
MANUSCRIPT WORD LENGTH: 5000
MANUSCRIPT COPIES: 4
PUBLICATION LAG TIME: 2-9 months
EARLY PUBLICATION OPTION: Not cited
ACCEPTANCE RATE: 5%
AUTHORSHIP RESTRICTIONS: No

PAGE CHARGES: Not cited
STYLE REQUIREMENTS: AA
STYLE SHEET: Yes
REVISED THESES: Not cited
STUDENT PAPERS: Yes
REPRINT POLICY: 12 free

SUBSCRIPTION ADDRESS: Western Journal of Nursing Research
1330 South State College Boulevard
Anaheim CA 92806
ANNUAL SUBSCRIPTION RATE: Individuals: $15 Institutions: $26
FREQUENCY: Quarterly CIRCULATION: New journal
AFFILIATION: Western Council on Higher Education for Nursing
INDEXED/ABSTRACTED IN: INI, CINAHL

JOURNAL TITLE: Women & Health

MANUSCRIPT ADDRESS: Helen I. Marieskind, DrPH
ESRD Network Coordinating Council #2
Box 33790, Seattle, Washington 98133
TYPES OF ARTICLES: Research, theoretical, commentaries

MAJOR CONTENT AREAS: spouse abuse, family planning, health promotion,
maternal/child nursing, public health, quality of
life, stigma, stress, women's issues

TOPICS PREFERRED: Issues in the health care of women, health/illness
patterns of women
INAPPROPRIATE TOPICS: None cited

REVIEW PROCEDURE: Editorial board and external review
REVIEW PERIOD: Not cited
MANUSCRIPT WORD LENGTH: 5000
MANUSCRIPT COPIES: 3
PUBLICATION LAG TIME: Not cited
EARLY PUBLICATION OPTION: Not cited
ACCEPTANCE RATE: Not cited
AUTHORSHIP RESTRICTIONS: Not cited

PAGE CHARGES: No
STYLE REQUIREMENTS: AMA, Own
STYLE SHEET: Yes
REVISED THESES: Not cited
STUDENT PAPERS: Not cited
REPRINT POLICY: 10 free

SUBSCRIPTION ADDRESS: Haworth Press, Subscription Department
28 East 22nd St.
New York NY 10010
ANNUAL SUBSCRIPTION RATE: Indiviudals: $20   Institutions: $36
FREQUENCY: Quarterly   CIRCULATION: Not cited
AFFILIATION: None cited
INDEXED/ABSTRACTED IN: EM, HLI, PA, SocA, WSA, AHCMS, API, CC(SBS, SSCI

◆

JOURNAL TITLE: World Health

MANUSCRIPT ADDRESS: The Editor
World Health
1211 Geneva 27, Switzerland
TYPES OF ARTICLES: Articles on public health themes. Most
articles are specially commissioned in advance.
MAJOR CONTENT AREAS: Community/public health nursing, health promotion, health sciences, health policies, primary
care

TOPICS PREFERRED: Broadly, public health--especially primary
health care and community health
INAPPROPRIATE TOPICS: None cited

REVIEW PROCEDURE: Editorial board
REVIEW PERIOD: 1-4 weeks
MANUSCRIPT WORD LENGTH: 2000
MANUSCRIPT COPIES: 1
PUBLICATION LAG TIME: 2 months
EARLY PUBLICATION OPTION: No
ACCEPTANCE RATE: 1%
AUTHORSHIP RESTRICTIONS: No

PAGE CHARGES: No
STYLE REQUIREMENTS: Own
STYLE SHEET: No
REVISED THESES: No
STUDENT PAPERS: No
REPRINT POLICY: 10 free

SUBSCRIPTION ADDRESS: The Editor
WHO, Avenue Appia
1211 Geneva 27, Switzerland
ANNUAL SUBSCRIPTION RATE: $15.00
FREQUENCY: 10 times yearly   CIRCULATION: 130,000
AFFILIATION: World Health Organization
INDEXED/ABSTRACTED IN: CINAHL

202

JOURNAL TITLE: World Hospitals

MANUSCRIPT ADDRESS: The International Hospital Federation
126 Albert Street
London NW1 7NX England

TYPES OF ARTICLES: Research, case studies, review, commentaries,
theoretical, unsolicited book reviews

MAJOR CONTENT AREAS: change theory, communication, continuing
education, continuity of care, health promotion,
sciences & policies, hospitals, inservice
education, primary care, professionalism, systems
theory, teaching/learning, testing/ measurement

TOPICS PREFERRED: Planning, management and administration of health
services

INAPPROPRIATE TOPICS: Medical and engineering topics

REVIEW PROCEDURE: Review by editor or director general
REVIEW PERIOD: 1 month
MANUSCRIPT WORD LENGTH: 2500
MANUSCRIPT COPIES: 2
PUBLICATION LAG TIME: 6-12 months
EARLY PUBLICATION OPTION: No
ACCEPTANCE RATE: 50%
AUTHORSHIP RESTRICTIONS: No

PAGE CHARGES: No
STYLE REQUIREMENTS: Own
STYLE SHEET: Yes
REVISED THESES: Yes
STUDENT PAPERS: No
REPRINT POLICY: Free journals

SUBSCRIPTION ADDRESS: The International Hospital Federation
126 Albert Street
London NW1 7NX England

ANNUAL SUBSCRIPTION RATE: $24
FREQUENCY: Quarterly   CIRCULATION: 3,000
AFFILIATION: International Hospital Federation
INDEXED/ABSTRACTED IN: CINAHL

◆

APPENDIX A
LIST OF MAJOR CONTENT AREAS

abuse (child/spouse)
accidents
adaptation
adolescence
adulthood
aging and aged
alcoholism & drug abuse
allied health personnel
anatomy & physiology
anesthesiology
anthropology
biochemistry
biofeedback
biology
biomedical research
biorhythms
body image
cancer
change theory
children
chronicity
circulatory diseases
clinical nurse specialties
communication
community/public health nursing
compliance
continuing education
continuity of care
counseling
crisis intervention/theory
critical care nursing
cultural diversity
death & dying
dependency
discharge planning
eating disorders

emergency services
epidemiology
ethics
family planning
fatigue
genetics
geriatric nursing
groups
growth/development
handicapping conditions
health policies
health promotion
health sciences
hospitals
human behavior
human sexuality
immunization
inservice education
instructional technology
leadership
life span
loss/grief
marriage & divorce
maternal/child nursing
medical surgical nursing
medicine
mental health/illness
mental retardation
microbiology
midwifery
natural science
neurological nursing
nursing assessment
nursing audit
nursing care
nursing diagnosis

nursing education
nursing history
nursing homes
nursing philosophy
nursing process
nursing research
nursing science
nursing service administration
nursing theory
nutrition
occupational health nursing
office nursing
operating room nursing
orthopedic nursing
pain
parenting
pathology
patient teaching
pediatric nursing
perception
pharmacology
physical therapy
physics
primary care

professionalism
psychiatric/mental health nursing
psychology
psychopathology
public health
quality of life
rehabilitation
relaxation
research methodology
respiratory diseases
retirement
safety/first aid
school nursing
sensory deprivation
sleep
sociology
stigma
stress
suicide
systems theory
teaching/learning
testing/measurement
trauma nursing
women's issues

APPENDIX B
RECENT FINDINGS

In an effort to provide accurate profiles of the journals included in this book, the editors checked information on titles, subscription, and manuscript submission addresses early in 1982. Title changes, cessations, and titles of new journals are listed below. A dagmar (†) identifies journals within the text which have had title changes or which have ceased publication.

CESSATIONS

Allied Health and Behavioral Sciences
EMT Journal
Nursing Dimensions

TITLE CHANGES

ARN Journal *is now* Rehabilitation Nursing
Association for the Care of Children's Health Journal *is now* Children's
    Health Care
Children in Contemporary Society *is now* Journal of Children in
    Contemporary Society
Family Health *is now* Health
Health Care in Canada *is now* Health Care
Health Practitioner and Physician Assistant *is now* Physician Assistant and
    Health Practitioner
Journal of Nurse-Midwifery *is now* Journal of Nurse-Midwives
Journal of Psychiatric Nursing and Mental Health Services *is now* Journal
    of Psychosocial Nursing and Mental Health Services
Life and Health *is now* Your Life and Health
Man & Medicine: Journal of Values & Ethics in Health Care *is now* Values
    & Ethics in Health Care
Nursing Law & Ethics *is now incorporated in* Law, Medicine & Health Care
Supervisor Nurse *is now* Nursing Management

NEW JOURNALS

AUAA Journal: Official Journal of the American Urological Association
    Allied
American Health

DCCN: Dimensions in Critical Care Nursing
Discharge Planning Update
Executive Health
Focus (AACN)
Health Care Horizons
Infection Control
Law, Medicine & Health Care

Medical Electronics
Nephrology Nurse
Nursing Life
Nursing Networks
Occupational Therapy in Mental Health
Physiotherapy
World Health Forum

SUBJECT, TITLE, AND KEYWORD INDEX

This Index will refer the reader to the page numbers on which journals are listed. Journals are listed by title, subject, and key words within their title.

In addition, if a journal's editor indicated a clear preference for certain types of manuscripts, these "manuscript preference subject areas" are also included as indexing terms. The reader will therefore be able to search for appropriate journals for article submission according to the general subject areas in which his or her article falls.

O

P